COUPLE-BASED INTERVENTIONS
FOR MILITARY AND VETERAN FAMILIES

Also from Douglas K. Snyder and Candice M. Monson

FOR PROFESSIONALS

Cognitive-Behavioral Conjoint Therapy for PTSD:
Harnessing the Healing Power of Relationships
Candice M. Monson and *Steffany J. Fredman*

Helping Couples Get Past the Affair:
A Clinician's Guide
Donald H. Baucom, Douglas K. Snyder,
and *Kristina Coop Gordon*

Treating Difficult Couples: Helping Clients
with Coexisting Mental and Relationship Disorders
Douglas K. Snyder and *Mark A.Whisman*

FOR GENERAL READERS

Getting Past the Affair:
A Program to Help You Cope, Heal, and Move On—Together or Apart
Douglas K. Snyder, Donald H. Baucom,
and *Kristina Coop Gordon*

COUPLE-BASED INTERVENTIONS FOR MILITARY AND VETERAN FAMILIES

A Practitioner's Guide

Edited by
Douglas K. Snyder
Candice M. Monson

THE GUILFORD PRESS
New York   London

©2012 The Guilford Press
A Division of Guilford Publications, Inc.
72 Spring Street, New York, NY 10012
www.guilford.com

Printed in the United States of America

This book is printed on acid-free paper.

Last digit is print number: 9 8 7 6 5 4 3 2 1

The authors have checked with sources believed to be reliable in their efforts to provide information that is complete and generally in accord with the standards of practice that are accepted at the time of publication. However, in view of the possibility of human error or changes in behavioral, mental health, or medical sciences, neither the authors, nor the editors and publisher, nor any other party who has been involved in the preparation or publication of this work warrants that the information contained herein is in every respect accurate or complete, and they are not responsible for any errors or omissions or the results obtained from the use of such information. Readers are encouraged to confirm the information contained in this book with other sources.

Library of Congress Cataloging-in-Publication Data is available from the Publisher.

ISBN 978-1-4625-0540-1

About the Editors

Douglas K. Snyder, PhD, is Professor of Psychology and Director of Clinical Training at Texas A&M University. He is coauthor of two books on evidence-based interventions for couples struggling with issues of infidelity (*Getting Past the Affair* and *Helping Couples Get Past the Affair*) and coeditor of two books on couple- and family-based interventions (*Treating Difficult Couples* and *Emotion Regulation in Couples and Families*). Dr. Snyder has served as Editor of the *Clinician's Research Digest* and as Associate Editor of the *Journal of Consulting and Clinical Psychology* and the *Journal of Family Psychology*. He has been funded by both the National Institute of Mental Health and the U.S. Department of Defense for research on couple-based interventions. In 1991 he was recognized by the American Association for Marriage and Family Therapy for Outstanding Research Contribution, and in 2005 he received the American Psychological Association's Award for Distinguished Contributions to Family Psychology.

Candice M. Monson, PhD, is Professor of Psychology and Director of Clinical Training at Ryerson University in Toronto. She is also an Affiliate of the Women's Health Sciences Division of the U.S. Department of Veterans Affairs National Center for PTSD, where she previously served as Deputy Director. Dr. Monson is one of the foremost experts on intimate relationships and traumatic stress and the use of conjoint therapy to treat posttraumatic stress disorder (PTSD). She has published extensively on the development, evaluation, and dissemination of PTSD treatments more generally, as well as gender differences in violence perpetration and victimization. She has been funded by the U.S. Department of Veterans Affairs, the National Institute of Mental Health, the Centers for Disease Control and Prevention, the U.S. Department of Defense, and the Canadian Institutes of Health for her research on interpersonal factors in traumatization and couple-based interventions for PTSD. Dr. Monson is coauthor of *Cognitive-Behavioral Conjoint Therapy for PTSD: Harnessing the Healing Power of Relationships*.

Contributors

Donald H. Baucom, PhD, is Richard Simpson Distinguished Professor of Psychology at the University of North Carolina at Chapel Hill. For more than 35 years, Dr. Baucom has developed and evaluated couple-based interventions from a cognitive-behavioral perspective. He and Norman Epstein have published two books on couple therapy, the more recent titled *Enhanced Cognitive-Behavioral Therapy for Couples: A Contextual Approach*. He, Douglas Snyder, and Kristina Gordon have coauthored two books about infidelity (*Getting Past the Affair* and *Helping Couples Get Past the Affair: A Clinician's Guide*). Dr. Baucom has received several teaching, mentoring, and clinical supervision awards.

Kevin S. Beasley, LCSW, is a clinical social worker for the U.S. Department of Veterans Affairs (VA) and works as a member of the Posttraumatic Stress Disorder Clinical Team at the Frank Tejada Outpatient Clinic in San Antonio. He previously served 4 years in the U.S. Air Force and, prior to his role at the VA, worked as a Family Violence Therapist for the U.S. Air Force. He has presented on conjoint therapy, family violence, and the military culture both nationally and internationally.

Pamela S. Collins, LCSW, is Treatment Program Manager for the U.S. Air Force Family Advocacy Program. She is the clinical consultant and training coordinator to over 200 family violence treatment providers at 75 Air Force bases throughout the world. Ms. Collins presents in various forums across the country on the Air Force response to domestic violence and child abuse.

ix

Ellen R. DeVoe, PhD, is Associate Professor at the Boston University School of Social Work. Her scholarship has focused on the impact of trauma on young children, parents, and families, and interventions designed to mitigate these effects. She has been Principal Investigator on several federally funded grants, including a study of the impact of the 9/11 attacks on New York City families. Currently, she is Principal Investigator of an award from the U.S. Department of Defense to develop and test a home-based program, Strong Families Strong Forces, for military parents returning from Iraq or Afghanistan who have children 5 years old or younger.

Brian D. Doss, PhD, is Assistant Professor at the University of Miami. His research focuses on developing and testing interventions for couples' difficulties, including couple therapy, web-based programs, and interventions during the transition to parenthood. He has been the Primary Investigator on several grants from the National Institutes of Health, including a 5-year grant to develop and test *OurRelationship.com*. His research has been cited on the *Today* show, CNN, MSNBC, *The New York Times*, *The Miami Herald*, and elsewhere. He has served on the editorial boards of the *Journal of Consulting and Clinical Psychology* and the *Journal of Family Psychology*.

Steffany J. Fredman, PhD, is a clinical psychologist in the Department of Psychiatry at Massachusetts General Hospital and Instructor in Psychiatry at Harvard Medical School. Dr. Fredman's clinical and research interests focus on research on posttraumatic stress disorder (PTSD) and related conditions within a couple or family context, with a focus on understanding ways that partner or family involvement in treatment optimizes outcomes for those with these conditions. She is coauthor of *Cognitive-Behavioral Conjoint Therapy for PTSD*.

Matthew J. Friedman, MD, PhD, is Executive Director of the VA's National Center for PTSD and Professor of Psychiatry and Pharmacology at Dartmouth Medical School. He directs the consortium, extending from New England to Honolulu, with a Congressional mandate to advance the understanding and treatment of traumatic stress through research and education. His research emphasizes clinical trials of psychotherapy and pharmacotherapy, focusing on complex PTSD comorbid with other psychiatric diagnoses, chemical abuse/dependency, or traumatic brain injury. He has received numerous honors, including the 1999 Lifetime Achievement Award and the 2009 Public Advocacy Award from the International Society for Traumatic Stress Studies.

Shirley M. Glynn, PhD, is a Research Psychologist in the Department of Psychiatry and Biobehavioral Sciences in the Semel Institute at University of California, Los Angeles, and a clinical research psychologist for the VA

Office of Mental Health Services and the VA Greater Los Angeles Health-care System. Dr. Glynn has extensive experience conducting psychosocial intervention trials to improve outcomes in serious psychiatric illness and trauma and has been funded by the VA, the National Institute of Mental Health, and the McCormick Foundation for her research. Dr. Glynn currently helps develop policy regarding families and their mental health in the VA and oversees VA national trainings in family interventions.

Kristina Coop Gordon, PhD, is Associate Professor of Psychology at the University of Tennessee. Her primary interests emphasize how couples respond to and recover from major relationship traumas and betrayals. She is coauthor of two books (*Getting Past the Affair* and *Helping Couples Get Past the Affair: A Clinician's Guide*). Dr. Gordon is a member of the Association for Behavioral and Cognitive Therapies Couple Research and Therapy Special Interest Group and the American Psychological Association's Society for Family Psychology. She recently received the Society's Distinguished Service Award for chairing their task force on Empirically Supported Couple and Family Treatments.

Richard E. Heyman, PhD, is Professor in the Department of Cariology and Comprehensive Care at New York University. Dr. Heyman has received 37 grants and contracts from major U.S. funding agencies on a variety of family-related topics, from anger escalation in couples to the impact of family violence on children to community-level prevention of family maltreatment, substance problems, and suicidality. Dr. Heyman has written over 100 scientific publications focused on couple dysfunction, partner abuse, and child maltreatment, and their risk factors and consequences.

Jamie M. Howard, PhD, is Project Director of the Strength at Home couples program in the VA Boston Healthcare System. Dr. Howard's clinical and research interests target the effects of PTSD on family functioning, particularly parent-child and intimate partner interactions. She has coauthored several articles and presented at multiple national conferences on the effects of trauma on families.

Shelley M. MacDermid Wadsworth, PhD, is Professor of Family Studies at Purdue University, where she is also Director of the Center for Families and Director of the Military Family Research Institute. Her research emphasizes the relations between work conditions and family life, with a specific interest in research about and for military families. Her research has been supported by a range of foundations, endowments, and governmental awards. Dr. MacDermid Wadsworth has received the Work Life Legacy Award from the Families and Work Institute and is a Fellow of the National Council on Family Relations.

Alexandra Macdonald, PhD, is Project Director of the Strength at Home men's program in the VA Boston Healthcare System. Dr. Macdonald's clinical and research interests focus on identifying and treating the effects of PTSD on relationship functioning, particularly intimate partner interactions. She has coauthored multiple articles, presented at national conferences, and co-led several workshops on the effects of trauma on individuals and relationships.

James A. Martin, PhD, is Professor of Social Work and Social Research at Bryn Mawr College and a Licensed Independent Clinical Social Worker with more than 40 years of practice experience. His scholarship, teaching, and public service focus on behavioral health issues impacting individuals, families, and communities, and his research and civic engagement address military and veteran populations. A retired Army Colonel, his military experience includes clinical, research, and senior management (command) and policy assignments. A combat veteran, he was the senior Social Work Officer in the Persian Gulf Theater of Operations during Operation Desert Storm.

Candace M. Monson, PhD (*see* "About the Editors").

Timothy J. O'Farrell, PhD, ABPP, is Professor of Psychology in the Department of Psychiatry at Harvard Medical School and Director of the Families and Addiction Program and the Counseling for Alcoholics' Marriages (CALM) Project at the VA Boston Healthcare System. His clinical and research interests focus primarily on couple and family therapy in alcoholism and drug abuse treatment and various aspects of substance abusers' family relationships, including partner violence, child functioning, and sexual adjustment. His books include *Behavioral Couples Therapy for Alcoholism and Drug Abuse* and *Treating Alcohol Problems: Marital and Family Interventions*.

Ruth Paris, PhD, is Associate Professor and Director of the Family Therapy Certificate Program at Boston University School of Social Work. Dr. Paris has evaluated and developed interventions serving diverse families of young children, including military service members, immigrant/refugee mothers, and parents in residential treatment for substance abuse. Dr. Paris has practiced clinical social work extensively with families in a variety of settings, including Massachusetts General Hospital, Kaiser Permanente, and community mental health.

David S. Riggs, PhD, is Executive Director of the Center for Deployment Psychology and Research Associate Professor at the Uniformed Services University of the Health Sciences. Dr. Riggs's research and clinical work examine trauma, violence, PTSD, and their impact on families. He has published over 60 articles and book chapters, coedited the book *Risk and*

Resilience in U.S. Military Families, and presented papers and workshops on such topics as PTSD, domestic violence, and behavior therapy. Dr. Riggs oversees the development and delivery of programs to train behavioral health professionals to care for service members and veterans and their families.

Abigail Ross, MSW, MPH, is a doctoral student at the Boston University School of Social Work and Project Director of the Strong Families Strong Forces program, a 4-year study funded by the Department of Defense to develop a home-based reintegration program for Operation Enduring Freedom/Operation Iraqi Freedom (OEF/OIF) veteran parents with young children. Her previous work has emphasized development and adaptation of family-based prevention, including a family-based intervention for suicidal adolescents and a depression prevention program for Latino populations at Children's Hospital Boston.

Steven L. Sayers, PhD, is Associate Professor of Psychology in the Department of Psychiatry, Perelman School of Medicine, University of Pennsylvania. At the Philadelphia VA Medical Center he is Director of the Advanced Fellowship Program in Mental Illness Research and Treatment. Dr. Sayers has published numerous articles regarding the role of family members and other social supports in mental and physical health. In 2008 he presented testimony to the Senate Committee on Veterans Affairs regarding his research with veterans and their family members.

David M. Scheider, DMin, is Director of the Family Life Chaplain Training Center at Fort Hood, Texas. He is a Licensed Marriage and Family Therapist and an American Association for Marriage and Family Therapy (AAMFT) Approved Supervisor. Dr. Scheider is a U.S. Army Chaplain (Lt. Colonel) and previously served as deputy garrison chaplain in Grafenwoehr, Germany.

Jeremiah A. Schumm, PhD, is Staff Psychologist at the Cincinnati VA Medical Center and Assistant Professor of Clinical Psychiatry at the University of Cincinnati. He has dual interests in the areas of substance use disorders and trauma-related disorders. He has authored over 20 peer-reviewed publications and 10 book chapters spanning these areas. Dr. Schumm has a particular interest in the application of conjoint treatments in treating these disorders and has developed an integrated couple-based treatment for veterans with co-occurring alcohol use disorder and posttraumatic stress disorder.

Michelle D. Sherman, PhD, is Clinical Professor at the University of Oklahoma Health Sciences Center and Director of the Family Mental Health Program at the Oklahoma City VA Medical Center. She is also a researcher with the South Central Mental Illness Research, Education and Clinical Center. Dr. Sherman has dedicated her career to understanding and supporting families affected by mental illness and trauma/PTSD. In her personal life, she also writes books for teens whose parents have experienced mental illness, trauma, and military deployment (*www. SeedsofHopeBooks.com*). She is a Fellow of the American Psychological Association's Society for Family Psychology.

Philippe Shnaider, BA, is a graduate student in clinical psychology at Ryerson University. His research interests include understanding therapeutic processes that predict treatment outcomes. He has contributed to a longitudinal study examining the interpersonal and intrapersonal risk and resilience factors in PTSD.

Laurie B. Slone, PhD, is Associate Director for Information and Communication at the VA's National Center for PTSD. She oversees the PTSD website *www.ptsd.va.gov.* Her research emphasizes barriers to care, social support, and community-based networks, as well as epidemiology. Dr. Slone is also Assistant Professor in the Department of Psychiatry at Dartmouth Medical School and a member of the International Society for Traumatic Stress Studies, and has been recognized with the Vermont Commendation Medal from the Vermont National Guard in 2007.

Lance Sneath, MS, is former Director of the Family Life Chaplain Training Center at Fort Hood, Texas. He is a Licensed Marriage and Family Therapist, an AAMFT Approved Supervisor, and a Diplomate in both the American Association of Pastoral Counselors and the College of Pastoral Supervision and Psychotherapy. Chaplain Sneath is a Lt. Colonel (Retired) in the U.S. Army, a veteran of Operation Iraqi Freedom, and has 25 years of active military service, including 4 years in the Air Force.

Douglas K. Snyder, PhD (*see* "About the Editors").

Casey T. Taft, PhD, is a staff psychologist at the National Center for PTSD in the VA Boston Healthcare System and Associate Professor of Psychiatry at Boston University School of Medicine. Dr. Taft serves as Principal Investigator on several funded grants focusing on understanding and preventing partner violence. He received the 2006 Chaim Danieli Young Professional Award from the International Society for Traumatic Stress Studies and the 2009 Linda Saltzman Memorial Intimate Partner Violence Researcher Award. He serves on several editorial boards of journals in the areas of clinical psychology, trauma, and the family.

Barbara Thompson, MS, is Director, Office of Family Policy/Children and Youth, Office of the Secretary of Defense. Her responsibilities emphasize programs and policies that promote military families' well-being, readiness, and quality of life. Ms. Thompson has been recognized as a leader in the field of early childhood education as one of only 11 Harris fellows to participate in Zero to Three's prestigious Leaders for the 21st Century program.

Valerie Vorstenbosch, MA, is a doctoral student in clinical psychology at Ryerson University. Her research interests include evidence-based assessment and treatment of anxiety disorders, including PTSD, obsessive–compulsive disorder, specific phobia, and social phobia.

Sonya G. Wanklyn, MA, is a graduate student in the clinical psychology program at Ryerson University. Her research interests include the process of recovery from trauma exposure, malingering of PTSD, risk and protective factors for criminal offending, and the intersection of intimate relationships and violent behavior.

June Behn Watts, MS, is a marriage and family therapist for the U.S. Department of Veterans Affairs at the Indianapolis Veterans Center. She served 8 years in the Indiana Army National Guard, and as a Mental Health Specialist with the 76th Infantry Brigade in support of OEF from 2004 to 2005. Her clinical and research interests focus on the impact of combat deployment on couples and family functioning. She is a member of the AAMFT and has presented at multiple conferences both nationally and locally on the effects of combat on intimate relationships.

Thomas C. Waynick, MS, is former Director of the Family Life Chaplain Training Center at Fort Benning, Georgia. He is a Licensed Marriage and Family Therapist, an AAMFT Approved Supervisor, and a Diplomate in both the American Association of Pastoral Counselors and the College of Pastoral Supervision and Psychotherapy. Chaplain Waynick is a Lt. Colonel in the U.S. Army and a veteran of OIF.

Mark A. Whisman, PhD, is Professor and Director of Clinical Training in the Department of Psychology and Neuroscience at the University of Colorado at Boulder. His research focuses on couple functioning and mental and physical health, with an emphasis on the onset, course, and treatment of depression. He is editor of *Adapting Cognitive Therapy for Depression: Managing Complexity and Comorbidity* and coeditor of *Treating Difficult Couples*, is Associate Editor of the *Journal of Family Psychology*, and serves on the editorial boards of several journals in clinical psychology.

Contents

COUPLE-BASED INTERVENTIONS
FOR MILITARY AND VETERAN FAMILIES

PART I

Empirical and Conceptual Foundations

CHAPTER 1

Couple-Based Interventions for Military and Veteran Families

Evidence and Rationale

Candice M. Monson and Douglas K. Snyder

At the writing of this book, over 2 million U.S. service members have been deployed in service to the conflicts in Iraq and Afghanistan since 2001, and many other troops have been deployed from other countries as part of the Multinational Forces. Based on data indicating that each U.S. service member has an average of 1.5 eligible dependents (i.e., spouses, children, adult dependents) this means that approximately 3 million family members have been directly affected by military deployment (U.S. Department of Defense, 2007). These estimates do not take into account the many extended family members, such as grandparents, aunts/uncles, siblings, and adult children, who have also been affected by the reverberations of deployment and the mental health problems and physical disabilities that may result from experiences during deployment. The most recent conflicts have brought heightened awareness of the effects of deployment and mental health issues on couples and families that arise during the course of military service. As a result, the U.S. Departments of Defense (DoD) and Veterans Affairs (VA), as well as veteran service organizations, have come to recognize the pressing need for family support services and interventions. Yet many clinicians within and outside of these organization are not well-versed in family theory and interventions, the military subculture that influences individual and relational functioning, or the best ways to incorporate family members in assessment and treatment when problems develop. Our overarching goal is to address this gap between the substantial family needs and clinician knowledge and skill to deliver high-quality couple and family interventions.

BRIEF HISTORY OF FAMILY RESEARCH WITH PRIOR VETERAN COHORTS

The effects of combat and combat-related mental health conditions on family functioning and vice versa have been well-documented, dating back to at least World War II, when researchers and clinicians noted the changes in family roles and functions that accompanied long deployments, and the adaptations that needed to occur for veterans to reintegrate into their families. For example, labor shortages resulting from the number of men deployed and the casualties of World War II brought women into the workforce in record numbers, leading to transitions in family functioning regarding child care and roles for women within and outside of the home. Those veterans who returned home, as well as their families, were forced to adapt to a new set of roles and, for many, to confront mental health issues that were not well understood or treated at that time. As a result, most of the documentation on service members' and veterans' families was epidemiological (e.g., rates of increased divorce, as well as increases in the birthrate—a.k.a. the "baby boom") or clinical descriptions of the types of struggles and transitions in family roles and functioning. Less was written about the associations between mental health conditions and their effects on the family or the role of the family in promoting individual veteran mental health, because much less was known about combat-related mental health sequelae at that time.

The Vietnam War brought a surge of empirical research and heightened public and professional recognition of individual combat-related mental health problems. In fact, Vietnam veterans and their posttraumatic reactions were a major impetus to the inclusion of the posttraumatic stress disorder (PTSD) diagnosis in the third edition of the *Diagnostic and Statistical Manual of Mental Disorders* in 1980. There was also more empirical attention paid to the association between PTSD and a range of psychosocial impairments, including its effects on couple and family functioning, as well as the individual mental health of spouses and children.

A landmark study of U.S. veterans' families came out of the congressionally mandated National Vietnam Veterans Readjustment Study (NVVRS; Kulka et al., 1990). The larger NVVRS comprised 1,200 male and 432 female veterans who served during the Vietnam War at least 15 years prior to the study's completion. A subsample of the overall NVVRS sample was involved in a study focused on the intimate partners and children of these veterans and their family relationship functioning. This substudy has yielded a number of substantial contributions to the understanding of the role of military service, combat exposure, and combat-related mental health problems in the context of family functioning. For example, the seminal paper from this study (Jordan et al., 1992) documented that the elevated rates of couple distress, divorce, parenting problems, and family violence found in these veterans was attributable to the psychopathology associated with combat trauma exposure (e.g., PTSD) versus combat trauma exposure per se. In fact, combat trauma exposure without a PTSD diagnosis was associated with *less* risk for perpetrating domestic violence. The rates of the various couple and family problems found in the NVVRS in those who were trauma exposed but without a PTSD diagnosis were comparable to the general population. Follow-up studies have found behavioral avoidance and emotional numbing symptoms to be more specifically implicated in the association between PTSD and intimate partner problems, as well as veterans' relationships with their children. The hyperarousal symptoms found in PTSD, which significantly overlap with symptoms of depression (e.g., irritability, sleep disturbance, attention/concentration problems), have been particularly associated with the perpetration of family violence in veterans. Studies with other samples of U.S. veterans and veterans serving other countries have found similar results (see Monson, Taft, & Fredman, 2009, for review).

A few studies regarding service members/veterans and their families have been conducted since the research focus on Vietnam veterans, to include studies with peacekeepers serving in various areas (e.g., Bosnia) and those serving in the first Iraq War. However, the current wars in Iraq and Afghanistan have led to the largest proliferation of studies on service members and veterans and their families during and after deployments. This focus on couple/family functioning is heartening given the well-documented effects of deployment, and especially combat deployments, on families (these effects are described by Beasley, MacDermid Wadsworth, & Watts, Chapter 4, and Snyder & Monson, Chapter 13). In addition, this recent research is more rigorous methodologically, because it is occurring during and more immediately following the deployments and, in some cases, is being conducted longitudinally to better understand the effects of deployment and deployment-related health problems on families over time.

In addition to these methodological improvements, there are characteristics about the current wars that may differentially affect families compared with prior conflicts. Specifically, in contrast to Vietnam, there is an all-volunteer military fighting force involved in these wars. Because the current cohort of service members is older, includes more women, and is more likely to be married and to have children compared with prior veterans, one could anticipate different individual and relational outcomes. In 2009, nearly 70% of enlisted troops were in their 20s, and most officers were in their 30s. About 50% of service members were married, and more than 25% had dependent children. Women also represent the fastest growing demographic of service members and veterans, and women's roles in the military and combat have evolved significantly since prior conflicts. Also, compared with prior peacekeeping and combat missions, there is an unprecedented reliance on the Reserve and National Guard components of the DoD which, as described by Martin and Sherman (Chapter 2) and Slone, Friedman, and Thompson (Chapter 3), are without many of the institutional resources and supports to which active duty service members and their dependents are entitled. Service members and their families are typically facing not a single deployment, but rather multiple deployments, with some having weathered five or six deployments already. These deployments are sometimes extended beyond the expected time frame, and this time variance can be highly disruptive to service members and their families. Furthermore, the insurgency warfare and guerilla tactics (e.g., improvised explosive devices, suicide bombings) being used in Iraq and Afghanistan have brought different wide-reaching effects on the physical and mental health of this most recent cohort of veterans compared with cohorts in prior eras. Advances in medical technology have significantly decreased the number of service members who die as a result of these and other war-related tactics, but the number of long-term physical and mental disabilities resulting from these injuries has significantly increased. Partners and extended family members often are required to provide varying levels of assistance and care for those with these disabilities. Finally, technological advances have radically changed the landscape of contact between deployed service members and their families, which is in marked contrast to the experience of deployed service members and their families in years past. The ability to be in contact in real time, with audio and video capabilities in many cases, carries with it a number of potential advantages and disadvantages to the adjustment of service members and their families during deployment.

LANDMARK FAMILY FINDINGS RELATED TO THE WARS IN IRAQ AND AFGHANISTAN

Alongside traumatic brain injury, we believe that the "signature wound" of the wars in Iraq and Afghanistan is the combat-related mental and physical health issues that adversely impact couple and family functioning. Epidemiological research indicates that approximately 20–35% of service members who served in combat deployments to Iraq or Afghanistan evidence clinical levels of PTSD, depression, general anxiety, or alcohol misuse, with rising rates of these problems over time (e.g., Hoge et al., 2004). In addition to documenting the high and increasing rates of veterans with mental health problems, an important point to highlight from this research is the even greater rise in reported interpersonal problems. In a longitudinal study of over 88,000 soldiers who served in Iraq, Milliken, Auchterlonie, and Hoge (2007) found a fourfold increase in reported interpersonal problems from the first to second waves of assessment (a median of 6 months). Others have found that more than 75% of married/partnered veterans who screen positive for mental health problems in VA outpatient treatment clinics report difficulties with partners or children.

Studies of Iraq and Afghanistan veterans, like those of prior veterans, have documented positive correlations between symptoms of PTSD, depression, sleep disturbance, dissociation, and alcohol use disorder and intimate relationship discord and parenting problems (e.g., Gerwitz, Polusny, DeGarmo, Khaylis, & Erbes, 2010). Extending this research to examine potential mechanisms accounting for the associations, partners' perceptions of service members' combat exposure have been found to influence the strength of the association between PTSD and relationship dissatisfaction. More specifically, when female partners perceive their husbands to have experienced relatively low levels of combat exposure and their husbands report high levels of PTSD symptoms, the association between PTSD symptoms and wives' discord is stronger (Renshaw, Rodebaugh, & Rodrigues, 2010). By contrast, when wives perceive their husbands to have experienced high levels of combat exposure, husbands' self-reported PTSD symptoms no longer predict their wives' relationship satisfaction; that is, wives appear to be less distressed if their husbands' PTSD symptoms can be understood as the result of combat exposure or other consequences of war. Wives' perceptions of caregiver burden for their veteran partners have also been found to be a mediator in the association between mental health problems and intimate relationship problems. Ultimately, over time the effects of PTSD on veterans' intimate relationships are likely to take a toll, but the meaning that caregivers give to their partners' symptoms can potentially serve either to soften or exacerbate that impact.

Rising rates of suicide by service members and veterans have been of great concern to the military and VA, and the role of interpersonal and family factors in precipitating suicidality and preventing attempts has become a focus of research and clinical attention. In the general suicide literature, relationship conflict emerges as a consistent and strong risk factor for suicidality. Other significant family risk factors include relationship separation or termination, as well as domestic violence in the relationship. Another important familial risk factor from the suicide literature is the veteran's or service member's own perception of being a burden to his or her family. Irrespective of type of mental or physical health condition, it is important for providers to remember the salient role of family relationship functioning in assessing and managing suicidality in veterans and service members. This is more fully discussed by Whisman and Sayers in Chapter 9.

A study on the role of couples' communication during deployment provides some initial empirically informed guidance about the best means and frequency of communication with regard to service members' mental health functioning, and thereby their combat readiness (Carter et al., 2011). This study revealed that overall frequency of communication was not associated with the male soldiers' severity of PTSD symptoms. However, there was a significant inverse relation between frequency of communication and PTSD severity for those soldiers who had high levels of relationship satisfaction. In other words, more frequent communication among satisfied couples was protective against PTSD symptoms. The authors examined the speed of communication as well, including delayed (i.e., e-mail, letters, care packages) and interactive (i.e., instant messaging, phone calls, video messaging) methods. Relationship satisfaction was even more important in the association between delayed communication and PTSD symptoms. More frequent delayed communication was associated with less PTSD symptom severity in couples with high levels of relationship satisfaction and more PTSD symptom severity in couples with low levels of relationship satisfaction.

A disconcerting finding that has emerged in this newest cohort of service members is a sex difference in the rate of divorce. The Pentagon has reported that female service members, in general, are twice as likely as their male counterparts to divorce. Enlisted women are three times more likely than male enlistees to divorce (Karney & Crown, 2007). The various reasons offered for this sex difference include the fact that female service members are more likely to be married to male service members, which causes increased tension from balancing family and mission demands, and greater sacrifices for these dual-career couples. In addition, women's roles in the military and combat have evolved and expanded, which has resulted in increased expectations of women, and these service-related demands are not being offset with changes in the routines and responsibilities for women at home. Research with female service members documents that the expectations for household upkeep and child care have been maintained in spite of women's greater work demands and likelihood of deployment. Furthermore, it is a more common expectation for women to stay at home to single-parent and maintain family life than for men to manage these demands while their wives deploy. Future empirical research into the reasons for this disparity will help to inform support and intervention strategies for women service members and their at-risk marriages.

Several studies investigating the mental health and overall functioning of female partners and children of deployed service members have revealed the stressful effects of deployment on these individuals left at home. A medical record review of over 250,000 U.S. Army wives, with over 6.5 million outpatient visits, revealed that those wives with a deployed husband were significantly more likely to be diagnosed with, and receive services for, a mental health condition compared with wives who did not have a deployed husband. The rates of the wives' mental health diagnoses increased even more as husbands' length of deployment increased (i.e., longer than 11 months; Mansfield et al., 2010). Similarly, as elaborated by DeVoe, Paris, and Ross in Chapter 5, rates of childhood behavioral and emotional problems can increase with the deployment of a parent. Although military families and dependents evidence a great deal of resilience under the pressures of military service, and deployments specifically, these studies point to the larger mental health effects of deployment on military dependents.

INTEGRATION OF FAMILY MEMBERS IN INTERVENTIONS

All of the family-oriented studies discussed earlier have concluded that there is a pressing need to increase family support and intervention efforts for veterans and service members and their families. Several studies have also specifically addressed the desire of veterans and their families to be involved in these interventions. A large majority of veterans seeking mental health treatment have indicated that they recognize that their mental health problems affect their families and want their family members to be involved in treatment (e.g., Batten et al., 2009). Spouses have also indicated their desire to be involved in assessment and intervention efforts, with many of them expressing a sentiment that their struggles and sacrifices have been overlooked.

There also seems to be greater societal recognition of the need for family involvement in mental health prevention, assessment, and treatment services in order to improve treatment efficacy and expand the benefits of the treatment. For example, in 2003, there was a specific call by the President's New Freedom Commission for family-centered services and treatments. In 2008, the VA was provided authority by Public Law 110-387, the Veterans' Mental Health and Other Care Improvement Act, to include marriage and family counseling as a service for family members of *all* veterans eligible for care. As a result, clinicians with expertise in couple and family therapy were hired, and training and dissemination efforts were initiated to increase staff capacity to deliver evidence-based couple and family interventions. Similarly, the DoD has initiated several training programs for its mental health, family advocacy, and chaplaincy staff on evidence-based interventions to prevent couple discord and to address couple distress, when it develops, and specific couple-level problems, such as infidelity and domestic violence. Snyder, Baucom, Gordon, and Doss

(Chapter 6) and Hayman, Taft, Howard, Macdonald, and Collins (Chapter 7) address these important problems. There have also been efforts to train staff in couple therapies that address specific, individual mental health conditions that are commonly found in veterans and service members and have the added benefits of enhancing couple functioning and improving the health and well-being of partners. Couple therapies for these conditions are presented, featuring interventions for PTSD (Monson, Fredman, & Riggs, Chapter 8) depression (Whisman & Sayers, Chapter 9) alcohol and other substance abuse (Schumm & O'Farrell, Chapter 10), traumatic brain injury (Glynn, Chapter 11), and grief and loss (Scheider, Sneath, & Waynick, Chapter 12).

We consider this book to be an extension of these important efforts, as we aim to facilitate preparation of the myriad providers that serve veterans, service members, and their families. We hope to widen the scope of these training efforts to include the many clinicians who see these individuals and couples outside of military and veteran healthcare settings in the community, and providers in other countries who may not yet have access to training in these evidence-based practices. We have aimed to make this book as user-friendly and clinically relevant as possible. Toward this end, the reader will notice that the chapters include case examples to illustrate more fully the concepts presented. Each chapter concludes with a list of "Resources" also cited in the text of the chapter rather than a full bibliography of references. We asked each contributor to identify those key resources so that busy providers could easily discern and access those materials if more information is desired.

In order to promote a solid theoretical and practical foundation for providers, Part I of this book presents chapters focused on helping providers be culturally competent regarding the social context that surrounds military and veteran families (Martin & Sherman, Chapter 2), and thinking about matching available resources and family needs (Slone, Friedman, & Thompson, Chapter 3). There is also a focus on the normative transitions and adjustments to and from deployment as they affect military and veteran families (Beasley, Wadsworth, & Watts, Chapter 4). Part II of the book (Chapters 5 to 12) focuses on best practice and evidence-based couple interventions for specific couple-level problems and individual mental health conditions most common to military and veteran couples, as well as their children. Each of these chapters includes reproducible handouts to facilitate relevant interventions. (Larger versions of these handouts can also be downloaded from the book's page on The Guilford Press website.)

Part III examines implications of the previous chapters for institutional policies and clinical practice in both the military and civilian communities (Snyder & Monson, Chapter 13). The book concludes with appendices of resources specifically developed for veterans' and service members' families, as well as an overview of military ranks, structural organization, and common terms that providers may encounter in the course of clinical work.

SUMMARY

The wars in Iraq and Afghanistan have brought unprecedented professional and public attention to our need to support families as they face deployment and redeployment, and to address the collateral damage that deployment-related mental and physical health problems can have on the families of veterans. Likewise, we are beginning to appreciate the powerful role that couple and family relationships can play in sustaining health and preventing longer-term problems when the inevitable stress of combat deployment comes. Service members, veterans, and their spouses have expressed their desire to have greater family involvement in the planning and provision of interventions to enhance treatment efficacy and the breadth of improvements when mental health conditions arise. To help meet these crucial needs, this book provides a comprehensive "go-to" resource for facilitating the health and resilience of service members, veterans, and their families—a group richly deserving of the best possible care and support that can be provided.

RESOURCES

Batten, S. V., Drapalski, A. L., Decker, M. L., DeViva, J. C., Morris, L. J., Mann, M. A., et al. (2009). Veteran interest in family involvement in PTSD treatment. *Psychological Services, 6,* 184–189.

Carter, S., Loew, B., Allen, E., Stanley, S., Rhoades, G., & Markman, H. (2011). Relationships between soldiers' PTSD symptoms and spousal communication during deployment. *Journal of Traumatic Stress, 24,* 352–355.

Gerwitz, A. H., Polusny, M. A., DeGarmo, D. S., Khaylis, A., & Erbes, C. R. (2010). Posttraumatic stress symptoms among National Guard soldiers deployed to Iraq: Associations with parenting behaviors and couple adjustment. *Journal of Consulting and Clinical Psychology, 78,* 599–610.

Hoge, C. W., Castro, C. A., Messer, S. C., McGurk, D., Cotting, D. I., & Koffman, R. L. (2004). Combat duty in Iraq and Afghanistan, mental health problems, and barriers to care. *New England Journal of Medicine, 351,* 13–22.

Jordan, B. K., Marmar, C. R., Fairbank, J. A., Schlenger, W. E., Kulka, R. A., Hough, R. L., et al. (1992). Problems in families of male Vietnam veterans with posttraumatic stress disorder. *Journal of Consulting and Clinical Psychology, 60,* 916–926.

Karney, B. R., & Crown, J. A. (2007). *Families under stress: An assessment of data, theory, and research on marriage and divorce in the military.* Arlington, VA: RAND Corporation.

Kulka, R. A., Schlenger, W. E., Fairbank, J. A., Hough, R. L., Jordan, B. K., Marmar, C. R., et al. (Eds.). (1990). *Trauma and the Vietnam War generation: Report of findings from the National Vietnam Veterans Readjustment Study.* New York: Brunner/Mazel.

Mansfield, A. J., Kaufman, J. S., Marshall, S. W., Gaynes, B. N., Morrissey, J. P., & Engel, C. C. (2010). Deployment and the use of mental health services among U.S. Army wives. *New England Journal of Medicine, 362,* 101–109.

Milliken, C. S., Auchterlonie, J. L., & Hoge, C. W. (2007). Longitudinal assessment of mental health problems among active and reserve component soldiers returning from the Iraq War. *Journal of the American Medical Association, 298,* 2141–2148.

Monson, C. M., Taft, C. T., & Fredman, S. J. (2009). Military-related PTSD and intimate relationships: From description to theory-driven research and intervention development. *Clinical Psychology Review, 8,* 707–714.

U.S. Department of Defense. (2007). *Demographics 2007: Profile of the military community.* Retrieved October 9, 2011, from *www.militaryhomefront.dod.mil/12038/project%20documents/militaryhomefront/reports/2007%20demographics.pdf.*

Renshaw, K. D., Rodebaugh, T. L., & Rodrigues, C. S. (2010). Psychological and marital distress in spouses of Vietnam veterans: Importance of spouses' perceptions. *Journal of Anxiety Disorders, 24,* 743–750.

CHAPTER 2

Understanding the Effects of Military Life and Deployment on Couples and Families

James A. Martin and Michelle D. Sherman

Jeanne, age 35 and a married mother of two children, ages 8 and 10, has been a member of the U.S. Army National Guard for the last 5 years, prior to which she served on active duty in the Army for 10 years. Jeanne recently returned from a 12-month deployment to Iraq as a noncommissioned officer (NCO; a Sergeant) in a transportation unit responsible for moving supplies by truck across very dangerous areas. Although she kept in touch with her husband and kids via the Internet and real-time voice and video communication, Jeanne missed them terribly and hated being absent from birthdays, holidays, basketball games, school musicals, and just hanging out together on weekends. While in Iraq, she was shot at and her unit encountered improvised explosive devices (IEDs) a number of times. In one of these incidents, three of her fellow soldiers were killed. She didn't tell her family about these deaths or the personal danger she felt during the deployment, because she didn't want them to worry about her. Her entire family greeted her enthusiastically with signs, flags, and hugs at the Welcome Home celebration, and for a while, things seemed to be okay. Now, a few months later, she's not quite sure where she "fits in" in the family. While she was gone, her husband pretty much ran the family by himself, and the kids now look to him for support, decisions, and discipline. Jeanne finds herself getting angry at little things that her kids do—stuff that would never have bothered her before. She occasionally has nightmares about events in Iraq. Jeanne had been promised she'd get her job back at the shipping company where she worked before the deployment. Now that she is ready to return to work, she's heard rumors that some National Guard members have experienced difficulty getting their jobs back, and she is nervous about talking to her former boss. The kids have changed so much, and she's not the same person she was before the deployment. It's going to take some time to reconnect as a family.

This chapter provides an important context for this book by describing the people and the unique military life experiences of current and former military members and their families. In order to work effectively with these individuals and their families, it is imperative to understand and appreciate the significant personal and family life sacrifices that are inherent in military service across the life course spectrum, from entry into the Armed Forces through and beyond reintegration into civilian life as a veteran (including the sacrifices made by members of the National Guard and the other Reserve Components and their families). The opening vignette about Jeanne and her family highlights the fact that today's military members and veterans differ considerably from a stereotypical image. Current military members and recent veterans represent an all-volunteer force that is well educated and racially and ethnically diverse across all ranks and occupational specialties. Many are veterans of combat, having served tours of duty in Afghanistan or Iraq. In this case, Jeanne represents one of the many female combat veterans and National Guard members who have been deployed in support of these wars.

Our goal in this chapter is to enhance awareness of military culture and military life experiences, and provide the groundwork for acquisition of culturally informed practice skills described in subsequent chapters. We also hope to encourage clinicians' interest in providing services to military/ veteran clients and their families. Whereas military life and duty can be risk factors for significant behavioral health and relationship problems, these experiences can also enhance personal and family resilience and are often a source of strength.

The first section of this chapter addresses issues related to Active and Reserve Component members. The second section discusses the veteran population, with a specific focus on recent veterans from the wars in Afghanistan and Iraq. Both sections identify a range of health and behavioral health issues associated with these wars, including the specific recognition of combat-related stress and trauma, and the associated prevalence of posttraumatic stress disorder (PTSD) and traumatic brain injuries (TBIs). It is also important to acknowledge the presence of other behavioral health conditions such as suicide, alcohol, tobacco, and drug use, and a variety of dangerous thrill-seeking behaviors that are in some way connected to duty and military life experiences. Finally, clinicians need to be aware of the prevalence of issues such as military-related sexual trauma (MST) for women and men, as well as the relationship difficulties that may emerge from any of these conditions and disrupt personal, family, school, or work functioning.

All providers need to understand the distinction between the Active and Reserve Components of the U.S. Armed Forces. The Active Component is made of five separate services: Army, Marine Corps, Navy, Air Force and Coast Guard—a part of the Department of Homeland Security. The Reserve Component is made up of the Army and Air National Guard and five other reserve services: Army Reserve, Marine Corps Reserve, Navy Reserve, Air Force Reserve, and Coast Guard Reserve. The National Guard and the other Reserve Components represent the tradition of the "citizen soldier" that dates back to the Revolutionary War. Unlike the Active Component, whose members serve on a full-time basis and come from communities all over the country, most National Guard and other Reserve Components consist of units that are regionally based, and their members are typically recruited from local areas.

The roles and responsibilities of the Reserve Components have changed dramatically in response to the challenges presented by the wars in Afghanistan and Iraq. The National Guard is the domestic "911" force, responding immediately to a wide array of local, state, and even national emergencies (e.g., Hurricane Katrina). Today, the Reserve Components have an important national defense role. No longer are they just an emergency "strategic force" to be used just in a national emergency; they are now an "operational force" designed to support ongoing, worldwide military missions. Members of the Guard and the other Reserves can expect to be mobilized for federal service on a regular basis (e.g., 1 year in every 5) to serve critical functions in support of our nation's national defense strategy.

Veterans, including those who continue to serve in the National Guard or the other Reserves after returning from a period of active duty, bring with them to civilian life an array of important duty and military life experiences. For some there are duty and military life exposures, as well as physical and mental injuries, that may be risk factors for a range of difficulties. Although these veterans receive care and services in a variety of community settings, the U.S. Veterans Administration (VA) is the largest provider of physical and behavioral healthcare specifically for this population. The VA also administers disability entitlements for those whose physical and mental health issues are defined as having been caused by their military service, or "service-connected disabilities."

OUR 21st-CENTURY ARMED FORCES AND THE CHANGING NATURE OF MILITARY SERVICE AND FAMILY LIFE

Beyond having a basic awareness of the structure of our Armed Forces, it is important for clinicians to have a fundamental appreciation of the people and the changing nature of military service and family life in the 21st century. In the following, we describe the people, their duties, their careers, and some important quality-of-life issues impacting military members and their families. Each of these domains of the 21st-century military continues to evolve within an array of social, legal, political, economic, and technological issues that have a profound influence on the military life course. For example, policies such as the much-debated "Don't Ask, Don't Tell" represent important personnel considerations, and like the military's racial integration policy of an earlier era the recent change in this policy represents both challenges and opportunities for enhancing our Armed Forces. Enlistment criteria, such as the requirement for high school completion and policies about waving civil legal involvements and certain criminal convictions, also reflect social considerations with potential long-term effects for the nature and quality of the Armed Forces. Advances in our understanding, treatment, and policies for compensation for injuries such as PTSD and TBI can have a profound impact on individual service members, veterans, and their families. All of these contextual factors represent important influences on the people, their duties, their careers, and their quality of life across the duty and military life course and into their transition and lives as veterans.

The People

The demographic trajectory of our Armed Forces has changed significantly since the adoption of the all-volunteer military concept in 1973 and the Department of Defense (DoD) emphasis on creating and sustaining a relatively small, well-trained, highly professional volunteer military. Today less that 1% of our population serves in the military. Although this rate has reached as high as 12% (contrasted with World War II, when 56% of the men eligible for military service on the basis of age actually served in the Armed Forces), it has always been less than 1% in peacetime and, other than World War II, has never risen above 5% during any major war.

The important change that has occurred with the adoption of today's all-volunteer force concept is that the Armed Forces are now a fundamental part of the education and labor markets and compete with higher education and civilian employers for young adults.

A second important demographic change during this period has been the expansion in the number and roles of women in the Armed Services. Women now make up about 14% of the military and percentages vary by service, with the Air Force having the highest percentage of women and the Marine Corps the lowest. Whereas current laws and military regulations still prohibit women from being assigned to ground combat units, women serving in Afghanistan and Iraq have been exposed to combat environments while serving in support roles such as truck drivers, medics, military police, helicopter pilots, and so on. As of 2010 women have served nearly 200,000 tours of duty in Afghanistan and Iraq, and about 3% of all combat causalities have been women.

Up-to-date military demographic information is easily accessible on the Internet from a variety of government and public sources. Table 2.1 provides a brief general overview of some basic and relatively stable demographics of the Armed Forces.

Approximately 70% of all Active Component military members and their families reside in the local civilian community near a military installation, and 30% live in government (or government-leased) housing on a military installation. In contrast, National Guard and other Reserve families are scattered across all 50 states and territories—many at a great distance from any military installation. These members and their families live in every American community, large and small, urban and suburban, and in particular, rural communities where "service" in the National Guard has a strong tradition and often provides an economic supplement to low wages or marginal employment.

During a deployment, the families of more senior and older Active Component military members typically remain in their current home or near the installation. Some younger spouses, especially those married to junior-ranking service members, return to their home communities and seek the support of their families and friends. Most National Guard and other Reserve families are already "grounded" in their civilian community and do not relocate; however, during a deployment, these families do not typically have the benefit of being on or near a military installation, and they generally lack the support of other military families.

Finally, as a context for this brief demographic profile, the U.S. military currently operates more than 800 military installations in 39 countries. On a typical day, approximately 90,000 Sailors and Marines are deployed at

TABLE 2.1. Demographic Profile of the Department of Defense (2009)

	Active Component	Guard/ other Reserve Components
Service members		
Total number	1,387,674	846,248
Ratio of officers to enlisted	1 to 5	1 to 6
Percent women	14%	18%
Percent minorities	36%	30%
Percent 25 years old or younger	46%	34%
Percent with bachelor's degree or higher	18%	19%
Percent married	55%	48%
Percent in dual-military marriages	7%	3%
Families		
Number of family members	1,897,913	1,121,868
Number of spouses	693,662	403,411
Percent with children	43%	42%
Average age at birth of first child	25	27
Number of adult dependents	8,501	1,958
Percent of children age 0 to 5	42%	26%
Percent single parents	5%	9%

Note. There are 3.5 million military members (this includes 1.4 million active duty members, 1 million Reserve Component members, and approximately 850,000 civilian employees). The data are from the latest DoD public demographic profile (2008). All percentages have been rounded to the nearest whole number. Source: Military Homefront Reports. Adapted from *http://cs.mhf.dod. mil/content/dav/mhf/qol-library/pdf/mhf/qol%20resources/reports/2009_demographics_report. pdf.*

sea away from their home and family. America's military is a global force, dispersed on every continent.

Their Duties

Josie and Rico, ages 20 and 21, respectively, had been high school sweethearts and were married right after high school graduation. Rico immediately joined the Marines and now, after completing his second year as a Marine, is deployed in Afghanistan. This is the fifth month in what is expected to be a 7-month deployment. Josie is proud and supportive of Rico's service, but she had never thought about his being sent so far away. They have a 2-year-old son and are expecting a baby girl in 3 months. They have a small apartment in the civilian community near the base. Like many young military families with limited financial resources, Josie and Rico have found it difficult to take advantage of the many support and socialization opportunities available on base. They are also 500 miles away from both of their families.

For the first few weeks after Rico left, Josie did well. She made a few friends among the other young Marine spouses in the same complex, and occasionally these wives got together at the playground with their children. She attended a few Family Readiness Group (FRG) meetings in Rico's unit, where she met some of the other unit wives, but most were older and their husbands were more senior in rank than Rico. Sometimes Josie felt a bit out of place at these meetings. As time passed, she stopped attending, although the wife of Rico's platoon sergeant calls her every Sunday to "check in." Lately Josie has felt overwhelmed, exhausted, and sad. She seldom is able to sleep through the night. With Rico gone, she has to do *everything*—not only all her usual household chores and caring for a very active 2-year-old, but also managing day-to-day decisions—car repairs, balancing the checkbook, and planning for the new baby. She is entering her third trimester and is increasingly tired. Rico is supportive when they talk on the phone, but it does not help much. Every day she feels more overwhelmed, and it's a struggle just to get through the day. Josie doesn't want to burden Rico with her feelings, because she knows he needs to focus on his mission in Afghanistan. She misses him terribly, feels so alone, and cannot wait for him to come home.

Josie's and Rico's experiences reflect the reality of life for many of today's military families. The long, repeated combat deployments, the high operation tempo, high rates of exposure to traumatic events in the war zone, and the considerable physical and emotional consequences of these deployments continue to take an enormous toll on the physical, psychological, and social well-being of military families. Our country's simultaneous requirements of fighting two major combat operations, while meeting all of the other national defense requirements, have placed great strain on each of the branches of service. Although all of the services are burdened, this is especially true for the Army and Marine Corps, which have carried the heaviest load in the ground wars in Afghanistan and Iraq.

When describing our nation's 21st century military forces, it is important to recognize that "deployment" is the fundamental role for military units, and it is what soldiers, marines, sailors, and airmen are trained and prepared to do. Military deployments encompass the "spectrum of military operations," ranging from humanitarian operations (e.g., the military's response after the earthquake in Haiti) to peacemaking and peacekeeping operations (e.g., military efforts in the Balkans), to major combat operations (e.g., Afghanistan and Iraq). Deployment requirements reflect day-to-day national defense policy decisions and the associated requirements for positioning forces around the globe. Whereas this "deployment burden" varies by component and service, as well as by the service members' specific military occupational skills, every service member understands the concept of "military readiness" and the importance of being prepared for deployment. The extent of deployment-induced stress for each military member can vary considerably, as the impact is usually a complex interaction among (1) the nature of the deployment exposures, (2) the individual's actual and perceived deployment experiences, (3) the duration of the deployment, (4) time home between deployments, (5) the number and frequency of deployments over time, and (6) other family issues that arise at home during the deployment (e.g., Josie's pregnancy during Rico's deployment).

Deployed service members have some buffer against daily family-life issues. They are less exposed to the direct intrusion of home or family expectations and demands on their duties. However, this separation is changing with advanced communication technologies (phone, Internet, and real-time video communication), which can present a dual-edge situation. Media advances support service members and families in maintaining important connections, and families can now provide support in a timely, frequent manner as never before. However, the ability to focus on battlefield duties can be diminished when the service member is preoccupied with family issues back home. Josie's experiences also remind us that the spouse at home often experiences the same "information intrusion and overload" when the minute-to-minute combat experiences of services members are constantly streaming into continuous "24/7" media outlets. Spouses and other family members need to learn how to avoid this information overload, especially excessive visual information exposures in the absence of any power to protect their loved ones from harm.

Their Careers

Dona and Jim, ages 40 and 45, respectively, have been married for 20 years. Like most couples, they've weathered many ups and downs as a Navy family, including Jim's 1-year unaccompanied assignment to Korea early in their marriage and two 4-year assignments with the entire family—the first in Guam and the second in Italy. They survived some financially tough times early in their marriage and succeeded in rearing two sons who are now preparing for college. Jim, a senior NCO in the Navy, has just returned from his third deployment at sea in the last 5 years, and the strain on this marriage is evident. Dona has been faithful to

Jim throughout his deployments, but recently she has been wondering about his fidelity. Even when home, Jim has traveled a lot as part of his Navy duties and has always worked extremely long hours, limiting their time together.

Now, when they do have a rare evening together, Jim just wants to watch television, and he avoids Dona's attempts at intimate communication. Although they had enjoyed a good sex life early in their marriage, Jim seems to have lost interest, so they are rarely physically intimate anymore. Dona feels like she's living with a roommate, not a husband. Jim has started to talk about retiring next year, and Dona is worried about finances with two children entering college and the financial and support needs of their own parents, who are in poor health. Mostly, Dona is worried that their marriage won't survive what she knows will be a very stressful transition for her husband from the Navy into civilian life. She fears the obvious economic uncertainties and the stress she expects the transition will cause Jim and, most importantly, that she will not be able to reestablish the intimacy she once enjoyed in their marriage.

The experiences of Dona and Jim reflect a range of common career military life experiences—overseas assignments, unaccompanied tours of duty, frequent deployments, and duty demands that often place strains on marriages at every phase of the military and family life course. Despite these challenges and a demanding lifestyle, most military families do well. In fact, many thrive, benefiting from the stimulating life experiences that are often associated with military life, such as living and traveling overseas, and the personal satisfaction and pride that typically come with successfully meeting challenging experiences, and the belief that one's service and sacrifice are important and valued.

Even when military marriages are successful, there can be emotional and relationship "residue" that remains when military duty or life challenges are profound or these military challenges occur in the context of other personal or family life challenges (e.g., death, injury, or illness in a family member or friend). For some military members and their families, duty demands, military life, and family life challenges are too great, such that they are not able to complete their military service obligation successfully and their spouses are not willing to continue in the marriage and remain in military life. While the military divorce rate has been relatively steady even in the post-9/11 period, about 3% per year, there is obvious stress on military marriages associated with the frequent, lengthy deployments to Afghanistan and Iraq.

Some military members, especially those in their initial enlistments, do not succeed in military service for a variety of reasons, ranging from medical discharges to those based on disciplinary actions. While beyond the scope of this chapter, clinicians need a basic understanding of the types of military discharges and the basic entitlements and consequences of each. A discharge or separation should not be confused with retirement; career military members who retire (typically after 20 or more years of service) are not discharged or separated; rather, they enter the Retired Reserve and may be subject to recall to active duty. The vast majority of those leaving the service after successfully completing an initial enlistment are actually "separated" rather than "discharged". A discharge completely alleviates the veteran of any unfulfilled military service obligation, whereas a separation (which may be voluntary or involuntary) typically leaves an additional unfulfilled military service obligation that is carried out in the Individual Ready Reserve (IRR). During the past few years a number of individuals, who had never thought that they would be "called back" to duty from their civilian life (i.e., members of the IRR), have found themselves back in uniform and back in combat.

There are also important distinctions between an "honorable" discharge (typically the individual has met or exceeded required standards of duty performance and personal conduct and completed their service obligation), and those in the categories of General, Other than Honorable, Bad Conduct, and Dishonorable. The latter types of discharges have negative or punitive characteristics, as well as significant benefit limitations. In the case of a dishonorable discharge, there are also severe limits on fundamental rights associated with citizenship.

In summary, military duties and the military lifestyle are challenging, and not everyone is suited for these demands, nor will everyone succeed. The same can be said for military couples and families. The DoD and the military services have made considerable efforts to provide couples and families with primary, secondary, and tertiary support to enrich, sustain, and support marriages and family life in recognition of these duty and military life challenges. And while some are not successful balancing the challenges of personal and family life with duty and military life demands, many individuals, couples, and families complete their military experience, whether it is one enlistment or a career, having gained important life skills and a sense of pride and accomplishment.

Their Quality of Life

The quality of life for military families has changed dramatically since the adoption of the all-volunteer force concept. As of 2010, the DoD is spending more than a billion dollars a year in support of military families, and this allocation for families has continued to rise in response to the obvious immediate and long-term needs associated with the wars in Afghanistan and Iraq. These entitlements and benefits reflect the reality that in order for military members to perform their duties successfully, it is necessary that they know that their families will be provided for, especially in a time of need. Without this commitment, the Armed Forces would likely not be able to recruit, sustain, or retain the quality and number of personnel required to meet national defense requirements.

In a 2009 DoD review of military quality of life, 19 major initiatives were highlighted in current efforts to improve the quality of life of service members and their families. These include programs such as installation Family Services, Family Advocacy, and Family Counseling programs designed to address a wide variety of family life issues, including the relationship stresses between husband and wife. Healthcare and the commissary/military exchange programs provide for day-to-day living needs, while efforts to support education benefits and financial security are geared toward the ongoing well-being of service members and their families. Other programs, such as the Wounded Warrior program, are geared toward service members who have experienced psychological or physical injuries from combat. The newest addition to the military's efforts to support members and families is called "Military OneSource," which encompasses many innovative outreach efforts, including a 24/7 hotline call center and website providing information, referral, and in some situations, direct services for the service member and family.

A major challenge now faced by the DoD (as well as the VA) is to move to a set of comprehensive, integrated, and evidence-based programs and services linked to outcomes that support recruitment, readiness, retention, and successful reintegration into civilian life. These programs and services must meaningfully benefit member and family quality of life and, at the same time, be integrated with both public and private sector programs and services. As the Secretaries of the DoD and the VA have publically noted, the capacity to support and sustain the nation's military members, veterans, and their families must include the participation of the entire community.

THE EVOLVING CHALLENGES OF REINTEGRATION AND SUSTAINMENT: TRANSITION TO VETERAN STATUS AND SUCCESSFUL ADAPTATION IN CIVILIAN LIFE

According to the National Center for Veterans Analysis and Statistics, there are over 23 million military veterans (92% of whom are male) and approximately 33% receive benefits and services within the VA healthcare system. Although approximately 40% of the entire veteran population is over age 65, thousands of men and women veterans have served in our military in the post-9/11 era and are now accessing the VA system. As of the end of 2009, of the more than 2 million men and women who have served in the wars in Afghanistan and Iraq, more than 1 million had left active military service and were eligible for VA services. Forty-six percent, more than 500,000, of these new veterans have already sought VA healthcare. Thus, these new, typically young veterans are entering a healthcare system that until recently was principally designed and funded to serve an older generation of male veterans.

Today's veterans are a unique amalgamation of men and women from all walks of life, parts of the country, and demographic backgrounds. These veterans brings unique military and personal life experiences back into civilian life—their personal and family relationships, school or employment, and their participation as community members.

Approximately 8% of all military veterans in the United States are women, and women comprise a greater percentage of this new generation of veterans than in previous cohorts. As opposed to their roles and the relatively safe settings they often occupied in previous conflicts (primarily medical and other support services), today women serve in a wide array of military roles and in settings where they are often exposed to danger, including combat operations. Our knowledge base about the experience of female veterans is still relatively small, with major questions remaining about how deployment and exposure to combat trauma uniquely affect women. Some have also speculated about how repeated separations from their children and the experience of combat may subsequently affect their mothering role in ways that are qualitatively different than that of fathers. Additionally, over 20% of all women veterans (and approximately 1% of men) have experienced sexual trauma and rape while in the military (MST; Kimerling, Gima, Smith, Street, & Frayne, 2007). The actual number of men who are victims of MST, corresponding to the much larger percentage of men in the military population overall, is greater than the number of women victims. For both men and women, the aftermath of MST involves ripple effects in all parts of the veteran's life, including relationship difficulties, possible PTSD, and increased risk of homelessness. As these victims transition into veteran status, they bring these challenges from their military service into their personal and family relationships, as well as their work and community life.

More than half of the current generation of veterans is married and many still have young children spanning the entire developmental spectrum, from infants to young adults. Families are adjusting to the reintegration of the veteran across a wide variety of family constellations. Both marital and parenting roles can provide important support to the veteran, as well as being a source of strain and family life challenges. The social support available through family relationships can function as an important buffer during the reintegration process, and the role of parent can provide an immense sense of identity and importance. However, reintegrating into the role of spouse/partner and parent, as well as reintegration into civilian community roles, can pose significant challenges.

Will and Danielle, ages 28 and 25, respectively, have been married for 2 years and are expecting their first child. Will and Danielle met, had a very brief courtship, and married shortly before the end of Will's last enlistment. Will, a military policeman in the Air Force Reserve, has a community college background with an Associate's Degree in law enforcement. He has served 4 years in the Air Force and was deployed on two combat missions to Iraq. Both deployments were stressful, and in Will's role as a military police officer, he encountered numerous confrontations with Iraqi civilians. In the last deployment he was exposed to many civilian deaths and injuries from suicide bombings in the urban areas where his unit operated. When Will decided to leave the Army, the couple moved to Minnesota to be near his family, because Danielle, as the only child of divorced parents, was not close to either of her parents.

Will is not happy with the low-paying security guard job he accepted in his home town and he recently has decided to use his military educational benefits to go back to school. He is considering a small local college where he can obtain a 4-year degree in law enforcement, which he hopes will provide employment opportunities that have not been possible with only an Associate's Degree. This young couple is still adjusting to their marriage, as well as a new community and new set of family and friendship relationships for Danielle. Although Danielle knows that Will is unhappy and suspects that some of their relationship problems have something to do with Will's experiences as a military police officer in Iraq, she just can't get him to talk to her about Iraq. The transition to being a full-time civilian and a part-time Reservist, as well as going back to college, and their soon-to-arrive baby will present additional challenges for Will, Danielle, and their marriage. Will likes being a military policeman but is not eager to return to a combat environment. Danielle fears that this is bound to happen at some point, and she fears raising their baby alone.

One of the hallmarks of the wars in Afghanistan and Iraq is the recognition of the large number of service members and veterans experiencing behavioral, health, substance abuse, and associated relationship problems as they attempt to reintegrate to family and community life. Of note are the large numbers of service members who are experiencing clinical and subclinical PTSD and mild to moderate TBI. This is in addition to the service members who have been evacuated from the war zone with serious physical or psychological injury, many of whom subsequently transition as veterans into the VA system of care. Awareness, assessment, documentation, and assistance for these difficulties are more available now than ever before, and tremendous efforts are being made to reduce the stigma surrounding accessing care. However, when describing this cohort, it is essential to highlight that many do live with PTSD and TBI, often described as the signature wounds of these conflicts, and these conditions can have long-term biopsychosocial consequences. Although some of these wounds are severe, for many more these injuries represent an unrecognized or untreated condition of varying severity that can represent a continued burden for veterans, their families, and their communities.

The Transition Challenges for New Veterans

The journey to veteran status can take many different routes, including retirement after a military career or release from the service after completing one or more enlistments or a period of commissioned service as a military officer. As noted earlier, for some individuals, the separation from service is premature and represents an unplanned discharge due to the consequences of an injury, illness, or personal misconduct. In the case of severe misconduct, this may result in a *less than honorable* or even a *dishonorable* discharge and the reduction or loss of veteran status and associated entitlements and benefits. The meaning and emotional residue of these kinds of discharges are distinct, and clinicians need to understand what the departure from service means to the individual client. For some, it's a time of pride and celebration of a successful career; others experience great sadness, and still others experience shame and guilt for their inability to continue serving with their peers.

An obvious transition for those not retiring more generally is entry into the civilian workforce. Many new veterans find comfort and a sense of belonging in various government positions, including positions in the VA healthcare system. Although many guidelines assure National Guard and Reservists that they will be able to return to their prior civilian job upon homecoming, anecdotal evidence suggests that this process is often not as smooth or guaranteed as one would hope. Transition into civilian status can be especially challenging for veterans who have incurred physical or emotional injuries during their military service. These men and women may have lost greatly valued skills and abilities that may render return to their previous line of work difficult or impossible.

Although tremendous efforts are being made to assist this new generation of service members in transitioning as veterans to the VA, the experience can be daunting, and for some overwhelming. The VA is an enormous system that comprises more than 150 medical centers and over 800 community-based outpatient clinics providing many outpatient services and located in more rural areas to improve access. Also more than 230 Vet Centers offer readjustment-focused counseling for veterans who have served in a combat zone and their families, many of which provide individual mental health services to family members as well as veterans. Veterans of the wars in Afghanistan and Iraq have 5 years of eligibility to initiate access to VA care after their military discharge from active duty status and, like all veterans, individuals whose conditions are determined to be service-related are entitled to continuing care. The same is true for members of the National Guard and the other Reserve Components who transition from active to reserve status after completing a tour in a combat theater of operations. For all veterans VA health benefits consist of medical care and financial compensation based on degree of functional disability due to service-related injury.

Navigating the complex VA hospital, clinic, and benefits procedures can be time- and energy-consuming, and can require persistence and patience. The VA website (*www.va.gov*) has a tremendous amount of information that can assist veterans and families, and all VA medical centers have patient advocates and customer service staff who can provide guidance.

The VA system has made considerable strides in contacting new veterans, welcoming them into the VA system, providing case managers at every hospital and clinic to assist with the transition to VA care, and using veterans of the Afghanistan and Iraq Wars as outreach workers to promote community awareness about VA services. In the past several years, the VA system has strengthened its mental health services by establishing many new mental health positions and promoting the adoption of evidence-based therapies. All VA hospitals now have at least one Suicide Prevention Coordinator, Local Recovery Coordinator, and Case Manager who assist newly returning veterans in accessing and coordinating their care. Specific multidisciplinary programs have been created to meet the unique needs of veterans who incur multiple traumas during service. Congress also recently mandated that all VA medical centers provide marital and family therapy. National training programs and ongoing consultation are being provided in many domains relevant to this new generation of veterans, including evidence-based treatment for PTSD (prolonged exposure and cognitive processing therapy), couple therapy, and cognitive-behavioral therapy for a range of relevant conditions (e.g., depression, insomnia). In addition, considerable efforts have been made to decrease the waiting time for veterans who apply for disability entitlements, resulting in quicker notification of possible benefits.

Changed Relationships with Family and Community

Veterans who have deployed to Afghanistan or Iraq universally describe themselves as "different" or "changed." Parents, spouses/partners, children, other family members, and communities have also changed during the service member's absence, so the reconnection process takes time, patience, and effort by everyone involved. The changed relationships can be conceptualized as three concentric circles, starting with the veteran defining a new sense of self as the innermost circle. As the veteran charts a new chapter in life, many opportunities exist for a fresh start. Some veterans find this period of time exciting and hopeful. Even basic elements of oneself can change, such as the ability to let one's hair grow longer, wear civilian clothes, and create one's own schedule marked by greater flexibility and personal choice. Some veterans embrace their new identity and become involved in veteran organizations and socialize with other veterans. Others experience the change as abrupt and difficult. The uncertainty of civilian life can produce anxiety and trepidation. Because many service members take great pride in their military identity, the loss of this identity can be painful. Military culture demands strict adherence to routine, and the sudden loss of this structure may leave a veteran struggling. Without such clear guidance, some veterans struggle and the journey from service member to veteran can be challenging and painful.

The next circle contains the veteran's immediate family and close friends. Military members and their families may have moved a number of times while on active duty. A return to civilian life provides an opportunity for some geographic stability and the veteran's presence at home can provide an opportunity for greater relationship intimacy and participation in family life. For some families, difficult interpersonal concerns that could be ignored during the service member's absences now are center stage in the family. Family members who have grown accustomed to running the family without the veteran's presence need to be flexible as they reintegrate the veteran into family routines and schedules. Couples and families can face challenges in many household domains such as finances or budgeting, intimacy, parenting, division of labor of household chores, and preferences for socializing. Such renegotiations can become more complicated for veterans also struggling with physical or emotional problems.

Reconnecting with children is an important reintegration task for military members and new veterans, who have missed important developmental changes in their families. Veteran parents may have looked forward to this special time with their children, only to feel insecure in their role as parent, hurt at their children's distance, and confused as to how to relate to their children. Veterans can benefit from basic information about child development and encouragement to be patient in connecting with their children. Fortunately, most children respond quickly to an available, nurturing parent, so bonds can be formed and strengthened when the parent can avoid guilt, remorse, or frustration and commit time and energy to his or her parenting role.

The outermost circle is the veteran's broader community, which may include the job, church, school, or even a basketball league or fitness club. Veterans who have experienced deployments often complain that their civilian peers "just don't get it." Veterans may lack empathy for friends who become emotionally distraught about seemingly minor issues (e.g., a burned meal at a restaurant, a bad grade on a test), when veterans have faced life-and-death situations in a combat zone. Many veterans feel offended by a peer's intrusive, inappropriate questions (e.g., "How many people did you kill?"). Veterans who have these experiences may withdraw or limit their socializing to other veterans, or avoid social contacts altogether. Although affiliation with others who share the experience is powerful and may be therapeutic, restricting oneself to such groups can limit opportunities socially, professionally, and academically. Therefore, it is important for veterans to negotiate these new relationships, setting limits and giving feedback when appropriate, and to reenter their communities as places to belong and to contribute.

The Many Strengths of the New Veterans

Although a considerable number of service members are entering the civilian sector with physical, emotional, or other cognitive challenges, it is important to identify and celebrate the strengths this generation of veterans brings to our communities. Many of these new veterans have faced hardships, including extended tours away from home, and most have a strong sense of pride in their country. They have demonstrated courage, selflessness, and resilience. Most have acquired skills and gained life experiences that will serve them well in school, jobs, and communities. For example, military life often instills in service members a commitment to the team or mission, wherein people rise above their individual needs to work for the greater good of their comrades. Service members are taught to be organized, structured, and dependable—all good qualities in employees and family members. The military places value on education, and many service members avail themselves of opportunities to further their training, bringing completed certifications and degrees into their roles as civilians. It is incumbent on healthcare providers, employers, mental health professionals, and communities to recognize and draw on these many assets in our newest cohort of veterans.

SUMMARY

It is important that clinicians understand the effects of military life and deployment on service members and their families. Many service members have experienced wonderful opportunities and positive life experiences during their military service. Many have also encountered an array of personal and family challenges that have profoundly impacted their lives and relationships, sometimes in adverse ways. Many of these men and women returning from deployment bring with them the physical, emotional, social, and spiritual aftereffects associated with combat or other traumatic exposures. Our hope is that all service members and veterans, especially those who need assistance, will find their communities to be "caring places" that are both willing and equipped to offer requisite compassion and care.

RESOURCES

Bowling, U. B., & Sherman, M. D. (2008). Welcoming them home: Supporting soldiers and their families in navigating the tasks of reintegration. *Professional Psychology: Research and Practice, 39*, 451–458.

Chandra, A., Lara-Cinisomo, S., Jaycox, L. H., Tanielian, T., Burns, R. M., Ruder, T., et al. (2010). Children on the homefront: The experience of children from military families. *Pediatrics, 125*, 16–25.

Friedman, M. J. (2010). Prevention of psychiatric problems among military personnel and their spouses. *New England Journal of Medicine, 362*, 168–170.

Hoge, C. W. (2010). *Once a warrior always a warrior: Navigating the transition from combat to home.* Guilford, CT: Globe Pequot Press.

Hoge, C. W., Castro, C. A., Messer, S. C., McGurk, D., Cotting, D. I., & Koffman, R. L. (2004). Combat duty in Iraq and Afghanistan, mental health problems, and barriers to care. *New England Journal of Medicine, 351*, 13–22.

Institute of Medicine. (2010). *Returning home from Iraq and Afghanistan: Preliminary assessment of readjustment needs of veterans, service members, and their families.* Washington, DC: National Academies Press.

Kimerling, R., Gima, K., Smith, M. W., Street, A., & Frayne, S. (2007). The Veterans Health Administration and military sexual trauma. *American Journal of Public Health, 97*(12), 2160–2166.

Mansfield, A. J., Kaufman, J. S., Marshall, S. W., Gaynes, B. N., Morrissey, J. P., & Engel, C. C. (2010). Deployment and the use of mental health services among U.S. Army wives. *New England Journal of Medicine, 362*, 101–109.

RAND Center for Military Health Policy Research. (2008). *Post-deployment stress: What families should know, what families can do.* Santa Monica, CA: RAND Corporation.

Sherman, M. D., & Sherman, D. M. (2009). *My story: Blogs by four military teens.* Edina, MN: Beavers Pond Press. Available at *www.seedsofhopebooks.com.*

Tanielian, T., & Jaycox, L. (Eds). (2008). *Invisible wounds of war: Psychological and cognitive injuries, their consequences, and services to assist recovery* (RAND Health and the RAND National Security Research Division, Document MG-720-CCF). RAND Corporation.

CHAPTER 3

A Framework for Accessing Resources for Military and Veteran Couples and Families

Laurie B. Slone, Matthew J. Friedman,
and Barbara Thompson

Since 2002, over 2 million U.S. service members have been deployed to war in Afghanistan and Iraq (Tan, 2009). Because on average each service member has 1.5 eligible dependents (i.e., spouses, children, adult dependents) this means that approximately 3 million family members have been directly affected by military deployment. This number increases when we consider the extended family, friends, and community members of these service members who are impacted. Grandma and Grandpa might have been caring for their two grandchildren over the past 13 months, the offspring of their daughter who is returning from Afghanistan next week. Uncle David fears for his nephew's safe return from Kuwait. The Human Resources manager at a retail store may be searching to find a temporary replacement for the store manager who is deploying with his Guard unit in September.

Service members and their families each deal with their own issues before and during the deployment (see Martin & Sherman, Chapter 2, and Beasley, MacDermid Wadsworth, & Betts, Chapter 4, this volume). Even after deployed loved ones return home, the honeymoon phase can be short-lived. Almost all service members will deal with common reactions that occur during reintegration, such as nightmares, financial readjustments, couples getting reacquainted, young children meeting their parent for the first time, and more. Following trauma experienced during war, most of those who return from deployment will readjust without complications, but a minority of service members will develop mental health problems.

As a provider, it is important to understand the characteristics of these service members and their families, as well as the full range of issues and challenges they may face.

We are becoming increasingly aware of how much need there is for assistance. Of those who have returned and deactivated from military service, over half have sought care from the Department of Veterans Affairs (VA; VA Office of Public Health and Environmental Hazards, 2011). This is in spite of the fact that we know that many are reluctant to seek care (Hoge et al., 2004). More than the mere absence of mental disorders, successful readjustment involves mental *health*. Readjusting into civilian life takes time, and successful reintegration involves regaining overall well-being. Recent research delineates the broad spectrum of needs of this cohort (Sayer et al., 2010). It involves readjusting to day-to-day challenges with hopes of a secure job, strong relationships, doing well in school, successfully handling finances, and being a productive member of society. Some of the stressors that complicate the lives of these individuals can be alleviated with existing resources and services. The challenge is matching service members, veterans, and families in need to those available resources.

Mental health professionals provide counseling and support targeting readjustment issues and mental health problems. It is also imperative that we are able to help veterans and families access the full range of resources and services that they might need. Because there are a multitude of extensive resources and services, it can be difficult to figure out how to navigate it all. Counselors and clinicians may know little about the resources that exist outside of mental health. Or they might know enough to be intimidated. How do you choose where to refer someone for what he or she needs? To meet the full range of needs that commonly occur, providers may need to rely on the skills of others. Counselors, social workers, clinicians, family readiness members, human resource managers, and chaplains cannot be expected to be specialists in dealing with the entire spectrum of challenges that impact mental, emotional, and physical well-being. But to help a veteran, one may need to provide career assistance, help with child care, or referral to assistance with refinancing a home. The goal is that no matter where or to whom veterans and family members turn for help, there should be no "wrong door."

In the United States, resources and services exist to help with all aspects of reintegration to civilian life following deployment to war. This chapter provides a framework based on six categories. This framework simplifies navigating these extensive resources, so that providers can make these services easier to access. Community providers and others can make use of this framework to help ensure that service members, veterans, and their families take advantage of all the services they need.

Given the full spectrum of needs, a broad range of services is necessary to the well-being of service members, veterans, and their families: from day-to-day living (giving the kids a ride to activities, finding employment, and financial assistance) to inpatient psychiatric care. In addition to mental health care, children's issues, communication problems, attending to career and education struggles, housing needs, and more, are all important issues to address. The focus in this chapter is on the *when, how,* and *where* to find needed resources.

Assessment is needed to determine *when* additional resources are needed and how to match the correct resource to a client. Assessment of service members or veterans requires understanding the context that surrounds individuals and their family members, including military culture, the screening processes in place, discovering the particular stressors affecting individuals and their families, and understanding the unique barriers to care that this cohort of veterans must overcome. Understanding the population and the individual will also help determine what type of resources this person might be interested in using.

The second part of this chapter deals with knowing *how* and *where* to refer. We provide a categorical framework to use following assessment, which will help match those in need with the proper services. Together with follow-up to ensure that adequate service has been obtained, this is the formula that can make a difference in the life of a service member or veteran and his or her family. Knowledge about the existence of various resources and services will help to a degree. However, to provide optimal assistance it is best to understand the needs, the context, the potential barriers, and the resources.

ASSESSING TO UNDERSTAND IF AND WHEN TO REFER

In order to understand the meaning of any assessment, one needs to be able to view the individual in context. To best serve our service members/veterans and their families, it is helpful to understand the military subculture (see Martin & Sherman Chapter 2, this volume). Although the experience of being in the military can be challenging, it also brings many positives: pride, patriotism, problem-solving skills, self-confidence and self-reliance, strength of character, and responsibility. Military members often take pride in being strong and able to handle things on their own; so do military families. Seeking assistance in time of need should be framed as good problem solving.

In addition to standard assessment for mental health issues, we assess to understand the challenges that military families face, the context, the potential barriers to care, and any issues that may be exacerbating problems. This will help to identify which resources are needed and to ensure that the formats of identified resources are appropriate in a given situation. For example, if a veteran has no phone, providing a hotline phone number to him or her will not be useful. Does the veteran have Internet access? This is important to know when providing veterans with a website containing important information. Alternatively, a family may find that watching a video together for psychoeducation is preferable to printed handouts. Asking questions will also help to identify and overcome any potential barriers to care.

It is important to ask questions, but it is equally important to know one's own limits. Asking to hear about traumatic events that are beyond one's capacity to help process, or saying "yes" to viewing combat-related photos even though the pictures might be upsetting, will ultimately not be of benefit to clients. When asking questions, be prepared to handle the answers or to refer someone in need. Asking the right questions about financial, educational, employment or other needs, is easier when the counselor is prepared to help find a resolution.

The Importance of the Military Subculture

In order to build rapport, knowing something about the person with whom one is trying to connect is integral. Focus group input and survey results indicate that service members believe it is critical to understand their military affiliation. For example, identifying their branch of service and how long they have served helps service members feel as though they are better understood. Other inquiries include how many times they have been deployed and how long ago, whether they served with their unit or as an Individual Augmentee (i.e., an individual who fills shortages or meets special needs in a unit), and whether they expect to be redeployed. It is helpful to know the difference between the National Guard and the Reserves, the rank structure, and that there are different terms to describe the service member based on branch of service (e.g., *soldier* usually refers to Army, *airmen/women* to the Air Force; see Martin & Sherman, Chapter 2, and

Shnaider, Vorstanbosch, & Wanklyn, Chapter 13, this volume). Someone who has not had any direct military experience should not be afraid to acknowledge what he or she does not know, while committing to learning more over time.

Screening and Referring

The majority of returning troops are regularly screened for mental and physical health problems to help identify areas of concern and encourage early treatment. All troops must complete the Post-Deployment Health Assessment (PDHA) when they return from deployment. This contains screens for posttraumatic stress disorder (PTSD), traumatic brain injury (TBI), alcohol use, and other potential problems. Research shows that new problems emerge, especially for National Guard and Reserve personnel, after service members have been back for a period of time (Milliken, Auchterlonie, & Hoge, 2007). To avoid overlooking problems, several months later they complete the Post-Deployment Health Reassessment (PDHRA). In addition, veterans entering the VA for any type of care are screened for a similar set of problems. Currently, there is no mandatory screening of military family members.

It is important to keep in mind that screening instruments are *not* diagnostic assessments. Screens are used to help reduce the burden of completing full assessments on every individual. They are indicators to identify at-risk individuals and are used to determine whether more formal assessment is needed. A positive screen for PTSD or TBI does not mean that the individual has PTSD or TBI. Care should be taken not to inadvertently alarm a client with inaccurate interpretation of a screen. Screening should lead to further assessment as indicated. If the provider administering the screen is not prepared to conduct a more in-depth assessment, then a referral should be made at that time. After further assessment is conducted, the individual should be provided appropriate care or referral to such care as needed.

Barriers to Assessment and Care

Even though screening measures help identify those who are more likely to have problems requiring treatment, if those positively screened do not gain access to further evaluation, screening is ineffective. Members of our Armed Forces are trained to be self-sufficient and competent. This strength of character may make it difficult for service members to admit there is a problem (Stecker, Fortney, Hamilton, & Ajzen, 2007). Many service members are concerned about stigma, about being perceived as weak, and about job security (Pietrzak, Johnson, Goldstein, Malley, & Southwick, 2009). They need to be reminded that part of problem solving involves knowing when it takes more than one person to come up with the best course of action. Pride and fear of stigma can prevent veterans from initiating care or staying in treatment.

Other barriers to care are institutional or operational in nature. For example, veterans and families in the workforce need convenient clinic hours and assistance with child care so that they can maintain other responsibilities in their daily lives. Because a majority of veterans tend to be geographically dispersed, assistance with transportation can be important. All forms of access to services are relevant. For example, even online services can be difficult for some to use; although workplaces may have Internet access, many homes in more rural areas still lack this service. Another barrier to care is a prevailing lack of knowledge about the effectiveness and the nature of treatment for common mental health problems during and following military service (Pietrzak et al., 2009). Effective treatment for PTSD exists, and this cohort needs to be informed about what treatment entails and that treatment works.

Mental health problems can make it more difficult to seek assistance. These same barriers may inhibit requests for other types of resources. Extra steps, such as helping someone in distress to make that first call or following up on referrals provided, can make a big difference.

Matching Individuals to Relevant Resources

Even after a topic or issue is identified, matching a person to the proper resource is not simple. There are multiple dimensions to consider. What is meant by *type* of resource? The type of resource may come from identifying a topic, for example, that the person needs care for PTSD or depression, or assistance finding a job or child care. Yet *type* can also mean the format of the information (e.g., an online self-help module, a phone line, printed materials, a training course, counseling or therapy). Does the resource provide one service or multiple services, and to whom? Veterans? Service members? Families? For example, if a provider is contacted by a family in need of financial assistance, the provider might ask: Is the status of this family active duty or is the service member now a veteran? Do the family members need information about financial planning or are they at the point that they need financial counseling? Do they have Internet access so that they can contact someone or find information online? Our framework for thinking about resources involves all of these. Hence individuals must be matched to resources according to audience, category or topic of resource sought, format, and resources also vetted.

Audience

Some resources and services target a specific group. The primary audience addressed for purposes of this chapter includes service members, veterans, and their families. However, a resource might specifically target veterans and not service members who are still on active duty, or vice versa. There are also differentiations among different groups of military members, such as branch and component (i.e., Reserve, Guard, active duty). Some services that are available to military members are also available to their families, but what constitutes "family"? A spouse and dependent children are usually included, but what about parents of service members? Siblings, grandparents, or extended family? Girlfriends, boyfriends, or ex-spouses?

In addition to resources and services that specifically target military populations, many agencies that serve the public at large also provide the same services to veterans, active duty service members, and their loved ones. These same social, occupational, and health services are there for this group that might now have emergent need. Many state and community resources fall into this category.

Other resources target the providers who care for those who have served in the military, including not only counselors and clinicians but also leaders, employers, college personnel, and others. Educational materials and training are available to help providers learn more about working in this sector. For providers who want to donate services, there are mechanisms in place to do so (e.g., Give an Hour, Hard Hats across America, and state- or community-based networks).

Materials, services, or information targeting these various audiences differ in their level of accessibility. We should be sure that the resources provided target the audience we are trying to serve.

Categories

The topics or categories of interest of various resources and services sought by service members, veterans, and their families can be divided in many ways: financial assistance, employment resources, mental health care, deployment information, child care, housing, education, and more. To simplify the wide-ranging scope of resources, we suggest a framework involving six categories: *the Basics* or *megaresources*—key organizations and resources that provide referral assistance for a variety of needs; *crisis resources* and hotlines; resources that provide *educational information*; resources that provide *social support; day-to-day life resources and services*; and resources that provide *mental health services*. This categorization is described in more detail in the section on how and when to refer.

Format of Information

The method of providing a given resource can be labeled "format." Is the service or resource provided via phone, website, reading material, or videos? Is it a hotline, a chat group, or a place to obtain an appointment? What is the delivery method for the information or service—for example, the Web in text format, video, or an online course; in person or on the phone? Other format characteristics include reading level, time to complete, how engaging or thorough the material is, the level of depth versus breadth of the materials, and administration via an individual or group. One size does not fit all, and format characteristics should be taken into consideration when options are provided. We point out these different characteristics to highlight the elements to consider when providing a specific referral or resource, and the various ways one can approach thinking about resources.

Vetting

Given the extensive resources and services that exist, vetting is an important issue. As with making any decision, the more information available, the better, and many factors need to be weighed against one another. As a general rule of thumb, authoritative sources, trusted peers, and expert-produced materials and resources are the best materials to utilize. Using information and services provided by VA, Department of Defense (DoD), and state agencies, although not always ideal, may be the easiest guideline to follow. Overall, research-based interventions are best, but whereas these interventions are beneficial for the majority, not all services work for everyone.

Different choices and a range of alternatives are often helpful to individuals and families in need. However, to avoid overwhelming veterans and their families and to encourage action, be careful not to offer *too* many choices. If given too many options from which to choose, individuals may not be able to discern how to select one, and this could result in their doing nothing at all (Iyengar & Lepper, 2000). It may be preferable to suggest the best several alternatives available.

HOW AND WHERE TO REFER

The DoD has long recognized that military service to our nation places a heavy demand on service members and families, and that support to military families can be accomplished in a variety of ways. To help military families cope with the current levels of stress, anxiety, and uncertainty, the DoD has redesigned and augmented existing family readiness programs and activities, as well as launched new programs over the past several years.

VA has also expanded its efforts and is designing programs to handle a variety of family needs.

A key goal is to ensure *that the right program gets to the right person at the right time* to support and strengthen military families. Below we outline a few services organized according to this categorical framework, as an introduction to the broad array of available services. These recommended resources are nationally recognized services, and most are government or government-sponsored programs. This book also contains Appendix A with extensive resources.

Basic Resources for Helping Professionals

Knowledge of a few basic or "mega" resources for service members, veterans, and their families is essential. The DoD and VA both have a long history in dealing with the types of stressors and trauma that service members and veterans have had to endure. These two large organizations are the foundation, providing overarching resources and services across a variety of domains. The defining line between veterans (served mainly by VA) and service members (served mainly by the DoD) can be difficult to determine. Reserve Component members deploy to combat zones, return as veterans, but continue to be in the military under deactivated status. The affiliation and status of the person or persons one is working with will help determine which path is best to take; however many of the available resources and services are offered to both of these groups.

For families, the DoD provides extensive family support at military installations and in the community to reach the Reserve and Guard Components and military family members who do not live on military bases. Military Family Assistance Centers are located in every state (the number of centers is based on the numbers of deployed personnel) and serve all branches of both the Reserve Component and Active Duty. Historically, VA has focused on the veteran; however, VA is now beginning to do more for families, including counseling at Vet Centers and training clinicians to provide evidence-based couple and family therapy.

An excellent online resource to support wounded, ill, and injured service members, veterans, their families, and those who support them is the *National Resource Directory*. Developed jointly by the DoD, VA, and the Department of Labor, this site aims to provides one-stop-shopping access to services and resources at the national, state, and local levels to support recovery, rehabilitation, and community reintegration. State services are also available to assist this cohort. Every state has an Office, Department, or Bureau of Veteran Services, and many state health and human services are available to members of this cohort who are also state residents. State

Offices of Veterans Affairs help with a variety of benefits and advocacy. Agencies or Departments of Health and Human Services are offered by each state to all citizens, including military personnel, veterans, and families.

Crisis Resources

Although knowing about megaresources to which we can refer a service member, veteran, or family member is essential, knowing crisis numbers is even more critical. Local resources can also be invaluable during a crisis. Suicide, domestic and sexual violence, and homelessness are some of the most pertinent crises warranting assessment and intervention. Tragically, suicides are occurring more frequently among members of our Armed Forces. Therefore it is important to know how to identify potentially suicidal service members and veterans, whom to call, and what to do. Service members and veterans are also at greater risk for intimate-partner aggression and for homelessness. Specific crisis resources for service members and veterans are included in Appendix A.

Informational Resources

Understanding the problem is often half of the solution; therefore, information is key. Sometimes the type of resource a person needs is information about what to expect, what is normal, and what indicates more serious problems. This is true not only for service members, veterans, and families but also for care providers in need of education and training. The megaresources already described contain rich and extensive educational information for a range of audiences. Other key online resources providing educational materials in a variety of formats include *afterdeployment.org*, *ptsd.va.gov*, and *Myhealthevet.va.gov*. Some educational materials are specifically tailored to providers, but most are for general audiences.

Social Support Resources

Because of the potential challenges that deployment brings, alternative sources of social support are essential. Social support is the most important protective factor against developing PTSD (Brewin, Andrews, & Valentine, 2000). The symptoms experienced by people who suffer from mental health problems affect others and, in turn, the reactions of loved ones affect those who are struggling to cope. The reciprocal nature of these issues makes social support even more vital.

Sometimes it is easier for military personnel to confide in someone who has been through similar experiences. For years, VA has provided group peer-to-peer sessions to allow these connections to be made, and VA continues to foster recovery in this manner. VA also now has a Veteran Combat Call Center, where veterans can talk 24/7 with another combat veteran. Veterans service organizations (VSOs) are places where veterans can come together to stay connected.

The two largest sources of family support are covered in the mega-resources: Family Support Centers located on military installations, and Military Family Assistance Centers located across each state. Many of these family programs offer family support groups, as do some VA Medical Centers.

Communities can help support military members, veterans, and families where they live. Several states have established community-based networks of support, or collaborations to increase awareness of the issues that service members and their families face due to deployment, as well as existing resources and services to help (Slone, Friedman, & Pomerantz, 2009). Many resources exist, and these partnerships help to increase awareness and communication. These networks have the goal of bringing communities together and making sure that service members, veterans, and families know that they are not alone.

Resources for Day-to-Day Living

Daily living can create high levels of stress in general, and the challenges of readjustment after deployment amplify these stressors. The megaresources from the DoD, VA, and individual states can provide assistance with most of the daily living experiences that can become problematic, including employment, college and educational needs, legal issues, and children's needs. Programs have been created to help with job training, placement, and security. Some veterans may be looking for civilian jobs for the first time. Others will need new employment to match their skills set or because a job no longer exists. A large percentage of recent returnees are, or will be, enrolled in higher education. Veterans in college may find the transition into a classroom challenging, because symptoms of readjustment may include problems with concentration. Adjustment challenges can also lead to trouble with the law (e.g., drinking problems, aggressive driving, anger, interpersonal conflict), so sometimes legal assistance is needed.

Other issues that arise for returning service members/veterans and their families and affect day-to-day life include sleep problems, anger management, funding for college, financial and housing problems, and relationship problems. Interpersonal conflict and relationship issues are of great concern. The DoD has developed programs to help support military families and couples with these relationships.

Mental Health Resources (and Training)

In this section we provide some basic information about existing mental health services. In addition, we include several training resources to help interested providers improve care for those dealing with mental health issues following time in a war zone. The DoD and VA provide a wide spectrum of formal mental health treatment for PTSD, depression, substance use disorders, TBI, and other problems.

There are a number of effective evidence-based treatments for these problems, and joint VA/DoD clinical practice guidelines have been outlined for each disorder (see Appendix A for relevant websites). For example, first-line treatments for PTSD include prolonged exposure therapy (PE), cognitive processing therapy (CPT), eye movement desensitization and reprocessing (EMDR), and certain medications (e.g., selective serotonin reuptake inhibitors). The VA has established a rollout program to train mental health practitioners in the use of PE and CPT. At the time of this writing, over 7,000 mental health clinicians have received such training. Furthermore, a parallel training initiative is occurring for DoD therapists.

Mental Healthcare within VA

VA Medical Centers provide a full range of mental health services, and many of VA's community-based outreach clinics do as well. There is a PTSD program or PTSD specialist at each Medical Center, as well as a Military Sexual Trauma Coordinator and a staff member trained to deal with comorbid PTSD and substance abuse disorder. Vet Centers supplement these services and extend care to family members. They also provide bereavement counseling to surviving parents, spouses, children, and siblings of service members who die while on active duty. Finally, there are online Program Locators to help find VA PTSD and substance use Treatment Programs nationwide.

DoD Programs for Psychological Health

In addition to mental health providers on bases and the aforementioned DoD resources, the Military Family Assistance Centers in each state have a Director of Psychological Health (DPH), who coordinates the psychological support for Guard members and their families, mitigating the National Guard's unique challenges. These challenges include the fact that armories and wings are community-based, locations are seldom near a military treatment facility, and some Guardsmen are not provided healthcare and treatment via the military. The DPH helps find alternate sources of care.

Community-Based Care

Private practitioners and providers at Community Behavioral Health facilities in each state also offer mental health care services for veterans, service members, and families. It is helpful to seek out providers who have experience in working with trauma survivors and dealing with the military subculture, and those who can apply evidence-based treatments for mental health issues that commonly occur in this population, such as PTSD. Several organizations facilitate the provision of free mental health services for service members or their families, such as Strategic Outreach to Families of All Reservists (SOFAR) and Give an Hour. See Appendix A to learn more or volunteer.

Chaplains

Often, service members faced with mental health issues first speak with a chaplain. Chaplains within both the DoD and VA are available for grief and spiritual counseling. There is often less reluctance on the part of service members and veterans to seek support from these professionals, because chaplains are usually the most accessible source of mental health support during deployments, and they can guarantee confidentiality both in DoD and VA settings.

Training Resources

Providers can obtain training specific to various disorders affecting service members and veterans from a variety of online resources. Examples include the following:

- *PTSD 101:* A Web-based curriculum that offers a range of relevant and timely topics related to PTSD and trauma. The goal is to develop or enhance practitioner knowledge of trauma and its treatment. It is free, taught by expert researchers and clinicians, and continuing education credits are available.
- *CPT Web:* A free, 9-hour, Web-based, multimedia education course for mental health professionals seeking to learn CPT for PTSD.
- *Pdhealth.mil:* An online resource designed to assist clinicians in the delivery of postdeployment healthcare by fostering a trusting part-

nership between military men and women, veterans, their families, and their healthcare providers to ensure the highest quality care.

- *Clinician's Trauma Update–Online (CTU-Online):* This Web-based resource includes brief updates on the latest clinically relevant trauma research emphasizing assessment and treatment. It is delivered six times per year via e-mail subscription.

SUMMARY

Many forms of support and services are both needed by, and available to, service members and veterans. Effectively drawing upon these resources requires an overall conceptual framework and familiarity with services that vary in their intended audience, as well as their focus and format. Service members and veterans need and deserve a full continuum of care. All providers of services—regardless of specific professional background or setting—should become knowledgeable about existing resources to ensure that no matter where the service member or veteran turns for assistance, there will be an open door.

RESOURCES

Brewin, C. R., Andrews, B., & Valentine, J. D. (2000). Meta-analysis of risk factors for posttraumatic stress disorder in trauma-exposed adults. *Journal of Consulting and Clinical Psychology, 68,* 748–766.

Hoge, C. W., Castro, C. A., Messer, S. C., McGurk, D., Cotting, D. I., & Koffman, R. L. (2004). Combat duty in Iraq and Afghanistan, mental health problems, and barriers to care. *New England Journal of Medicine, 351,* 13–22.

Iyengar, S. S., & Lepper, M. R. (2000). When choice is demotivating: Can one desire too much of a good thing? *Journal of Personality and Social Psychology, 79,* 995–1006.

Milliken, C. S., Auchterlonie, J. L., & Hoge, C. W. (2007). Longitudinal assessment of mental health problems among active and reserve component soldiers returning from the Iraq War. *Journal of the American Medical Association, 298,* 2141–2148.

Pietrzak, R. H., Johnson, D. C., Goldstein, M. B., Malley, J. C., & Southwick, S. M. (2009). Perceived stigma and barriers to mental health care utilization among OEF-OIF Veterans. *Psychiatric Services, 60,* 1118–1122.

Sayer, N. A., Noorbaloochi, S., Frazier, P., Carlson, K., Gravely, A., & Murdoch, M. (2010). Reintegration problems and treatment interests among Iraq and Afghanistan combat veterans receiving VA medical care. *Psychiatric Services, 61,* 589–597.

Slone, L. B., Friedman, M. J., & Pomerantz, A. S. (2009). Vermont: A case history

for supporting National Guard troops and their families. *Psychiatric Annals,*
39, 89–95.

Stecker, T., Fortney, J. C., Hamilton, F., & Ajzen, I. (2007). An assessment of
beliefs about mental health care among veterans who served in Iraq. *Psychiatric Services, 58,* 1358–1361.

Tan, M. (2009). 2 million troops have deployed since 9/11. Marine Corps
Times. Retrieved November 1, 2011, from *www.marinecorpstimes.com/
news/2009/12/military_deployments_121809w/.*

VA Office of Public Health and Environmental Hazards. (2011). *Analysis of VA
health care utilization among Operation Enduring Freedom, Operation Iraqi
Freedom, and Operation New Dawn veterans, from 1st Qtr FY 2002 through
4th Qtr FY 2011.* Washington, DC: Author. Retrieved from *www.publi-
chealth.va.gov/docs/epidemiology/healthcare-utilization-report-fy2011-
qtr4.pdf.*

CHAPTER 4

Transitioning to and from Deployment

Kevin S. Beasley, Shelley M. MacDermid Wadsworth,
and June Behn Watts

John was feeling many expectations placed upon him as he prepared to deploy. He'd been told to put his affairs in order as if he were never coming back. He needed to reassure his family that he *would* be back and not to worry, when at the same time he wasn't sure that would be the case. He felt like he needed to be the strong one and not share his feelings and "drive on," while all these stresses were going on in the back of his mind. He didn't feel free to share his concerns with his buddies, because it would make the situation that much more real. Being in a leadership position, he felt particularly obligated to alleviate his soldiers' concerns, because he believed he was responsible for bringing them home safely. John had his gear in plastic bags and packed for field training only to find out that he was stuck at the mobilization (MOB) site for 3 months. The MOB site was only a few hours from home, but for John it may as well have been on the other side of the world. The assigned dates to actually deploy kept changing; everyone at the MOB site was just ready to go so that they could start counting down the days of deployment.

For educators and providers to begin the process of helping John and his family, it is imperative to understand the nature of military deployment. Research dating back to World War II provides important insights into deployment and the family processes that unfold around it. The best-known early study of deployment, marriage, and family life by Hill (1949) offered several observations about families as they reunited following men's service in World War II that are relevant to today's families. First, there was considerable diversity in the patterns of families' readjustment following reunion, including patterns of stable, improving, or declining function over time. Second, families' experiences during reunion were connected to their experiences prior to and during deployment. Some families functioned so well during deployment, for example, that they left little or no room for the absent member to reenter the family upon return, and subsequently experienced difficulty. Third, families' adjustment to each deployment-related transition occurred in stages. These early observations have continued to find empirical and clinical support across diverse wars and generations.

Several additional conclusions become evident upon reviewing more recent literature specifically related to intimate relationships and deployment. The first is that deployment is not a single event but a complex series of transitions and events that occur over an extended period of time. Service members usually depart for deployment after a period of hasty or prolonged preparation that might also include short separations for training, which we refer to as the "predeployment phase" (McCarroll, Hoffman, Grieger, & Holloway, 2005). They may spend several weeks in a domestic location away from their homes before traveling to the deployment location, a situation in which they feel like they have partially but not fully departed. There may be periods during the actual deployment when family members cannot communicate with one another or know one another's location. In the immediate wake of return during the postdeployment phase, reunion may occur in several steps, including a ceremony at the demobilization location, a parade at their home or duty location, and a series of reconnecting events with family and friends. Finally, there is a longer period of reintegration with networks of family, friends, and coworkers. Every deployment is both complex and distinct. Moreover, every couple or family responds to these various transitions in its own unique way.

In addition, modern-day military personnel are quite diverse and deploy in a variety of circumstances. For example, about 27% of service members deployed to Iraq or Afghanistan were members of the U.S. National Guard or the Reserves, who faced the added challenge of departing from and returning to civilian communities and jobs. Some service members are deployed as "Individual Augmentees" to fill gaps in units or branches of service other than their own, sometimes resulting in isolation for themselves and their families. Many families also face logistical, financial, and emotional challenges associated with dealing with service members' physical or psychological injuries (Castaneda et al., 2008; MacDermid Wadsworth, 2010).

A second conclusion is that deployment-related separations can be stressful and difficult, and combat-related deployments appear to be especially so (MacLean & Elder, 2007). A substantial proportion of service members worry about the physical challenges of deployment, such as heavy workload; psychological challenges, including concerns about their families; and potential moral challenges related to their own actions during deployment (McCarroll et al., 2005). Family separation has been more strongly related than any other concern to reports of mental health symptoms in the Mental Health Assessment Team studies (Mental Health Advisory Team [MHAT-V], 2008). Spouses also report psychological challenges such as worry and loneliness, logistical challenges such as being a "geographically single" parent, and economic challenges such as paying for tasks the military member would otherwise perform. It is also important to note, however, that service members and their spouses also reliably identify positive outcomes associated with deployment-related separations, including personal growth, refocused priorities, opportunities to develop new social support relationships, and increased self-efficacy (Castaneda et al., 2008; McCarroll et al., 2005).

Unlike civilian life, deployment and relocation are cultural norms for military families. Every military career starts with an experience that shares characteristics of deployment—military basic training. If the service member is married, this initial experience away is a test of two major relationships: not only the spouses' relationship with each other but also the relationship between the couple and the military. Deployment is a routine part of military life for service members and their families. Most military families have accepted this as "part of the job." Since September 11, 2001, however, the tempos of deployment cycles have dramatically increased for all branches of the military.

Recent findings regarding the impact of deployment on military families indicate that the relationships of military families are strained by deployments (Bowling & Sherman, 2008). In addition, some studies indicate that divorce rates among enlisted personnel and officers have increased since involvement in Iraq and Afghanistan, while divorce rates among civilians have been stable or declined during the same period. Moreover, the marriages of women service members, and especially those who are enlisted, appear to be more vulnerable than those of men. For both enlisted personnel and officers, women are more than twice as likely as men to divorce (Karney & Crown, 2007).

As a provider working with military families, it is crucial to avoid assumptions about the long-term effects of the current conflicts on relationship stability or the impact of deployment on the quality of the relationship for a particular couple. One must explicitly assess the role that deployment plays in a given couple's presenting problems. Furthermore, although most military members and their spouses or children do not report clinically significant psychological symptoms following return from deployment, there is clear evidence that when such symptoms do occur, they are associated with myriad corrosive influences on family life, including expressions of anger, hostility, withdrawal, and divorce (MacDermid Wadsworth, 2010).

PHASES OF DEPLOYMENT

As indicated earlier, it is best to think of deployment as a complex process in which couples and families experience a variety of different reactions, emotions, and interactions, rather than a linear process with uniformly defined stages and routine experiences. Similar to previous stage-based models of grief, we have come to know that people do not necessarily experience these stages in a prescriptive and sequenced manner, especially in a time of expected redeployment. Below we divide the deployment cycle according to operational phases used in the military, recognizing that couples' experiences of deployment vary widely within these operational phases.

Predeployment

Existing research indicates that the period prior to deployment is often quite busy and anxiety arousing, because couples and families are preparing legally and emotionally for the possibility that their loved one may not return from the deployment. Couples can begin not only to drift apart because of their respective tasks required to prepare for deployment but also to manage preemptively the anticipated loneliness and burden associated with maintaining the household and the additional demands that come with living alone or being a single parent (Pavlicin, 2003).

This is a period in which spouses often share pride in the service member's duty to country and sacrifice. However, couples may experience conflict over the military core value of "service before self." Partners may question or even be resentful if they believe that the service member is serving at cost to the couple and other family obligations. Deployments can be especially challenging to new marriages or relationships.

Deployment

> Once he finally deployed, John wrestled with how to stay connected with his wife Mary and their children back home. The phone banks and computers at the forward operating base (FOB) always had a long wait. He and Mary had agreed to talk once per week, but when missions kept him from holding to that schedule, Mary worried about whether he had been injured or worse

while outside the wire. John looked forward to hearing about day-to-day events back home, as if he were part of them, but it was tough, because Mary and the kids wanted to know about his days, too, and there were things he didn't want to share because they were too painful or would cause them to worry. John also realized that at times Mary would keep things from him as well—mostly minor crises involving the children or the house—and sometimes he resented this, but at other times he was glad Mary wasn't burdening him with home front problems the way some of the other spouses did with his buddies in the platoon. He and his platoon buddies had developed a strange kind of closeness that only comes from knowing that each has responsibility of helping the others stay alive. It was weird, because sometimes he felt closer to them than to Mary. And then he felt both guilty and sad, and angry about that at the same time.

Mary struggled as well. She admired John for his military service and had understood when the time came to redeploy. But once he actually deployed, everything changed. It was Mary alone, no teamwork on the home front, and she had to make sure that everything ran smoothly in his absence. She could handle the logistics well enough, but emotionally there was just a huge void. The first few weeks she cried herself to sleep every night but then realized she couldn't continue that way. Her family was an hour away—too far for frequent visits or daily logistic support. She had a friend nearby, but she was outside the military community and couldn't really understand Mary's experiences, though she tried. There were times when Mary resented John's deployment and all the forces that had brought it about. There were times she no longer wanted any part of the military lifestyle. And then she thought of John and all the sacrifices he had made for their family, as well as their country. And then she, too, felt guilty, sad, and angry—all of which she tried to hold at bay during those precious times when she and John actually got to talk by phone.

Deployment itself brings both challenges and benefits to military families, with differential effects on active duty and Guard or Reserve families (Castaneda et al., 2008). Military members worry about their relationships, and their relationships have a strong effect on their individual mental health. At the same time, service members report financial gain, a sense of pride and patriotism, and greater connection to their fellow service members through shared activities and a common mission during deployment.

While service members are deployed, their family members often experience a sense of confidence and independence. However, spouses often experience minimal personal time, too many responsibilities to juggle at home, changing marital roles, emotional distance from their partner, and sometimes parenting challenges due to children exhibiting problematic behavior at school and at home. Some partners also have to negotiate relocation to be closer to extended family members during deployments, which is accompanied by job changes and school transitions, if the couple has children. It is also important to consider economic challenges that may occur during the deployment phase related to the nondeployed partner rearranging employment or paying for child care or other household services usually performed by the deployed family member.

From an emotional perspective, spouses and children often report anxiety or depression, worry, loneliness, and sadness, especially if the deployment is hazardous. It is also common for families to experience an ambiguous loss of their deployed family member: He or she still has an emotional presence in the family but is not a full and participating member. Also, roles and boundaries between the nondeployed spouse and extended family, as well as children, commonly change. For example, caregiving and discipline are largely left to the nondeployed partner, and children may present more logistical and emotional demands when their parent is deployed.

Reintegration

As John's deployment drew to a close, both he and Mary experienced a surge of anticipation and excitement. The first few weeks back home were wonderful—the honeymoon reunion was even better than that after his first deployment. But eventually John was ready to resume some of the roles he'd had prior to the deployment—making decisions about household purchases, disciplining the kids, handling the TV remote! Some of those roles Mary was eager to share, but others she wanted to retain for herself, or at least to have equal say-so. Their youngsters had some difficulty adjusting as well—delighted to have their Daddy back home, but not being used to having another adult tell them what they could or couldn't do. Besides, John didn't seem to understand what a huge difference just 1 year could make in kids' lives. It required some pretty serious discussions and flexibility to figure out how Mary and John were going to adapt to being a couple again, and more than just two adults living under the same roof. And the possibility of another deployment lurking in the shadows sometimes just prolonged their feelings of being in transition.

Pincus, House, Christenson, and Adler (2001) propose that the reintegration process following deployment generally takes 3 to 6 months, beginning with an emotionally positive homecoming, followed by a honeymoon period, and ending with restabilization. The couple must renegotiate family routines, roles, and various changes that have occurred during the period of deployment. Spouses have to adjust to a loss of the independence they gained during the deployment and sometimes report increased needs for personal space. Partners often feel like they are getting to know each other again because of changes in each of them during the deployment period. Returning service members can feel like "outsiders" in their own families when they have children, because of the many subtle and sometimes major adaptations that have occurred while they were away. Finally, fathers frequently report the challenge of switching from the communication style they used during deployment to one that is suitable for use with their children. They also describe needing to reassure their children that they will not be immediately deployed again, while knowing that redeployment is likely.

It is important to note that reintegration can be a hazardous period for some couples. Some studies have shown a modest but significant relation between length of deployment and rates of subsequent intimate partner violence, especially if the service member suffers from combat-related mental health problems. Increases in rates of child maltreatment during this period have also been documented.

CONCEPTUAL UNDERPINNINGS TO UNDERSTANDING THE DEPLOYMENT CYCLE

Theoretical models of individual and family stress are often used to account for the deployment-related experiences of military families. For example, similar to models of stress specific to individuals, family stress theory predicts that crises occur whenever family demands are judged to exceed the resources families can use to respond (McCubbin & Patterson, 1983). To the extent that deployment-related stressors are highly disruptive or destructive, occur with little warning, cause prolonged feelings of uncertainty, or are part of an accumulation of challenges, they may constitute "catastrophic" stressors. For example, unexpected extensions to tours of duty have been associated with more problems with mental health, employment, marital communication, and household management (MacDermid Wadsworth, 2010).

A stress-producing contextual factor that takes on special significance during wartime is role ambiguity. As mentioned earlier, during deployment, service members are physically absent from their families yet psychologically present. That said, before and after deployment they may be physically present but psychologically absent, especially if the service member is experiencing deployment-related mental health or substance abuse problems. Moreover, the resources, skills, and specific military context for families are important to the couple's adaptation during the deployment phases (Karney & Crown, 2007). For example, service members and their spouses have reported better adjustment and more optimism about coping with deployment when they felt supported by military communities and leaders (MacDermid Wadsworth, 2010). These findings are consistent with family stress theory and other theories accounting for resiliency to stress and trauma. The key impetus of psychological strain involves threatened or actual loss of resources. From this perspective, resources relevant to marriage include individual characteristics such as optimism and hardiness, interpersonal factors such as social support or negative reactivity, and contextual factors such as chronic and daily stressors (Karney & Crown, 2007).

IMPLICATIONS FOR BEST PRACTICES
IN BUILDING COUPLE RESILIENCE

Although both civilian and government providers recognize that military members and their families face high levels of stress during deployment, they have offered few systematic programs and interventions to help. The Family Readiness Group (FRG), U.S. Army Social Work Care Manager Program, and the recent Web-based Tricare Assistance Program (TRIAP) are exceptions, although these programs generally have not been evaluated, and the few program evaluations that have been done yielded mixed results. So what can providers do when research does not fully inform clinical interventions? In the following sections we turn to existing data and best practices to inform services for military families related to deployment, while empirical examinations continue.

A framework developed for working with military families across the deployment cycle uses a combination of clinical experience from working with these families and contributions by Bowling and Sherman (2008), MacDermid Wadsworth (2010), and Walsh (2006) regarding family resilience.

Positive Outlook

Stress research indicates that individuals and families who perceive stressors as challenges to meet versus sources of defeat are more likely to report positive coping and growth as results of the adversity. In the couples context, the more that partners can join together to overcome the challenge as a unified front, the more likely they are to be capable of facing adversity and stronger because of it. In this vein, partners' shared sense of humor can offer a powerful source of positivity and a strategy for increasing cohesiveness. This positivity also helps to buffer the effects of stress at the individual level.

Shared Value System and Spirituality

Partners who share similar values are more likely to build consensus about the sacrifices that they are making for the military and their country. A shared value system also facilitates attributing a shared meaning to the stressors, which in turn further reinforces their joint experience in overcoming the challenges accompanying deployment. Moreover, shared religious or spiritual belief systems, often linked to values and social structures promoting the stability of couples and families, can be important sources of emotional and logistical support.

Emphasis on Family Accord and Effective Communication

Resilient individuals and families draw upon the nurturance of close relationships. Thus, lowering criticism and hostility, and encouraging harmonious, low-conflict interactions can build resilience in couples. Individual differences are tolerated and may even be seen as strengths to draw upon for more effective problem solving. Partners can learn effective communication skills to increase the likelihood that they can be clear, collaborative, and kind with one another in their communication, especially around difficult topics. These communication skills can be especially powerful when discussing the many "touchy" topics that arise when preparing for or coping with the actual deployment, and reacquainting themselves during reintegration. Effective communication can also be used by each partner to acknowledge the unique challenges of the other's experience during the deployment. This perspective taking achieves the goal of sharing to prevent growing apart, enhances social support, and increases empathy.

Flexibility in Roles

As indicated earlier, the absence of a partner changes family roles and expectations. The most adaptive couples comprise individuals with a flexible repertoire of behavior in relation to one another, within the broader family, and in relation to the broader military and community environment. Increasing the degree to which both partners can serve as a caregiver, consoler, protector, disciplinarian, housekeeper, financial manager, chef, and so on, will increase the couple's capacity to meet and grow from the challenges that deployment brings.

Recreation, Routines, and Rituals

Effective stress management strategies for the couple and family during deployment include maintenance of a regular schedule with routines and rituals. This may include day-to-day activities such as walking the dog, a routine bedtime, and evening meals, or less frequent but important rituals such as holiday gatherings, anniversary celebrations, and religious observations. Couples and families may need to adapt these rituals to fit the circumstances of deployment (e.g., Web-based videoconferencing of a birthday party), but regardless of specific adaptations, they should attend to the importance of staying connected.

ISSUES TO CONSIDER
IN PROMOTING COUPLE RESILIENCE

Below we consider military-specific considerations in implementing these suggestions for promoting couple resilience. These include consideration of family preferences within the military subculture, stigma related to seeking services, and the role of military command.

Family Preferences and Military Subculture

Service members and their families are a complex mix of ethnicities and cultures existing within a particular subculture of military life. Because of this diversity, the DoD Task Force on Mental Health (2007) states that "[mental health care] must be provided by professionals familiar with military life." It goes on to specify, "Psychotherapeutic services are best provided by a professional who fully understands the social and psychological context in which the patient functions. The military is a unique cultural context, and the psychological health problems experienced by service members and their families are inextricable from the unique experiences of military service" (p. 42). Keeping these caveats in mind, providers should be culturally competent and sensitive to the unique characteristics of military families, irrespective of whether the provider is in uniform (see Slone, Friedman, & Thompson, Chapter 3, this volume, for more information about military culture).

An important cultural value pertinent to deployment is the impact of the Armed Forces core values on military families. Military core values are an integral part of being successful as a military member. Across all branches, service to country comes before self. Military members have signed a contract with the government to serve their county, which translates to having less freedom. An example is that military members cannot give a 2-week notice and leave their job. Resigning from the military in the midst of an enlistment is not an option, without the possibility of criminal charges. Military families are also shaped by these core values. When a service member lives out "service before self," country demands outweigh not only individual desires but also family wishes. To create the flexibility needed to honor the military's core values, family priorities must be slanted toward the service member's career, which can cause power imbalances between spouses and within families. This does not necessarily mean that the military member has more actual power in the family. But it can and often does mean that the family prioritizes resources to support the military member, which can sometimes create resentment and hostility, either between partners or toward the military.

Stigma

Service members are in a unique situation regarding minimal boundaries between information about their physical or mental health and their employer. This lack of privacy is a major contributor to stigma about mental health services. Evidence of stigma surrounding mental health issues in the military is overwhelming, and this is likely to have a negative impact on service members and their family obtaining support and care during the deployment phases. Nearly 60% of soldiers and 50% of Marines surveyed have reported that leadership would treat them more negatively if they sought counseling. However, other studies indicate that significant numbers of military members are overcoming this perceived stigma and seeking care. A large epidemiological study found that within the first year after combat, 35% of Operation Iraqi Freedom military personnel sought military mental health services (Hoge, Auchterlonie, & Milliken, 2006). Providers need to understand that stigma persists at many levels in the military, requiring continuous education throughout the military community about the benefits of preventive and interventive care around the deployment cycle.

Military Command

Military command can play a major role in service members' and their families' accessing care during the deployment cycle. For example, commanders can either reduce or create obstacles to getting services by allowing time off from work (or not) for appointments. They also have a powerful role in establishing a unit culture that either encourages or discourages seeking care for any issue, at any stage of deployment. Providers are also influenced by command attitudes toward mental health education and treatment services. Recent MHAT-V findings of Behavioral Health staff stationed in Afghanistan found that 87% of personnel reported that they frequently talked with unit commanders, while only about half agreed that commanders respected patient confidentiality regarding these issues. In addition, only 50% agreed that commanders supported the providers' recommendations for medical evacuation out of the theater of action. The report goes on to state that military members tell providers that they believe seeking mental healthcare is seen in the military as "breaking" (i.e., being weak or unfit for duty).

An additional issue to consider is that, like service members, military command may see civilian providers as "outsiders." Although the outsider status of civilian providers does not necessarily preclude developing an effective working relationship with command, this comprises an additional possible hurdle for civilian providers to overcome. Finally, for many service members and their family members, the core values of service may seem at odds with treatment seeking. Service members may construe service before self as a reason not to prioritize mental health needs for self or family. This may be particularly true of higher-ranking military members, who may believe that making time for self- or family care takes time away from being a strong leader, especially during the predeployment and deployment phases.

Sergeant Burkholdt was a Mental Health Specialist for a brigade of 1,500 soldiers spread out across three base camps. Much of her time was devoted to helping soldiers struggling with relationship problems back home. Some complained of spouses who were spending all their money and of feeling powerless to intervene, because they had signed over power of attorney before deploying. Others had married just prior to deployment, in an effort to obtain benefits for partners they had known only a few months. Many of her soldiers suspected or knew of infidelity by their spouses back home; a smaller number confessed to their own infidelity downrange. Some described their spouses' suicidal behaviors or children with serious health problems, and reported finding it difficult to concentrate and stay focused on their mission. Other soldiers felt suicidal themselves. Because it was a combat environment, Sgt. Burkholdt was expected to keep the commanders informed if a soldier was potentially a danger to him- or herself or others. Some commanders welcomed Sgt. Burkholdt's input, but others worried about potentially weakening brigade strength by taking soldiers off the front lines for emotional problems. As a Mental Health

Specialist, it was difficult sometimes to discern who her real client was—the individual service member or the U.S. Army.

SPECIAL NEEDS POPULATIONS AND CONCERNS DURING THE DEPLOYMENT CYCLE

Many military families deal with deployment without crisis or problems. Others grow and learn from the process, even when traumatic events occur during deployment. Some couples, however, struggle and need formal support throughout the deployment cycle. Providers often find a mix of military members and family members presenting for care, and below are some unique populations and concerns to consider.

Single Parents

When s single parent in the military deploys, the stress on the parent and children can be particularly high when nontraditional caregivers (i.e., siblings, parents, or friends) assume temporary guardianship for the service member's children. Providers should be prepared to adapt services for these caregivers to the extent possible, because many of these caregivers may not be eligible for full mental health services.

Dual-Military Couples

Dual-military couples (with both partners serving in the military) are uniquely impacted by deployments. Both partners may be called upon to deploy at the same time, resulting in the same problems associated with single parents. Even if only one spouse is deployed, the other military member must fulfill his or her military duties while assuming full responsibility for running a household.

Nonmarried Partners

For nonmarried intimates, partners remaining at home have little, if any, support from the military health system. They may also live in areas where mental health providers do not understand the unique stressors associated with military life. Providers—whether on college campuses, military bases, or in a small town far away from a base—need to be aware of these intimate partners to help them receive the support they need. Nonmilitary providers, in particular, may encounter intimate partners who are gay, lesbian, or bisexual, because these partners currently cannot access care; even if the partners are married in a state that allows same-sex marriage, these marriages are not recognized by the federal government.

Suicide or Self-Harm

Some level of suicide ideation was reported by 10% of combat personnel and 11% of support personnel who responded to the MHAT surveys, indicating a high risk of suicide or self- harm behavior among service members during deployment. Providers also need to be alert to the potential for nondeployed family members to contemplate suicide or self-harm throughout the deployment cycle. Suicide and self-harm assessments are clinically warranted for all military family members presenting for care, including adolescents and children. Providers may also want to talk with military members and family members about how their partners are doing, because partners are often the first to hear suicidal statements made during separation. Providers must report these concerns to the appropriate military or civilian authorities as quickly as possible.

Drug and Alcohol Use

It is well documented that alcohol and drug use increase during times of stress, in general, and the time surrounding deployment is no exception. Recent research indicates that between 25 and 33% of service members and veterans screen positive for problematic substance use when assessed. Providers should recognize that nondeployed partners may also develop problematic alcohol or substance use while under the stress of the deployment cycle. For example, in a large study of U.S. Army medical records, wives of deployed husbands had modestly higher rates of alcohol- and drug-related disorders when compared with wives whose husbands were not deployed (Mansfield et al., 2010).

SUMMARY

Each deployment presents its own unique challenges to couples and families, as well as unique opportunities for individual and relationship growth. The mission for educators and counselors providing services to military consumers is to provide information, guidance, and support to maximize these growth opportunities and minimize the potential for maladaptive and enduring responses to the inherent stresses of deployment transitions. Many couples and families already master these challenges on their own with little or no outside help, demonstrating remarkable resilience. Others can benefit from prevention programs that provide information about individual and relationship stressors across the deployment cycle, contextualize common responses, and provide guidance that promotes preemptive strategies that facilitate anticipation, planning, and mastery of predictable challenges. And still others struggle more noticeably and require therapeutic interventions to ameliorate the adverse consequences of deployment stressors for their individual or relationship functioning.

Understanding this diversity of individual responses within the context of normative and predictable phases of the deployment cycle is essential to delivering effective services. Some providers may have an advantage of having experienced one or more roles related to deployment themselves—perhaps as a former service member or family member. Indeed, the vignettes offered in this chapter are informed, in part, by June Behn Watt's multiple roles as the spouse of a deployed service member, as a deployed Mental Health Specialist herself providing services to a brigade of 1,500 soldiers during service in Afghanistan, and currently providing services to veterans and their families in the United States. For educators and therapists without firsthand experience of deployment in one capacity or another, interactions with service members and their families provide an opportunity to learn—as well as to teach and to counsel. Listening to service members' personal stories of both resilience and vulnerability brings life to the theories and descriptive frameworks regarding the challenges of deployment transitions.

Finally, both prevention and intervention programs built around the deployment cycle will benefit from attention to those factors that reliably influence resilience and vulnerability. Some individuals present special challenges and needs—for example, those with prior emotional or behavioral difficulties or chaotic relationships. Identifying those individuals and families, and providing an additional layer of care both prior to and following deployment, may reduce the adverse consequences commonly associated with deployment. Similarly, some individuals demonstrate remarkable resilience. Identifying and then promoting those influences that facilitate adaptation and growth—including optimism, shared values, relationship and family accord, and flexibility in roles—offer opportunities for supporting and safeguarding those serving their country, and the individuals in their lives most dear to them.

RESOURCES

Bowling, U. B., & Sherman, M. D. (2008). Welcoming them home: Supporting service members and their families in navigating the tasks of reintegration. *Professional Psychology: Research and Practice, 39*, 451–458.

Castaneda, L. W., Harrell, M. C., Varda, D. M., Hall, K. C., Beckett, M. K., & Stern, S. (2008). *Deployment experiences of Guard and Reserve families.* Santa Monica, CA: RAND Corporation.

Department of Defense Task Force on Mental Health (2007). *An achievable vision: Report of the Department of Defense Task Force on Mental Health.* Falls Church, VA: Defense Health Board.

Hill, R. (1949). *Families under stress: Adjustment to the crises of war, separation, and return.* New York: Harper & Brothers.

Hoge, C. W., Auchterlonie, J. L., & Milliken, C. S. (2006). Mental health problems, use of mental health services, and attrition from military service after returning from deployment to Iraq or Afghanistan. *Journal of the American Medical Association, 295,* 1023–1032.

Karney, B. R., & Crown, J. S. (2007). *Families under stress: An assessment of data, theory and research on marriage and divorce in the military.* Santa Monica, CA: RAND National Defense Research Institute.

MacDermid Wadsworth, S. M. (2010). Family risk and resilience in the context of war and terrorism. *Journal of Marriage and Family, 72,* 537–556.

MacLean, A., & Elder, G. H. (2007). Military service in the life course. *Annual Review of Sociology, 33,* 175–196.

Mansfield, A. J., Kaufman, J. S., Marshall, S. W., Gaynes, B. N., Morrissey, J. P., & Engel, C. C. (2010). Deployment and the use of mental health services among U.S. Army wives. *New England Journal of Medicine, 362,* 101–109.

McCarroll, J. E., Hoffman, K. J., Grieger, T. A., & Holloway, H. C. (2005). Psychological aspects of deployment and reunion. In P. W. Kelley (Ed.), *Military preventive medicine: Mobilization and deployment* (Vol. 2, pp. 1395–1424). Falls Church, VA: Surgeon General of the Army.

McCubbin, H. I., & Patterson, J. M. (1983). The family stress process: The double ABCX model of adjustment and adaptation. *Marriage and Family Review, 6,* 7–37.

Mental Health Advisory Team V. (2008). *Operation Iraqi Freedom 06–08.* Washington, DC: Office of the Surgeon, Multinational Force Iraq, and Office of the Surgeon General, U.S. Army Medical Command.

Pavlicin, K. M. (2003). *Surviving deployment: A guide for military families.* St. Paul, MN: Elva Resa.

Pincus, S. H., House, R., Christenson, J., & Adler, L. E. (2001). The emotional cycle of deployment: A military family perspective. *Journal of the Army Medical Department, 2,* 15–23.

Walsh, F. (2006). *Strengthening family resilience* (2nd ed.). New York: Guilford Press.

PART II

Evidence-Based Interventions

CHAPTER 5

Enhancing Parenting in Military and Veteran Families

Ellen R. DeVoe, Ruth Paris, and Abigail Ross

Joe was on his second tour of duty in Afghanistan when the Humvee he was driving exploded after hitting an improvised explosive device (IED). One of his buddies was killed, and Joe sustained debilitating injuries to his legs. After surgery and rehabilitation, he returned home to his wife, Nora, and their three children (ages 16, 10, and 4). Joe had enlisted in the U.S. Army National Guard, with his wife's support, following the September 11, 2001, attacks. When he returned from his first deployment, the family adjusted well and the couple had their third child. Joe's adjustment to being home this time, however, was extremely difficult for all family members. In addition to being in pain, Joe thought constantly about his buddy and spent hours communicating on line with others from his unit. He had difficulty sleeping because of leg pain and nightmares but did not want to "talk to a shrink." During the day, he snapped at his family even though he wanted to be more patient. His 10-year-old daughter frequently asked Nora, "What happened to Daddy? He's not the same." His 16-year-old son seemed to understand his physical limitations and tried to join him in watching sports. Despite his son's efforts, however, Joe would eventually retreat to his bedroom when the kids were home because "it was all too much." Joe finally agreed to meet with a therapist when his wife asked him to stay at his mother's until he could "deal with the kids."

INCIDENCE AND IMPACT OF DEPLOYMENT ON MILITARY FAMILIES

Since the September 11, 2001, attacks, U.S. war operations related to Afghanistan and Iraq have relied upon a volunteer force of over 3.5 million members. Unlike conflicts of earlier generations in which military personnel were younger, typically single, and without children, a substantial number of active duty and Reserve military members serving in Operation Iraqi Freedom/Operation Enduring Freedom (OIF/OEF) are parents of dependent children. Of the more than 2 million children who have experienced the deployment of at least one parent, children ages birth to 5 years comprise the largest age group, followed by 6- to 11-year-olds, and 12- to 18-year-olds. Given the number of children and parents affected, combined with the potential effects and high operational tempo of these conflicts on service members, prevention and intervention strategies must take into account the totality of a service member's experiences and responsibilities, including family and parenting roles at home.

CONCEPTUAL AND EMPIRICAL UNDERPINNINGS

In this chapter, we offer a conceptual framework grounded in the developmental context of the child and family to understand the complexities couples face in maintaining parenting roles and parent–child relationships throughout the deployment cycle. Next, we examine the available literature on the impact of deployment-related separation upon military and veteran parents and their children. Finally, we suggest guidelines for assessment and intervention, along with practice principles for the provider who works with military couples who have children.

Developmental Ecology as a Conceptual Framework for Understanding Military Families

A developmental–ecological perspective serves as an integrating framework for understanding the range of responses among all family members to the specific experiences of parental deployment, absence, return, and the effects of deployment upon parent–child relationship. Accordingly, the impact of deployment separation and reintegration on children and adolescents and parent–child relationships is considered along multiple and interacting levels of risk and protection. At the first layer, the personal level, unique individual factors, including age, temperament, health, and developmental history are considered. Younger children, those with compromised health, or children experiencing mental health or developmental challenges are likely to need extra support during a parental deployment, which can further strain the at-home parent. A second layer of the family's ecology includes the immediate social/familial and ongoing context of deployment-related stress experienced by the child, each parent, and other members of the family. For example, deployment may be accompanied by financial stress, caregiver role burden, couple strain, and parenting challenges. At the most basic level, children, adolescents, and partners miss and may yearn for their deployed service member. Family members may also experience positive growth and development because of deployment, including increased sense of competence, success in new roles and responsibilities, and newfound independence. Because each deployment has its own unique characteristics, couple and parenting adaptations are likely to vary across families.

A third layer of the family ecology includes diverse factors that either buffer or stress the child or adolescent during deployment, including parental mental health, the quality of parenting and the parent–child relationship, and community influences. It follows that children whose parents are better able to respond sensitively to their emotional needs (even from theater of combat) and have a strong relationship as a couple, and whose siblings assist in emotional support will likely have healthier overall psychosocial adjustment. Finally, broad sociocultural values and belief systems affect a family's military and deployment experience. For example, currently, community beliefs about military service, support for the mission, and political attitudes regarding the OIF/OEF conflicts are important influences on families and vary significantly according to residence (e.g., military installation or community), region of the country, and social networks. All couple and child reactions throughout the deployment cycle can be understood through this holistic conceptual frame and remediation, and where needed, can be offered by a variety of providers at any one of the four ecological levels. For the couple and family provider specifically, it is important to identify whether and how co-parenting contributes to or is affected by a couple's core concerns.

PARENTING TASKS AND CHILD ADAPTATION ASSOCIATED WITH PHASE OF DEPLOYMENT

Given the dynamic nature of current military service, children's coping abilities and each partner's parenting ability fluctuate over the course of deployment and will be influenced by the family's position within the broader deployment life cycle. Logan's (1987) original conceptualization of the "cycle of deployment" is now used to describe a series of phases that service members and their families experience beginning with notification of an upcoming deployment, through postdeployment transitions (see Beasley, MacDermid Wadsworth, & Watts, Chapter 4, this volume, for fuller description; Logan, 1987; American Psychological Association Presidential Task Force on Military Deployment Services for Youth, Families, and Service Members, 2007). Each phase of the deployment cycle is accompanied by logistical and emotional tasks, and transitions for the service member parent and his or her partner and children, and can serve as an organizing framework for interventions with couples and families.

Predeployment Phase

The predeployment period is characterized by anticipation of separation and loss, which may be compounded by a narrow window of time between notification and departure (National Military Family Association, 2005; MacDermid, 2006). Family members and service members alike may respond with detachment, increased conflict, or difficulty communicating. National Guard and Reserve families may be especially challenged because of relatively shorter preparation time and limited access to the critical information, resources, and social supports that are available to installation-based families (MacDermid, 2006). Significant concerns for the at-home parent include anticipating how to manage the worry of chronic threat to the parent in theater and the practical demands of maintaining a household and caring for children. For the service member, a major source of tension during the predeployment period may be conflict between preparing for the mission and the pull to be with family and loved ones. Parents often struggle with how and when to communicate with their child(ren) about the impending departure and the service member's mission. Children of all ages, even babies and toddlers, perceive the changes in the immediate family environment during this time, even if they are not able to express their feelings. Older children and adolescents may put the pieces together before they are told about an upcoming deployment and should be supported as early as possible in managing the news. (See Handout 5.1, *What to Say and When to Say It: Preparing Your Children for Deployment*, at the end of this chapter.)

Deployment Phase: Parenting from the War Zone

A small body of literature has explored the experiences of fathers in managing their parenting roles during deployment. Early research described the deployed parent as "absent" from the child's life during deployment, a characterization that no longer applies due to 21st-century technology. However, the parenting role remains extremely complex for deployed parents even with greater ability for real-time communication with spouses and children from the site of deployment. Service members have emphasized that their parenting experiences directly influence their abilities to perform mission-related duties in theater. Specifically, service member fathers described the competing demands of ensuring the safety of their own troops and themselves, caring for young Iraqi children, and attending to their own children's needs from afar. Some fathers reported that these contradictory roles challenged their ability to focus on the mission and decreased their attention to individual and unit safety. (See also Handouts 5.2, *Creating a Parenting Plan for Deployment*, and 5.3, *When the Questions Get Harder: Talking with Your Child about War*, at the end of this chapter.)

Deployment Phase: Becoming a Single Parent at Home

At the point of departure, family members left behind may experience a period of emotional and even physical destabilization (Pincus, House, Christensen, & Adler, 2001). For some couples and families, there can be a sense of relief that the anticipation of the deployment is over, and new routines and adjustments can begin to form. Not surprisingly, some non-deployed spouses report feelings of sadness, anger, and anxiety, and can feel overwhelmed with financial, household, and parenting responsibilities (Pincus et al., 2001). There is also evidence that risk of maltreatment, primarily neglect, increases during deployment (Gibbs, Martin, Kupper, & Johnson, 2007), suggesting that many at-home parents are experiencing increased stress related to parenting roles during deployment. On balance, many at-home parents manage the demands of deployment successfully and are able to develop effective family routines and social supports. For spouses who may be vulnerable, engagement is enhanced when outreach and preventive intervention are initiated before the service member departs. For these families, the sequence of intervention may involve a period of support with an at-home spouse even though this represents a deviation from more traditional couple intervention models. After deployment the provider must then attend to alliance issues to enable the returning service member to join in the intervention.

Impact of Deployment on Children and Adolescents

Many studies indicate that the at-home parent's mental health significantly influences the children's ability to adjust to parental absence and is particularly important for the youngest children, who are highly dependent upon the parent–child relationship. Specifically, infants and toddlers may become more irritable, have more sleep disruption, and develop eating problems or separation anxiety when the at-home parent is suffering from depression or anxiety. Young children also may ask repeated questions about when the deployed parent coming home.

Several studies of school-age children and adolescents show that parental deployment is linked to a number of challenging outcomes, including depression and anxiety, behavioral problems, emotional dysregulation, and declines in academic performance. For many adolescents, the deployment period is also stressful because of possible relocation, school transfer, loss of peer group and extracurricular activities, and realigned family roles demanding increased responsibility (Pincus et al., 2001). The "ambiguous loss" that families struggle with may create barriers to adaptive coping for those at home and can manifest as depression or difficulties in family relationships. Specifically, an adolescent may express a feeling of disengagement from the deployed parent in tandem with yearning, because "He's still my dad but he may not come home." In a study of adolescents (ages 12–18) attending a summer program for military youth, participants reported missing routine day-to-day activities and boundary negotiation with parents about family roles during deployment and reintegration. Furthermore, adolescents reported increased depression, acting-out behavior, anxiety about the deployed parent's safety, and less involvement in extracurricular activities (Huebner, Mancini, Wilcox, Grass, & Grass, 2007). Dysregulated behavior, such as "lashing out," a commonly reported coping mechanism, was often invoked in response to circumstances that might not otherwise have been upsetting.

Deployment length exacerbates the strain on children and adolescents. Findings from a recent study of 11- to 17-year-olds reveal that length of parental deployment is associated with a number of challenges for youth during both deployment and reintegration (Chandra et al., 2010). Participants reported depression, anxiety, increased awareness of the dangers associated with deployment, and changes in school performance, with girls and older adolescents having more difficulty adjusting to the parent's return. With regard to multiple deployments, other researchers argue that the best predictors of an adolescent's overall ability to cope include a high-functioning at-home parent and family system, the adolescent's belief that there is public support for the wars, and the adolescent's perception that the deployed parent is making a meaningful difference.

Postdeployment Phase

In this period, both the service member and the at-home parent may experience stress around role negotiation related to parenting, and household and financial functioning. Returning parents describe difficulties reengaging in life at home, may seem detached or psychologically absent, and may perceive themselves to have less parental authority than the at-home parent during readjustment. Postdeployment adjustment may also be challenging for children and adolescents. Findings from a recent study of OIF/OEF families with at least one young child indicated that in the postdeployment period, very young children were more likely to have problems sleeping alone, to manifest more separation anxiety specific to the returning parent, and to be reluctant to seek comfort from the returning parent (Barker & Berry, 2009). Younger children may not recognize their service member parent, leaving the parent potentially hurt or at a loss as to how to relate to the child. Older children and adolescents may resist changes in rules or routines as the returning parent is reintegrated in the family. If children have been "in trouble" during the deployment, they may be fearful of the returning parent's reactions.

Resilience

Despite the challenges families face throughout military service, the majority of children with deployed parents cope well. Recent research on "resilience," described as positive adaptation in the face of adversity, suggests that military children and adolescents engaged in high levels of prosocial behavior and positive thinking strategies to cope with the stress of parental deployment. In Chandra and colleagues' (2010) study, school personnel reported that, overall, most youth adapt successfully to parental deployment, but that the parent's military branch and number of deployments make a difference in promoting or diminishing resilience. Factors that seem to promote resilience in adolescents, and most likely all children, include discussion about the deployment prior to departure, family stability, high-quality parenting by the at-home parent, and social support. Relatively few studies have explored resilience in babies, toddlers, and preschoolers, though quality of parenting has emerged consistently as the most critical element associated with adaptive coping and resilience in children of all ages.

In the remainder of this chapter, we present guidelines for the provider working with a military or veteran couple that is co-parenting. Because there are no specific intervention models in this arena, we describe principles of assessment and intervention, along with process elements to guide those providing services. A significant clinical challenge for the provider is to maintain an appropriate focus on, and balance between, couple-related issues and co-parenting concerns, and to develop the skills necessary to move between couple and broader family-related themes, as dictated by each individual couple.

DETAILED GUIDELINES
FOR CO-PARENTING ASSESSMENT

When a military or veteran couple seeks assistance for relationship or family concerns, it is critical for the counselor to learn whether the couple has children and, if they do, the degree to which parenting and parent–child relationship functioning is relevant to the couple's concerns or resilience. For couples who are parents, however, tension or conflict in the relationship can compromise parenting as well. For example, the stress of couple problems often leaves less energy and patience for each partner in parenting roles and, in the extreme, can contribute to maladaptive parenting practices, including neglect and abuse. Similarly, in cases where parenting is not a primary or presenting concern, the therapist needs to be mindful of the impact the couple's difficulties may be having on the children and the ability to co-parent. For instance, is the couple fighting in the presence of the children? Are the partners able to remain unified in their parenting in spite of their conflict, or do they undermine the other's parenting efforts? Regardless of the couple's core concerns, the provider should help the couple become aware of the interplay between couple difficulties and parenting practices and effectiveness.

Parent Assessment

The mental health status of each parent influences parenting. When couples present with parenting concerns, an important purpose of assessment is to gain insight into how each partner's mental health status diminishes or contributes to good parenting practices. In addition to conducting a comprehensive individual adult assessment, the provider should explore the level of agreement within the couple on the mental health functioning of each partner. For example, the provider might ask the wife of a service member with combat stress to describe the type and intensity of symptoms she observes in her partner. Similarly, the husband of a new mother may provide important information about his wife's postpartum functioning, which leads to more accurate planning and intervention. It is especially critical to assess the history of depression, including postpartum depression, anxiety and traumatic stress symptoms, substance use, and partner violence, given the potential impact of these disorders on couple functioning, parenting, and parent–child relationships.

If a military or veteran couple is experiencing difficulties in the parenting roles, the provider should initiate a structured discussion that focuses on current and past parenting challenges, concerns about a specific child, and hopes for change in the parenting realm. A comprehensive assessment includes an exploration of the couple's overall functioning as co-parents, changes in their co-parenting capacities over the course of military service, and what supports are available to bolster parenting. The provider also should explore each parent's roles in the family and household (e.g., who does what with and for the child(ren), who makes decisions about the child(ren), who handles discipline), the flow of typical days, activities the family enjoys, and amount and quality of time spent with children. Information regarding changes in family structure and parenting functions related to military service and transition out of the military to veteran status is essential in understanding parental stress. For example, many families move in with relatives or ask a grandparent to live-in during the deployment. While this type of arrangement can be extremely helpful, it can also create tension between generations and within the couple upon the service member's return. Children also may be cared for by a stepparent or partner of the service member during deployment. If this relationship is a long-term and ongoing one in which the child feels a level of trust and the partner is committed to the child, caregiving may be similar to that of a parent or relative. If not, care should be taken to address the child's potential feelings of abandonment by the primary caregiver.

Child-Focused Assessment

The child assessment yields information that can be used to facilitate parenting strategies that are most appropriate to individual children and the family's circumstances. This focus is on supporting parents in recognizing and addressing their children's needs. In the context of couple intervention, the provider should obtain each parent's perspective on the child's or children's status in order to assess whether parenting should be a focus of treatment, and whether children are having difficulties that parents do not yet recognize. In addition to obtaining developmental history, the provider should explore how the children have managed military service.

School performance is highly relevant, as children of all ages may respond to the stress of deployment and separation with academic declines, school refusal, or behaviors that interfere with school or child care functioning. Because peer relationships are an important source of support and growth for all children, parents can be asked about their children's best friends and prosocial activities, involvement in school and extracurricular activities, and whether they know other children in military families. For example, young children can become aggressive toward or withdraw from peers; school-age children can lose interest in friendships or have difficulty making new friends when the family has relocated. Adolescents react to deployment and reunion in diverse ways, ranging from anxiety about the deployed parent's safety to antisocial or risky behaviors (including drug and alcohol abuse) to competent adaptation. The provider is looking for changes, especially declines, in child or adolescent functioning that cannot be explained developmentally or by medical status, as well as other concerns, such as excessive worry or depression. The provider needs to become educated about the range of child and adolescent responses to stress, with the goal of accurately assessing child status and providing relevant information to military and veteran couples about their children's functioning and needs.

Children with special needs, such as developmental or physical disabilities, or medical conditions, often have particular care requirements that may draw family resources away from siblings, the parents' ability to engage in self-care, and the couple relationship. The provider should ask the couple to describe specific care needs and resources, developmental level, as well as unique ways in which the child may have been affected by a parent's military service. The impact of caring for a special needs child on couple functioning and satisfaction also may be an important area for exploration.

For some couples, the child assessment process alone will enhance their awareness of their children's needs and adaptations. For example, a parent might suggest that a child did not notice or has not been affected by parental deployment. In response, the clinician should carefully reinforce the notion that even though children and adolescents can be quite resilient, they are very aware of their parent's absence and always have reactions to the deployment and return of a parent. Other couples may be more attuned to specific challenges their children have had in response to deployment, and are seeking assistance in how best to support their children or "get them back on track." Still other couples have divergent perspectives regarding how their children have fared and how parenting should be approached. For example, a service member might comment that his 5- and 12-year-old daughters have handled his deployment "with no problem," while his wife reveals that both children had many sleepless nights during his deployment and are very anxious that he will leave again. Similarly, an at-home parent who has "run a tight ship" may be resentful of the returning parent's relaxed approach to discipline and family routines. For couples presenting with significantly diverse ideas about parenting, the provider should learn whether parenting differences are creating "couple" issues, and if so, will need to address these dynamics.

Parent–Child Relationship Assessment

Understanding parents' perceptions and interpretations of a particular child and their relationship to that child is central in considering whether parenting should be a primary focus of work. Assessing the specifics of each parent's relationship with each child is best accomplished through interview questions in combination with direct observation. Interview questions drawn from the Working Model of the Child Interview (Zeanah & Benoit, 1995) aim to access the parents' internal representations or working models of their relationship to their child. Questions can be focused on the child that parents are most concerned about or can be asked multiple times for all children in the family. The ways in which parents respond to questions are as important as the content of their statements. For example, it is important to note whether a parent avoids certain questions or becomes preoccupied with others. Similarly, the degree to which parental affect matches the content of the response provides valuable insight into relationship dynamics. In some cases, when a service member parent has only recently returned from deployment, the at-home partner may answer most of child-focused questions. Furthermore, when a service member parent has returned with combat stress or a physical disability, he or she may not feel confident in responding to child-focused queries. For veteran couples who have been home together, each parent may be able to offer an independent opinion about their children. When a parent is not able to offer a detailed picture of each child, the provider should explore possible explanations, including traumatic brain injury (TBI), posttraumatic stress disorder (PTSD), parental depression, as well as psychosocial or family-related dynamics.

Whenever possible, children should participate in a session in order to provide an opportunity for the therapist to observe directly family dynamics, the couple's co-parenting in action, and parent–child interactions. The overall goal of conjoint sessions is for the provider to observe interactions between parents and children. In particular, they afford the provider an opportunity to get to know the child and his or her style and to assess parenting behaviors between adult and child and within the co-parenting couple. The provider also can observe family rules, affective expression, degree of mutual pleasure, evidence of tension in relationships, and the ability of the parents to attune to children and respond to their moment-to-moment behaviors and moods. The structure and process of family sessions vary depending on the age of the child. Issues central to deployment and military service should be raised by the provider and included in the session in ways that are developmentally appropriate. Depending upon each child's developmental stage, the therapist should facilitate sharing of the child's specific experiences and understanding of parental deployment and reunion, if the child is comfortably and safely able to do so in the presence of the parents.

Parents of children under 1 year of age can bring their infant to the session, allowing the provider to assess both parents' comfort level and behavior in parent–infant interactions. Although in most couples the mother will have a well-established and, we hope, positive rhythm with her baby, mothers who are experiencing or have had a postpartum mood disorder or PTSD may not be optimally attuned to their babies. Similarly, returning fathers may be less comfortable or confident in interacting with their babies and toddlers because of lack of familiarity or mental health concerns, such as TBI or combat stress. Parents can engage in a play session with toddlers and preschool children with particular age-appropriate tasks suggested by the therapist, such as blocks, drawing, and imaginative play. School-age children can be brought into a session to identify challenges at school or home, and for structured discussion of parental deployment, when relevant. The provider can invite the parents to play with their school-age child using board games or art materials. Adolescents may need to be seen alone by the therapist for a brief time prior to a conjoint session with the parents. Similar to sessions with younger children, the provider should facilitate a conversation between the parents and adolescents about school or home life. Highly emotionally charged relationships between parents and adolescents are challenging for all involved parties, but the provider should attempt to observe the parents interacting with their son or daughter.

FACTORS INFLUENCING INTERVENTION

Although all military and veteran families in which a parent has deployed face the multiple strains of separation, ambiguous loss, and concern about the service member, each family's experience of the deployment cycle is unique. Several specific aspects of deployment may intensify or mitigate parenting stress, child distress, and adaptive coping by all members of the family. First, the type of deployment serves as a critical element in each family's experience. Although any relocation to a war zone inherently includes some risk to the service member, missions that put service members squarely in harm's way are likely to cause greater concern in partners, children, and family members. Second, to the extent that access to communication technology is affected, mission and rank may have an important but unintended impact on a couple's ability to maintain satisfactory and necessary communication throughout deployment. Third, prior deployments may serve to bolster family members' confidence in their ability to handle a future deployment, or multiple redeployments may be a breaking point for families. Finally, the current phase of the deployment cycle (e.g., whether a service member is preparing to deploy to a war zone or has returned home after deployment, or both) is a critical contextual factor that defines a family's needs and a couple's ability to seek help. In the next section, we suggest specific guidelines for the family provider on the basis of the phase of deployment.

INTERVENTION PRINCIPLES ASSOCIATED WITH PHASE OF DEPLOYMENT

Predeployment

Parenting tasks vary depending on the age of the child and the stage of the deployment cycle. As discussed earlier, during the predeployment stage the service member is preparing for mobilization, and family members are anticipating the loss. Young children may seem detached from the process, or older children may appear more dismissive or aggressive. All family members may be struggling with how to say good-bye. Often service members are at a loss as to how to describe where they are going and what they will be doing, particularly to very young children. Intervention with parents at this stage should address anticipatory feelings and anxieties, as well as strategies for how to talk with children in age-appropriate ways. Furthermore, how the family will communicate during deployment should be discussed, with specific guidelines for how the deployed service member wants to be involved in parenting, as well as the at-home parent's need for support from the service member and others. Children from preschool onward may benefit from a session in which parents and caregivers are assisted in discussing the upcoming deployment and engaging their children in conversation about possible concerns. (See Handout 5.1.)

Deployment

The remaining parent is typically the main source of support for children and adolescents of all ages. Because the at-home parent's ability to manage feelings and demands is crucial for a children's coping and resilience and for couple functioning, couple work may focus on supporting the nondeployed partner during the period of separation. While managing their own feelings of sadness, anger, or worry, at-home parents may simultaneously be overwhelmed with having to take over all the household and family responsibilities, as well as continue a job outside of the home. When meeting with the at-home parent, the provider should first inquire about ways of coping with the deployment, specifically focusing on parenting tasks. In addition, the therapist should ask about the child's behavioral and affective responses to the stress of the separation, with specific questions focused on how the child is managing daily tasks, sleep patterns, school, and communication with the deployed parent. As described earlier, children of all ages can become behaviorally symptomatic while struggling with anxiety about the service member's well-being, separation from a primary caregiver, the break in a standard routine, or witnessing the affective or functional difficulties of the at-home parent.

The provider should remain attuned to all of these factors, keeping in mind the couple's parenting plan. At this stage young children may not be able to talk on the phone, but they can see their parent on a webcam. Visual images of the deployed parent, whether in photographs, videos, or on the computer screen, can be helpful in keeping young children connected to a parent, although some may find it too emotionally challenging to manage. School-age children often enjoy the electronic contact with the deployed parent and can be engaged in sending packages, letters, or videos. Teenagers may choose to maintain their own communication with a parent when possible, although they should be encouraged to participate in family phone calls or webcam chats to maintain a sense of family continuity. The remaining parent has the challenging task of supporting communication strategies that can be beneficial for each child in the family and the deployed parent, and that also meet his or her own needs as a member of the parenting couple. (See Handout 5.2.)

Reintegration

Some children develop or continue to have difficulties even after a parent's return from deployment, which makes reintegration more challenging for all family members and may delay the returning parent's ability to regain a stable parenting role. For babies born during a deployment, the returning father must get to know his new son or daughter at the child's pace, which can be challenging or disheartening if the baby is slow to warm up to a new caregiver. Young children may not be able to relate to or remember the deployed parent; school-age children may have settled into new routines that they are hesitant to change. Subsequent separations from that parent, whether for drill weekends for members of the National Guard or Reserves, or separations connected to regular workday activities or trainings, may serve as triggers for a child's separation anxiety and should be addressed with consistent patience and information to the child who is distressed.

Co-parenting challenges during reintegration may include the returning parent's sense of alienation from parenting routines, lack of confidence regarding parenting practices, disagreement with how the spouse handled parenting during the deployment, unwillingness to discipline, and difficulties with pacing (e.g., taking over parenting authority before a child is ready; not following the child's lead or cues for interaction). The at-home parent may experience relief at "handing over" child-related responsibilities, resentment or frustration related to the returning parent's efforts to do things differently, or interest in collaborating with the returning parent, among other feelings. During the reintegration phase, each parent's experience and perspective can be built upon to renegotiate parenting roles and develop new family routines. Reintegration adjustments in family life, the couple relationship, and parenting, while often positive, may also present unexpected challenges to the couple. The couple therapist should support parents in considering together, during reintegration, how they would like to approach parenting and support each other in day-to-day parenting practices.

For families in which the service member has combat stress or other mental health concerns, it is critical that the provider assess how a service member's mental health or deployment-related experiences are affecting parenting, and support the couple in acknowledging and addressing these difficult dynamics. In this situation, one or both members of the couple may benefit from motivational interviewing strategies to gently raise awareness of a partner's distress or symptoms, and their impact on family functioning. When the couple is able to work from a shared understanding of the service member's specific symptoms, both couple-focused and parenting goals can be addressed more effectively. Specifically, it is essential to assist the couple in recognizing and managing trauma triggers as they relate to everyday household and family routines. For example, a toddler's normal play activities or an adolescent's basement rock band practice could serve as triggers for a service member parent with traumatic stress reactions. Similarly, a service member's avoidant behavior may be misinterpreted and very hurtful to both children and partners. Thus, when a service member is suffering from PTSD or other mental health symptoms, the provider should give basic psychoeducation regarding the symptoms and help parents to provide information at developmentally appropriate levels, so that children can better understand the returning parent's behavior. For the service member, outside referrals for individual services may be warranted.

OPTIONS FOR INTERVENTION:
WHAT DOES THE COUPLE NEED?

The main goal for the provider working with a military or veteran couple in which parenting is a core clinical concern is to determine the extent to which parenting interventions are necessary. Offering primary prevention, including developmental education, parenting support, and psychoeducation about the deployment life cycle, can be beneficial for most couples regardless of a child's age or adjustment. In addition, during reintegration, most parenting couples can benefit from discussions focused on balancing and readjusting parenting and couple roles and demands. For those couples with a child exhibiting worrisome affect or behaviors, the provider can use the assessment as a time to suggest referring the child for his or her own treatment. At the same time, couples whose children are clearly in need of a referral for treatment will benefit from work that focuses on managing children's behaviors or special needs and understanding how family or couple dynamics contribute to children's difficulties. Couple work can also assist the parents in understanding how problems with the child are affecting the couple relationship. Family therapy may be the treatment of choice when the provider determines that the parents need to be more involved in a treatment process that focuses on the family as a whole as opposed to the parenting couple. If a parent's physical illness, disability, or mental health interferes with optimal parenting practices, the provider can choose to remain with the couple and shift the focus to address these needs more prominently or refer the couple to a family therapist who focuses specifically on parenting.

Case Illustration

Joe and Nora attended their first session with the therapist after Joe had been home for 5 months. In their first session, Joe explained that he was concerned that "someone might find out" if he attended therapy. As the therapist explained the policies related to confidentiality, Joe seemed to relax somewhat, although he still seemed anxious. The therapist then asked what prompted the appointment. Nora reported, "Even though I know Joe loves the kids and they love him, he really can't handle being around them at all. He just hides in his room and barks at all of us when we're home. I've reached the end of my rope with him and don't know what to do, so I asked him to stay at his mom's till he figures it out." Nora also expressed some disappointment that "things aren't going better between us," but was most concerned about Joe's relationships with the kids. As Nora spoke, Joe put his head down and slumped on the couch. He said that he felt badly about how he was with the kids but couldn't help himself. He was just so tired, and everything seemed so loud when they were around that he just wanted to be in his room.

   Over the next two sessions, the therapist explored Nora and Joe's life before military service, during deployment, and in the reintegration period. Both Nora and Joe agreed that they had "weathered" the first deployment "pretty well," but it had been more difficult to find time together since the birth of their youngest daughter. Nora also had "begged" Joe to leave the military when Natalie was born, but he felt he "had to go back." The therapist also asked both Nora and Joe about their individual family health and mental health histories and current concerns. Nora stated that she had never really had any problems until Joe left for his second deployment. When he received his papers, she was so angry and resentful that she "tried to ignore him." After he left, she "worried all the time but tried to put on a good face for the kids." As the therapist encouraged Joe to say more about his day-to-day life since he returned home, Joe slowly revealed the extent of his trauma symptoms and depression. Nora added her observations of Joe, including his avoidance of their children, his withdrawal from her, and his "intense" irritability. She also knew that he was not sleeping, because she often awoke to an empty bed or to Joe's nightmares. The couple therapist gently suggested that Joe might be suffering from PTSD, and that there were treatments available that could help him manage and get some relief from his symptoms.

Joe and Nora agreed that taking care of their kids had gone well until Joe's second deployment. As they built a family, Nora had worked part-time and, when not deployed, Joe was a supervisor for the State Department of Transportation. During the first deployment, Nora had adjusted to being on her own, taking care of her two children, and maintaining her part-time job. She and Joe had weekly communication by phone, and they tried to "keep it light." When Joe returned, they were able to find a rhythm and ease into new roles. This time, however, the deployment was "much more stressful" for everyone. Nora pointed out that the kids were older and "more difficult to manage." Nora's anxiety was also "much worse," because Joe's mission the second time was more dangerous. She tried not to show her worry in front of the kids, but the older ones "figured it out and started asking a lot of questions about Daddy." Joe explained that on his last deployment, he really couldn't think about what was happening at home, because he would "get caught up in it" and lose focus on the job. He tried to be supportive on the phone and during web-based videoconferences, but he felt like he was "going through the motions." Since coming home, he has felt like "an outsider" in his family. The couple therapist reflected that the family is adjusting not only to Joe's return but also to typical developmental shifts in the children that will require different and flexible approaches to parenting for each child.

The couple therapist assessed with Joe and Nora their perceptions and observations of each child's relationship with each parent. Joe and Nora reported that they had very much wanted to have all of their children and used to enjoy spending time together as a family. Since Joe's return, however, "family time" had been so uncomfortable that Johnny always "has other plans" and Sam makes excuses to be unavailable. The couple agreed that Natalie was having the most trouble with Joe's return because she was "a little afraid" of her father, and was "very attached" to Nora and her big brother, Johnny. Natalie cried whenever Nora left the house without her and wanted Nora to sleep in her bed, like she did when Joe was deployed. Nora was frustrated with Joe's short temper with the children and thought that his avoidance was "hurting their feelings and making things worse." Although Joe was aware of his lack of patience with the kids, he was surprised to hear Nora's perspective on how the kids were affected by his behavior.

Throughout the treatment, the therapist simultaneously worked to help Joe acknowledge and address his PTSD symptoms and the difficulties they were causing in his family relationships. With much encouragement, Joe finally agreed to an individual assessment for his symptoms and made the intake call himself. Nora expressed great relief that Joe was willing to get more help for his PTSD. As Joe became involved in his own treatment, the couple therapist focused on working with Joe and Nora to identify and manage Joe's triggers, beginning with those involving the kids and everyday household routines. With Nora's support at home and increased awareness on the part of the children, Joe was able to be more involved in the family and to participate actively in his marriage and his relationship with each child.

SUMMARY

The current demographics of the U.S. fighting forces clearly demonstrate that the family is a defining concern for millions of military-connected and veteran families. As such, the centrality of parenting, the parent–child relationship, and the impact of prolonged separation must be recognized and supported in any service model for military couples who are parents. Providers who work with military and veteran couples are uniquely situated not only to attend to a couple's interpersonal and intimate dynamics but also to the parenting arena and its far-reaching implications. A developmental–ecological conceptual framework can help the provider keep in mind the layers of relevant interacting domains for military couples with children. A primary focus is to support couples in identifying and balancing the needs of the partner relationship with parenting responsibilities and practices throughout the deployment cycle in order to bolster couple, parent–child, and family resilience. Because many couple intervention models are not tailored to parenting couples, the guidelines suggested in this chapter offer multiple pathways to support the central role of children in contemporary military and veteran families, and to honor the complex realities that accompany parenting during a time of war.

RESOURCES

American Psychological Association Presidential Task Force on Military Deployment Services for Youth, Families, and Service Members. (2007). *The psychological needs of U.S. military service members and their families: A preliminary report.* Washington, DC: American Psychological Association.
Barker, L., & Berry, K. (2009). Developmental issues impacting military families

with young children during single and multiple deployments. *Military Medicine, 174*, 1033–1040.

Barnes, V. A., Davis, H., & Treiber, F. A. (2007). Perceived stress, heart rate, and blood pressure among adolescents with family members deployed in Operation Iraqi Freedom. *Military Medicine, 172*, 40–43.

Chandra, A., Lara-Cinisomo, S., Jaycox, L. H., Tanielian, T., Burns, R., Ruder, T., et al. (2010). Children on the homefront: The experience of children from military families. *Pediatrics, 125*, 16–25.

Gibbs, D. A., Martin, S. L., Kupper, L. L., & Johnson, R. E. (2007). Child maltreatment in enlisted soldiers' families during combat-related deployments. *Journal of the American Medical Association, 298*, 528–535.

Huebner, A., Mancini, J., Wilcox, R., Grass, S., & Grass, G. (2007). Parental deployment and youth in military families: Exploring uncertainty and ambiguous loss. *Family Relations, 56*, 112–122.

Logan, K. V. (1987, February). The emotional cycle of deployment. *U.S. Naval Institute Proceedings Magazine, 113*, 43–47.

MacDermid, S. M. (2006). Multiple transitions of deployment and reunion for military families. Retrieved 11/1/2011 from *www.cfs.purdue.edu/mfri/deployreunion.ppt*.

National Military Family Association. (2005). *Report on the Cycles of Deployment Survey: An analysis of survey responses from April–September, 2005*. Alexandria, VA: Author.

Pincus, S. H., House, R., Christensen, J., & Adler, L. E. (2001). The emotional cycle of deployment: A military family perspective. *Journal of the Army Medical Department, 20*, 615–623.

Zeanah, C. H., & Benoit, D. (1995). Clinical applications of a parent perception interview in infant mental health. *Child and Adolescent Psychiatric Clinics of North America, 4*, 539–554.

What to Say and When to Say It:
Preparing Your Children for Deployment

Instructions: Use these handouts together to think about how and when to tell your children about an upcoming deployment and how to say good-bye at the point of departure. As difficult as this conversation can be, both emotionally and logistically, it is critical to consider carefully how to inform and support your children in preparation for a parental deployment.

General Guidelines: What Does Your Child or Adolescent Really Want and Need to Know?

Children of all ages need to know who will take care of them, that both parents love them, and that they will be protected and cared for throughout the deployment cycle.

- Young and school-age children need to hear these messages concretely and with physical reassurance, such as hugs. Follow a "less-is-more" principle; that is, provide the information your child requests and assess whether more detail is necessary.
- Older children and adolescents may hear best through honest discussion and reassurance that you are still there to support them even though they are older. Provide information at a more sophisticated level and provide support to enable them to handle more difficult realities. For example, an older child or adolescent will understand that deployment to a war zone can involve dangers and risks. However, you can reassure your child that you are very well trained and that your goal is to stay safe and come home.
- Be direct and honest, even with young children, but do not give unnecessary or frightening details.

Before Deployment

Consider the timing of telling your children about an upcoming deployment. Although you do not want to prolong anxiety, do make sure you leave time for your family to process the event. Here are some suggested activities:

- Make "protected" time to announce the news and to respond to your children's reactions.
- Spend special time with each of your children before you leave for deployment.
- Write letters to your children before you leave; make videos or audios and create rituals that can serve as comforts and reminders to your children of how much you love them.
- Tell your children where you are going and what you will be doing. Keep it simple.
- Reassure your children that you will take very good care of yourself and be as safe as possible while you are away. Remind them to do the same.
- Tell your children you will miss them very much, and that you will think about them every day.
- Tell your children you are not leaving because of anything that they did/thought/said, because you don't love them, or because you do not want to be home with them.
- Encourage your children to ask questions and stop explaining when your children appear satisfied with your answers and explanations.
- Explain how you will communicate with your children during deployment (e.g., e-mail, telephone, webcam).

Say Good-bye!

Be sure you say good-bye in person to each child when you leave! Support your child regardless of how he or she reacts (e.g., with tears, anger, sadness). For example, if your child cries, tell your child that you are sad too and that's okay. If your child is angry, sympathize with him or her and say, "I can understand why you are angry—but remember that I love you no matter what."

HANDOUT 5.2

Creating a Parenting Plan for Deployment

Instructions: Use this handout to create a parenting plan for the period of deployment. Although it is difficult to anticipate every *parenting* situation that may arise during deployment, it is important to consider how best to take care of your children while one parent is deployed. The goal of this exercise is to put some thought into what your children need, based on their ages, personalities, and developmental abilities, and how each of you can best be supported by the other throughout this time. Ask yourselves these questions:

What Will Your Children Need during the Deployment?

In the largest sense, your children need to know that you love them, that you are there to support them, and that your family is safe. You know your children best, so consider how each of your children may respond to the deployment, and how best to meet their individual needs over time.

- "How do my children communicate with me? Given their ages and abilities, what kinds of communication will be most useful or meaningful to my children?"
- "What can I do before I deploy to keep communication going while I am away?"
- "What do I need from my partner to parent successfully during deployment?"

If You Are the Nondeploying Partner, Ask Yourself:

- "What do I need to take care of myself?"
- "What will make me feel most supported and appreciated in my efforts to parent while my partner is deployed?"
- "What is my 'style' of parenting and how will I be most effective on my own?"
- "What are my emotional and concrete resources? For example, who can I talk to while my partner is away? Where can I turn for concrete help, such as household maintenance?"

If You Are the Deploying Partner, Ask Yourself:

- "Given my mission, what is a realistic plan for communicating with my family?
- "How might I be affected by knowing what is happening at home with my kids?"
- "Are there child-related issues that my partner should not tell me about because it will be too distracting or upsetting?"
- "Will I do better if I know exactly what's happening at home?"
- "What can I do to keep the lines of communication open with my kids?"
- "How can I balance mission and family responsibilities during deployment?"

What Is Realistic for Your Family?

It is important that you and your partner are realistic about the challenges of parenting during deployment, and the constraints on your ability to communicate with each other in satisfying and useful ways. Thoughtful and realistic planning before deployment and open communication with each other throughout deployment will facilitate your ability to problem-solve and support each other and your children.

When the Questions Get Harder:
Talking with Your Child about War

Instructions: Use this handout with your partner to discuss how you would like to handle your children's questions and need for information about what really happens when a parent is deployed. Even very young children can and do sense when the family environment is stressful or when a parent is upset. As children get older, they begin to understand the potential dangers and actions required in war and peacekeeping, which can result in requests for more information about parental military service, mission, and the purpose of conflicts. As they get older, kids learn about deployment on their own through the Internet, TV, and other media outlets, and their friends. With all of this in mind, it is important for you and your partner to think about how you want to tell your own family's story of military service.

Are You Ready for Your Children's Questions?

- "What do our kids understand about military service at this point?"
- "What do we want them to know about deployment, war, and peacekeeping?"
- "What questions have our children asked? How did we answer?"
- "What are our concerns in giving our children more information?"
- "Do we have a family story of military service? What is it?"
- "What do we do when our kids start asking harder questions?"

Kids Are on a "Need-to-Know Basis"

Kids will typically ask for just enough information to deal with their current concerns. If you give them too much information, it can be overwhelming and confusing, especially for younger children. Make sure you know what they are asking. Support them no matter what they ask or how they react.

Tell the Truth

Kids are smart. What you want to do is let them know that you respect their right and desire to understand what is happening in your family, while also helping them handle new and deeper knowledge about military service.

We know children do better when the message from parents is positive, truthful, and unified. Imagine the different school and social contexts of your children. What is likely to emerge in these environments regarding your military service and deployment? Consider both positive and negative messages about military service and how you want to address your children's developing views, even if they are not the same as yours. The following topics are common themes to consider and discuss with your children in an age-appropriate manner.

- Service, sense of purpose, duty, courage, pride, patriotism
- Work, education, training in military service
- Political perspectives, including positive views and opposition to war
- Your specific mission and what you are/were required to do; what you witnessed
- What your service means for your children, your lifestyle, and your family

CHAPTER 6

Infidelity and Other Relationship Betrayals

Douglas K. Snyder, Donald H. Baucom,
Kristina Coop Gordon, and Brian D. Doss

He had been on his second deployment to Iraq only a month when Master Sergeant Steve Endicott became alarmed by the absence of communication from his wife Julie. Their time together since his return from his first deployment had been strained. During his prior deployment, Julie had struggled to manage the home front and care for their 3-year-old son. After he returned, Steve had initially attributed the distance between them to the challenges of becoming reacquainted and accommodating changes in their roles. But the emotional and physical distance persisted, and their bickering seemed to increase both in frequency and intensity. They had talked some prior to this second deployment about how to stay better connected, but Julie had seemed unenthusiastic and noncommittal. Her responses to his e-mails were brief and sometimes separated by several days. When Steve learned that a buddy back home had seen Julie riding around town with another man, Steve panicked. How could he save his marriage? How could he hold onto Julie when he was 7,000 miles and an ocean away? He couldn't eat, he couldn't sleep, and he certainly couldn't focus on his mission while on patrol. Another buddy he'd deployed with suggested that Steve talk to their unit chaplain. Although not particularly religious, Steve knew he needed someone to talk with, and Chaplain McIntire seemed like a safe bet. It ended up being one of Steve's better decisions.

THE INCIDENCE AND IMPACT OF INFIDELITY

Sexual infidelity occurs with high frequency both within the general U.S. population and among treatment-seeking samples. Representative community surveys indicate a lifetime prevalence of sexual infidelity in the United States of approximately 20–25%, with rates higher among men than among women. Broadening infidelity to encompass emotional as well as sexual affairs approximately doubles these rates. Although the incidence of infidelity among couples in which one or both partners serve in the U.S. Armed Forces is unknown, anecdotal evidence suggests comparable or higher rates compared to civilian samples. A 1992 national survey of more than 3,000 respondents showed that current or former military service members were twice as likely as their civilian counterparts to have had an affair, although the timing of the affair and the influences of military service were not determined (London, Allen, & Wilmoth, 2011). Soldiers tend to enlist young and marry young; just 1% of the civilian population under 20 is married, compared with nearly 14% of military members in the same age group—and marriage at a young age is a strong predictor of subsequent infidelity. Moreover, in the past decade, these marriages have been tested by the longest and most recurrent deployments in the history of the volunteer military. Among combat-exposed troops, the high incidence of stress-related mental health problems evidenced 3–4 months after returning from deployment (estimated by the U.S. Army's Surgeon General at 30%) further strains couples' relationships and renders them more vulnerable to infidelity. Indeed, among military couples seeking marital therapy from U.S. Army family life chaplains, roughly 50–60% seek assistance with issues of infidelity—a rate strikingly higher than that for the percentage of civilian couples in marital therapy (approximately 15%) (Atkins, Eldridge, Baucom, & Christensen, 2005).

Adverse individual and relationship consequences of infidelity are well-documented (Allen, Atkins, Baucom, Snyder, Gordon, & Glass, 2005). For persons recently learning of a partner's affair, research documents a broad range of negative emotional and behavioral effects, including partner violence, depression, suicidal ideation, acute anxiety, and symptoms similar to posttraumatic stress disorder (PTSD). Among persons having participated in an affair, similar reactions of depression, suicidality, and acute anxiety are also common effects—particularly when disclosure or discovery of infidelity results in marital separation or threats of divorce. Consequences of infidelity for a couple's relationship are equally well-documented. Infidelity is among the most frequently cited causes of divorce; a recent survey of 8,637 community respondents found that having an affair nearly doubled the likelihood of divorce (from 21 to 40%) in that sample.

Couple therapists working in civilian settings describe infidelity as being among the most difficult problems to treat. Several factors render working with military and veteran couples struggling with issues of infidelity potentially even more challenging. First, because of the deployment cycle, interventions may be difficult to implement when an affair is first disclosed or discovered; organizing interventions with partners separated geographically requires coordinating professional as well as technological resources. Second, issues of confidentiality assume special importance for some individuals, because infidelity remains a punishable offense under Article 134 of the Uniform Code of Military Justice (UCMJ). Finally, comorbid emotional and behavioral difficulties have increased prevalence among personnel exposed to combat—particularly emotional expressiveness and regulation deficits accompanying PTSD and other stress-related disorders—and may contribute to relationship vulnerability to infidelity or complicate the recovery process.

In this chapter we present a conceptual model and describe specific interventions for military and veteran couples struggling with infidelity, building upon the *only* treatment designed specifically for couples confronting an extradyadic affair that has been empirically evaluated and supported as efficacious (Gordon, Baucom, & Snyder, 2004). We describe overall treatment strategies and specific therapeutic interventions, then outline an eight-session adaptation of this treatment that lends itself particularly well to active military couples for which the deployment cycle or other factors may constrain the length and format of couple-based interventions. We offer an illustrative case study exemplifying selected components of the treatment protocol, describe means of tailoring the intervention to complicating individual or relationship characteristics, and discuss ways in which further adaptations of this intervention may assist in addressing a range of relationship betrayals other than infidelity.

CONCEPTUAL AND EMPIRICAL UNDERPINNINGS

Our intervention for couples struggling with issues of infidelity builds upon strengths of two empirically supported treatments for couple distress—specifically, cognitive-behavioral couple therapy (CBCT) and insight-oriented couple therapy (IOCT). CBCT is a skills-based approach emphasizing communication skills (e.g., emotional expressiveness and problem solving) as well as behavior change skills (e.g., constructing independent or shared behavior change agreements), with additional emphasis on cognitive processes (e.g., relationship beliefs and standards, expectancies, and interpersonal attributions) that moderate the initiation, maintenance, or impact of these relationship skills (Epstein & Baucom, 2002). IOCT is a developmental approach emphasizing the identification, interpretation, and resolution of conflictual emotional processes in the couple's relationship related to enduring maladaptive interpersonal patterns established in previous relationships (Snyder & Mitchell, 2008). Although theoretically grounded primarily in these two approaches to couple therapy, the specific interventions comprising our treatment are fully congruent with a broad range of alternative theoretical approaches fostering change in couples' problem-solving interactions (e.g., solution-focused therapy) and emotional responsiveness (e.g., emotion-focused therapy).

In addition to integrating empirically supported components from cognitive-behavioral and insight-oriented couple treatments, the affair-specific intervention outlined here also builds upon the empirical literature regarding recovery from both interpersonal trauma and relationship injuries. Specifically, infidelity is viewed as a traumatic event in the relationship that dramatically disrupts partners' assumptions about themselves and their relationship, causing both emotional and behavioral upheaval related to perceived loss of control and unpredictability of their future. Among other individual symptoms, reactions to infidelity frequently include intrusive and persistent rumination about the affair, hypervigilance to relationship threats and the partner's interactions with others, vacillation of emotional numbing with affect dysregulation, physiological hyperarousal accompanied by disrupted sleep or appetite, difficulties in concentration, and a broad spectrum of symptoms similar to those exhibited in PTSD.

Consistent with conceptualization of infidelity as an interpersonal trauma, this affair-specific intervention for couples also draws on literature regarding recovery from interpersonal injury, including an emerging empirical literature on stages and processes of forgiveness. Similar to trauma-based approaches, across diverse conceptualizations of recovery from interpersonal injury, a crucial component involves developing a changed understanding of why the injury or betrayal occurred and reconstructing a new meaning for the event. Preliminary evidence concerning interventions aimed at promoting recovery from interpersonal injury— heretofore developed almost exclusively from an individual- rather than couple-based perspective—indicates that such interventions can facilitate a more balanced appraisal of the injuring person and event, decreased negative affect and behaviors toward the offender, and increased psychological and physical health (Gordon, Baucom, & Snyder, 2005).

We organize our treatment for affair couples into three stages:

- *Stage 1: Dealing with the initial impact.* Partners are taught specific skills for managing emotions, and decision-making skills for addressing relationship crises precipitated by the affair and disruption of individual and couple functioning.
- *Stage 2: Exploring context and finding meaning.* Interventions

guide partners in examining factors from within their relationship, outside their relationship, and themselves that increased their vulnerability to an affair.

- *Stage 3: Moving on.* Interventions help partners explore personal beliefs about forgiveness and examine how these relate to recovery from the affair. Concluding interventions target specific means for strengthening the couple's relationship and protecting it from future threats to fidelity.

Detailed guidelines for clinical assessment and intervention—along with extended case examples and representative dialogues between therapist and partners—have been provided in a published clinician's guide (Baucom, Snyder, & Gordon, 2009), which also describes how to integrate a self-help book designed for affair couples (Snyder, Baucom, & Gordon, 2007) into treatment as a supplemental resource.

Evidence of Treatment Efficacy

Preliminary evidence for the efficacy of this treatment approach in a replicated case study design has been presented elsewhere (Gordon et al., 2004). Consistent with anecdotal literature, the majority of injured partners entering this treatment initially showed significantly elevated levels of depression and symptoms consistent with PTSD. Concern with emotional regulation and struggles to understand their betrayal dominated. Relationship distress was severe; feelings of commitment, trust, and empathy were low. By termination, injured partners demonstrated gains in each of these areas. Most importantly, gains were greatest in those domains specifically targeted by this treatment, such as decreases in PTSD symptomatology, gains in empathy, and increased relationship commitment. Treatment effect sizes were moderate to large and generally approached average effect sizes for efficacious couple therapies not specifically targeting couples struggling as a result of an affair, a noteworthy finding given that therapists rate this problem as being among the most difficult to treat.

Participating partners in this study also entered treatment with moderately high levels of overall dissatisfaction with their marriage and showed reductions in distress levels following treatment. Moreover, when describing the impact of treatment, participating partners noted that the treatment was critical to exploring and eventually understanding their own affair behavior in a manner that reduced likely reoccurrence, tolerating their injured partners' initial negativity and reexperiencing of the affair, and collaborating with their partners in a process of examining factors contributing to the affair.

In a recent study, Snyder, Gasbarrini, Doss, and Scheider (2011) examined issues of transportability and dissemination of this treatment—specifically evaluating the extent to which U.S. Army chaplains receiving a brief, structured training protocol would show gains in (1) knowledge about marital infidelity and its impact, (2) basic understanding of the composition and content of the brief structured intervention for affair couples, and (3) their ability to use that training to make preliminary decisions about how to intervene with couples presenting with particular issues at various stages of treatment. Findings affirmed that chaplains receiving either a 1- or 2-day training incorporating a detailed treatment manual, didactic presentation, and video-recorded exemplars of clinical interventions not only learned the information but also could apply it appropriately in analogue clinical situations.

Further evaluation of this treatment awaits a randomized clinical trial involving the full-length protocol as well as abbreviated adaptations. Adaptations of this intervention to partners separated by deployment have only recently undergone qualitative evaluation adopting case study designs. However, findings to date provide encouraging support for both the efficacy and dissemination of this treatment to couples in military and veteran settings.

GUIDELINES FOR ASSESSMENT AND INTERVENTION

Stage 1: Addressing the Impact of an Affair

Treatment Challenges and Strategies

Couples entering treatment following recent disclosure or discovery of an affair often exhibit intense negative emotions and pervasive disruption of both individual and relationship functioning that challenge even experienced couple therapists. One or both partners may report inability to complete the most basic daily tasks of caring for themselves or their children and may be unable to function effectively outside the home. Questions of whether to continue living together, how to deal with the outside affair person, whom to tell of the affair and what to disclose, how to attend to daily tasks of meals or child care, and/or how to contain negative exchanges and prevent emotional or physical aggression all need to be addressed early on to prevent additional damage to the partners or their relationship.

Effective intervention requires explicit, active interventions by the therapist to establish and maintain a therapeutic environment. Doing so requires establishing an atmosphere of safety and trust, and preparing the couple for therapy by providing a conceptual model for treatment. Increased safety and trust result from limiting partners' aggressive exchanges within sessions in an empathic but firm way. The therapist needs to provide a brief overview of the three-stage treatment model that conveys a clear vision of how recovery progresses and what is required of participants along the way. Presenting a trauma model facilitates partners' understanding of their own, and each other's, experiences. Allowing partners to describe how they have struggled thus far needs to be balanced by a structured process that limits domination by discussion of the affair details, intervenes in the crisis to help the couple determine how best to get through the coming weeks, and promotes a collaborative effort to understand more fully the context of what has happened in order to be able to reach more informed decisions down the road.

During Stage 1 it is important for therapists to avoid getting lost in the chaos of partners' own emotional turmoil; this requires slowing interactions, keeping discussions focused on the most urgent or immediate decisions, and containing negative exchanges during sessions. Therapists should refrain from either encouraging or supporting unrealistic commitments, which can set the couple up for further failure (e.g., never speaking again to an affair partner who works in the same office); they also should avoid trying to exert influence over persons not included in the sessions (e.g., the affair partner or extended family). Just as important as containing destructive negative exchanges is confronting some couples' "flight into health" as a way of avoiding distress in the short term; instead, the therapist should work to promote tolerance for examining the affair more intensively in order to promote more enduring resolution in the long term.

Therapeutic Components of Stage 1

Initial Assessment. The initial interview with a couple should elicit a brief history of the couple's relationship, including previous separations or treatment, information about any children and basic couple routines, and observation of the partners' communication patterns. Information about the outside relationship should also be obtained, including a brief history, the extent of any ongoing contact with the outside person, and knowledge of the affair by others. Partners' individual strengths and vulnerabilities should be assessed, including risks for self-harm and capacity for self-care. Additional outside stressors or support resources should be identified as these relate to interventions designed to contain initial emotional or behavioral turmoil. After completing an initial assessment, the couple should be provided an explanation of the stages of the recovery process and the trauma response conceptualization described earlier.

Boundary Setting. When a couple feels out of control and in crisis, providing healthy boundaries can help to create some sense of normality and predictability. Couples reeling from an affair often need immediate assistance in setting limits on their negative interactions. For some couples, this involves making agreements about when, how often, and what aspects of the affair they will discuss. The guidelines offered in Handout 6.1 (*Talking about the Affair*, at the end of this chapter) can assist partners in discerning which issues to pursue. For other couples, problem-solving strategies may be directed toward temporary solutions designed primarily for "damage control." For example, if a common cause of arguments is a wife's anxiety regarding her husband's whereabouts, then her husband may agree to be zealous in checking in with her until some trust or security has been reestablished.

In order for the injured partner to feel safe enough to engage in the therapeutic process, it is important for his or her partner to set strong boundaries on interactions with the outside third party. This is most easily achieved if the partner participating in the affair agrees to end the relationship with the third person, with no further contact. However, some partners are unwilling to terminate all interaction with the outside person when the affair is discovered; sometimes logistics make it impractical to have no interactions, at least immediately (e.g., when the partner and outside person work together); and at times, the outside person continues to contact the participating partner, despite being told not to do so. Because rebuilding trust is a crucial part of the therapeutic process, the therapist encourages the participating partner to be honest in stating what boundaries he or she is willing to set with the outside person at present, and how that will be carried out, along with agreements for how the injured partner will be informed of contact with the outside person. However, it is crucial that the couple eventually together set limits on interactions with the outside person, particularly if the outsider insists on intruding into their relationship.

Self-Care Guidelines. Another major target of Stage 1 involves helping both partners to take better care of themselves in order to have more emotional resources as they work through the aftermath of the affair. We offer partners basic self-care guidelines that encompass three areas: (1) physical care that includes aspects such as eating and sleeping well, decreasing caffeine, and exercising; (2) social support, with careful attention to what is appropriate to disclose to others and what is not; and (3) spiritual support, such as meditation, prayer, and talking with spiritual counselors, if doing so is consistent with the partner's belief system.

Time-Out and Venting Techniques. In light of the intense negative interactions between the partners at this stage in the process, most couples need strategies that allow them to disengage when the level of emotion becomes too high. "Time-out" strategies are introduced, and partners are instructed on how to recognize when a time-out needs to be called and how to do so effectively. Partners are also instructed in how to use the time-outs constructively—for example, to "vent" their tension through nonaggressive physical exercise, or to calm themselves through relaxation strategies.

Discussing the Impact of the Affair. A common need for an injured partner is to express to the participating partner how she or he has been hurt or angered by the affair. Often these interactions between the partners are rancorous and complicated by feelings of guilt on the part of the participating partner or bitterness about earlier hurts or betrayal in their relationship. We teach couples to use appropriate emotional expressiveness skills for both speaker and listener to help the injured person communicate feelings more effectively and the participating partner to demonstrate more effectively that she or he is listening. We may also facilitate the process of coming to an understanding of the affair's impact by encouraging the injured partner to write a letter exploring his or her feelings and reactions to the affair, then encouraging the participating partner to reflect his or her understanding of the injured partner's experience in a way that demonstrates both empathy and remorse for the injured partner's emotional distress.

Coping with "Flashbacks." A final but critical component in Stage 1 is the explanation of "flashback" phenomena and the development of a plan for how to cope with them. For example, a husband may discover an unexplained number on a telephone bill, which may then remind him of the unexplained telephone calls during the affair and trigger a flood of affect related to his wife's affair. We provide a set of guidelines for addressing flashbacks (these and other guidelines are included in the self-help book for couples). Within these guidelines, couples are taught to differentiate between upsetting events that reflect current inappropriate behavior and events that trigger feelings, images, and memories from the past, and to problem-solve together on more effective ways to cope as a couple when these flashbacks occur.

Case Illustration: Initial Interventions during Deployment

By the time Steve told Chaplain McIntire about events back home involving his wife Julie, he had already spent several sleepless nights debating what to do next. When Julie failed to respond to his first few e-mails, Steve's messages became more desperate and angry, and he threatened to reroute his paychecks to a hidden account and then pursue divorce and custody of their son upon his return. He feared and prepared for the worst. In talking with his chaplain, it became clear that although Steve didn't want his marriage to end, he recognized that his and Julie's relationship had been under duress for the past several years. Chaplain McIntire helped Steve to craft a different e-mail to Julie, acknowledging the difficulties they'd been having but expressing a wish to work through them. Steve also invited Julie to clarify her situation and any involvement with someone else.

After Steve's initial visit, Chaplain McIntire e-mailed one of the chaplains stationed at Steve's home base back in the States and, without disclosing the partners' names, explored the possibility of coordinating an intervention with the couple. Chaplain Taylor had been trained in the same affair intervention protocol as Chaplain McIntire, and the two had common handouts and other resources upon which to draw. In his second visit with Steve, Chaplain McIntire shared the other chaplain's contact information and suggested that Steve invite Julie to approach Chaplain Taylor to consider options for "facilitated discussions" long-distance.

In the following days Steve and Julie exchanged several e-mails and phone interactions via Internet, affirming mutual interest in trying to hold their marriage together but making little progress on their own. Both finally agreed to a videoconference facilitated by the two chaplains at their respective locations to reach some initial decisions about immediate steps to contain the current crisis, if possible. In their first videoconference, Julie admitted pursuing interactions with a mutual friend, Alex, over the past several months, but denied that there had been any physical involvement. She described resentment about having been dislocated to a part of the country far removed from friends and family, as well as frustration with Steve's alternating aloofness and emotional outbursts following his return from his first deployment.

Julie expressed little interest in a long-term relationship with Alex and with encouragement from Chaplain Taylor eventually agreed to suspend any further interactions with him. Chaplain McIntire suggested that Steve had possibly been struggling with undiagnosed symptoms of PTSD following his first deployment, and Steve agreed to consult with mental health staff at his base overseas to explore whether interventions targeting this now or following his return in 3 months were appropriate. The couple agreed to specific times to talk by phone twice weekly, with an additional videoconference once per week coordinated by Chaplains McIntire and Taylor. Neither partner was willing to commit to a final decision about their marriage, but they agreed to defer such a decision pending couple counseling following Steve's return from this current deployment.

Stage 2: Examining Context

After addressing the initial impact of the affair in Stage 1, the second stage of treatment focuses on helping the couple explore and understand the context of the affair. This second stage typically comprises the heart of treatment and demands the greatest amount of time. Injured partners (and sometimes partners participating in the affair) cannot move forward until they have a more complete and thoughtful understanding of why the affair occurred. Partners' explanations for the affair help the couple decide whether they want to maintain their relationship, what needs to change, or whether they should move forward by ending their relationship.

Treatment Challenges and Strategies

Couples need a road map for recovering trust and intimacy. Injured partners, in particular, need ways to restore emotional security and reduce their fear of further betrayals. Both partners often crave mechanisms for restoring trust—injured partners for regaining it, and participating partners for instilling it. Following an affair, couples who fail to restore security remain chronically distant and emotionally aloof, craft a fragile working alliance marked by episodic intrusions of mistrust or resentment, or eventually end their relationship in despair.

The overarching goal of interventions in Stage 2 is to promote a shared comprehensive formulation of how the affair came about. For injured partners this formulation facilitates greater predictability regarding future fidelity, and a more balanced and realistic view of their partner (either a softening of anger or addressing enduring negative qualities). For participating partners an expanded explanatory framework promotes more accurate appraisals of responsibility for decisions culminating in the affair. A comprehensive and accurate understanding of factors contributing to the affair prepares both partners for necessary individual and relationship changes aimed at reducing these influences.

Several challenges can undermine interventions during Stage 2 if not handled well by the therapist. First, it is important to emphasize to partners that "reasons" for the affair do not comprise "excuses"; that is, participating partners are always held responsible for their choice to have the affair, while delineating the context within which they made that decision. Second, when exploring aspects of the injured partner that potentially contributed to the relationship becoming more vulnerable to an affair (e.g., deficits in emotional responsiveness, excessive negativity, prolonged absences, or significant emotional or behavioral problems), it is important to examine such factors without blaming the injured partner for the participating partner's response of engaging in an affair. Either partner may exhibit characteristics that render collaborative exploration of contributing factors more difficult (e.g., poor emotion regulation that makes such discussions too threatening to pursue; inability to process or conceptualize psychological or interpersonal phenomena; or persistent externalization of responsibility for one's own behaviors). In such cases, couple-based interventions throughout Stage 2 need to be integrated with individual interventions targeting partners' own characteristics detracting from the goals and therapeutic processes essential to this stage.

Therapeutic Components of Stage 2

Exploring Factors Potentially Contributing to the Affair. Allen et al. (2005) have articulated a comprehensive organizational framework for exploring a diverse range of factors potentially contributing to the context of an affair or influencing one or both partners' subsequent responses. The major domains of factors to explore in Stage 2 include (1) aspects of the relationship, such as difficulty communicating or finding time for each other; (2) external issues, such as job stress, financial difficulties, or conflicts with in-laws; (3) issues specific to the participating partner, such as his or her relationship beliefs or social development history; and (4) issues specific to the injured partner, such as his or her developmental history or relationship skills. In each domain, these factors are considered for their potential role as predisposing or precipitating influences leading up to the affair, factors impacting maintenance of the affair and eventual discovery or disclosure, and influences bearing on partners' subsequent responses or recovery. Common influences listed in Handout 6.2 (*Potential Contributing Factors to Vulnerability to an Affair*, at the end of this chapter) help to guide this exploration process.

These sessions exploring the context of the affair typically are conducted in two ways. Depending on the partners' level of skills and motivation to listen to and understand each other, these sessions can take the form of structured discussions between partners as they attempt to understand the many factors that potentially contributed to the affair. The therapist intervenes as necessary to highlight certain points, reinterpret distorted cognitions, or draw parallels or inferences from their developmental histories that the partners are not able to do themselves. However, if the couple's communication skills are weak, if either partner is acutely defensive, or if the partners are having difficulty understanding each other's positions, then the therapist may structure the sessions to be more similar to individual therapy sessions with one partner, while the other partner listens and occasionally is asked to summarize his or her understanding of what is being expressed. For example, the therapist might begin a session exploring relationship factors this way:

> "The last time we met we agreed that today we would look at factors in your own relationship that may have increased your risk for becoming involved with someone else. You've both mentioned previ-

ously that you were having more arguments before Steve redeployed, but I'm curious to understand this better. What were your disagreements about and, more importantly, what happened when you tried to resolve them? Was this a change from how your marriage had been before Steve's first deployment? I'm also interested in whether there were any changes in your emotional and physical closeness. Let's consider these one at a time. Julie, could you begin with your description of how you and Steve tried to manage your differences between his first and second deployment?"

Similar guided discussions would be used to explore other potential contributing factors.

The therapist also looks for patterns and similarities between what the partners have reported in their individual histories and the problems they are reporting in their own relationship. It is in this exploration that the treatment borrows most heavily from insight-oriented approaches. Understanding how past needs and wishes influence an individual's choices in the present is a critical element to understanding why the individual chose to have an affair, or how the injured partner has responded to this event. For example, a partner who was repeatedly rejected sexually in early adolescence and young adulthood, and consequently sees him- or herself as unlovable and undesirable, may be particularly vulnerable to choosing a sexual affair to resolve enduring feelings of rejection or abandonment. Directing both partners to explore these influences helps them to gain a deeper understanding of each other's vulnerabilities and may help promote a greater level of empathy and compassion between them.

Constructing a Shared Narrative. After examining potential contributing factors across diverse domains, the therapist's task is to help the couple integrate the disparate pieces of information they have gleaned into a coherent narrative explaining how the affair came about. Achieving a shared understanding of how the affair came about is central to partners' developing a new set of assumptions about themselves, each other, and their relationship. This goal can be accomplished in several ways. One way is for the therapist to explain to the couple that this is the next task and to ask each partner to prepare for the next session by trying to "pull it all together," including a focus on the relationship issues, outside issues impacting their relationship, and individual issues related to either the participating or injured partner that contributed to the context within which the affair occurred. The couple and therapist then discuss their fullest understanding at the next session.

Alternatively, each partner can be asked to write a letter for the next session (similar to the task described earlier in Stage 1), in which each person describes now in a fuller and softened manner what he or she understands to be these relevant factors. As a result of such issues arising from discussion of the affair, the therapist and the partners discuss what aspects of their relationship may need additional attention and how this can be accomplished in order to help them avoid future betrayals. In this respect, the therapy begins to move from a focus on the past to a focus on the present and future of the relationship.

Stage 3: Moving On

Even after a therapist helps a couple to contain the initial negative impact of an affair, then guides them through a systematic appraisal of potential contributing factors, either partner can remain mired in the past or be indecisive about the future. Injured partners' hurt, anger, or fear of future betrayals may persist or episodically resurface in intense or destructive ways. Partners may also struggle with unrelenting guilt, unresolved resentments toward their partner that originally contributed to the affair, lingering attachment to the outside affair partner, or ambivalence about remaining in the primary relationship.

Treatment Challenges and Strategies

Once therapeutic efforts in Stage 2 have been completed or approach a point of diminished new information, the therapist needs to help partners move on emotionally—either together or apart. When therapists or couples talk about "moving on," "forgiving," or "letting go" they often mean different things—both in terms of what it would look like at the end and what it would take to get there. When helping couples to recover from infidelity we define "moving on" as comprising four key elements: (1) Each partner regains a balanced view of the other person and their relationship; (2) the partners commit to not letting their hurt or anger rule their thoughts and behavior toward the partner or dominate their lives; (3) each voluntarily gives up the right to continue punishing the partner for his or her actions or demanding further restitution; and (4) they decide whether to continue in the relationship based on a realistic assessment of both its positive and negative qualities.

Treatment strategies in Stage 3 emphasize helping partners examine their personal beliefs about forgiveness and how these relate to their efforts to move on from the affair. Additional strategies encourage integration of everything partners have learned about themselves and their relationship— well beyond the affair—to reach an informed decision about whether to continue in their relationship or move on separately. The guidelines offered in Handout 6.3 (*Factors to Consider in Reaching a Decision about Your*

Relationship, at the end of this chapter) assist in this decision process. For couples deciding to move on together, interventions emphasize additional changes partners will need to undertake either individually or conjointly to strengthen their relationship and reduce any influences that potentially render it more vulnerable to another affair in the future. If one partner or the other reaches an informed decision to end the relationship, the partners are helped to implement that decision in order to move on separately in ways that are least hurtful to themselves and others they love—particularly their children.

It is important during Stage 3 that therapists strike a balance between respecting partners' personal values and challenging ways in which partners' beliefs may interfere with moving on in an emotionally healthy manner. Some couples risk remaining ambivalent about their marriage or primary relationship for years—draining themselves of the energy required to nurture and strengthen their relationship, while avoiding the challenges of pursuing healthier alternatives either alone or in a different relationship. Therapists need to help partners actively engage in a complex process to reach decisions that allow them to move forward.

Therapeutic Components of Stage 3

Discussion of Forgiveness. Basic aspects of forgiveness are discussed with the couple, including (1) common beliefs about forgiveness, (2) consequences of forgiving and not forgiving, and (3) addressing blocks to forgiving or "moving on." For example, partners may report difficulty with forgiveness out of beliefs that forgiving their partner is "weak" or is equivalent to declaring that what happened is acceptable or excusable. Or partners may equate forgiving with forgetting, or with rendering oneself vulnerable to being injured in a similar way in the future. Addressing such beliefs by exploring whether one may forgive yet also appropriately hold the partner responsible for his or her behaviors may result in the couple developing a new conceptualization of forgiveness that feels more possible to achieve.

Similarly, the therapist often must explore issues that prevent the couple from moving forward. One such issue may be that one spouse is still dominated by anger about his or her partner—for example, because of perceived power imbalances following the affair or failure to regain an adequate sense of safety in the relationship. In such cases, the anger may serve a protective function for the angry spouse. Alternatively, the anger may point to unresolved relationship struggles that were not explored or resolved in earlier stages. Sometimes difficulty in moving beyond anger toward forgiveness reflects lingering resentments from the affair not based on current dynamics in the relationship. In such cases, it may be helpful to use motivational interviewing techniques to help the angry partner examine the costs and benefits of continuing in this position versus actively working to put the anger and the event behind him or her.

Exploration of Factors Affecting the Decision to Continue the Relationship. In this final stage of treatment, partners are encouraged to use what they have learned about each other and their relationship to decide whether their relationship is a healthy one for them. To this end, partners are encouraged to ask themselves separately—and then discuss together within the sessions—a series of questions that the therapist designs to help them evaluate their relationship. These questions focus on whether each partner is willing and able to make individual changes needed to preserve the relationship and help it be rewarding; whether, as a couple, the partners can work together effectively as a unit for the family; and whether they are willing to make needed changes in interacting with the outside world (e.g., patterns at work, with other people) that might be related to the affair.

Sometimes couples recognize enduring individual or relationship issues that could potentially benefit from continued therapeutic work. Alternatively, one or both partners may conclude that critical factors contributing to the affair cannot be resolved and decide that the best decision is to end their relationship and move on separately. When, after careful consideration of all the relevant information, either partner concludes that continuing the relationship is not in his or her best interests, we work to help the partners dissolve the relationship in a manner that is least hurtful to the two of them and to others involved in their lives—including children, other family members, and friends.

FACTORS INFLUENCING TREATMENT

As challenging as affair couples can be to treat because of their initial emotional and behavioral turmoil, recovery from infidelity can be rendered even more difficult by factors extending beyond the affair itself. We distinguish among three general classes of such exacerbating dynamics—specifically, those factors characteristic of the couple's relationship, the individual partners, and aspects of the outside partner.

In both our clinical and empirical work, we have found that couples having protracted histories of frequent or intense relationship conflict typically require more extensive treatment to develop better conflict management and resolution skills and address specific sources of distress—particularly if such conflicts have a history of escalating to physical aggression. Severe and intractable patterns of intimate partner violence render conjoint therapy ill-advised because of potential risks of inadvertently enabling or provoking further aggressive exchanges. However, given high rates of low-level physical aggression among distressed couples generally—and increases in violence associated with infidelity specifically—the incidence of aggressive exchanges between previously nonaggressive partners following disclosure or discovery of an affair should not preclude the conjoint treatment strategies described here. Instead, it is important to assess any threats or occurrences of physical aggression at any level during the initial assessment interview, as well as at the outset of subsequent sessions, particularly if the couple has demonstrated risk for aggression previously. This can be done in the context of inquiring about any critical incidents since the previous session—including not only physical aggression but also contact with the outside person or other disruptive experiences. Any concerns about partner aggression should assume treatment priority with designing and monitoring explicit no-violence agreements and time-out procedures.

Both the clinical and empirical literature indicates that coexisting individual emotional or behavioral difficulties render couple therapy more difficult (Snyder & Whisman, 2003), and this applies as well to treating affair couples. Given the increased risk for depression, suicidality, substance misuse, acute anxiety, and heightened emotional reactivity that generally follows revelation of an affair, these responses will almost certainly be aggravated in partners already predisposed to such difficulties. For example, major depression may preclude sustained exploration of factors contributing to the affair during Stage 2 of this intervention. Or generalized anxiety may exacerbate the tendency to dwell on the affair betrayal and disrupt efforts to restore trust and predictability. We have found two comorbid conditions to be particularly problematic for sustained recovery from an affair. The first involves emotion regulation deficits in either partner involving marked affective instability (e.g., intense episodic dysphoria, irritability, or anxiety) and difficulties in regulating anger. With such partners, treatment needs to incorporate a substantial focus on individual strategies for self-regulation (e.g., promoting self-care and more adaptive strategies for managing intense feelings, and expanding appropriate social support).

The second individual disorder suggesting a poorer prognosis involves the features of "antisocial personality." By definition, such features include deceitfulness, impaired empathy for others, limited frustration tolerance, resistance to assuming responsibility for one's own actions, and failure to anticipate the consequences of various behaviors. Oftentimes, such persons demonstrate a recurring history of poor relationship decisions with intimate partners, friends, or coworkers. Uncovering such patterns during Stage 2 of treatment should lead to focused questions during Stage 3 when reaching a decision about how to move forward. Specifically, injured partners should be encouraged to consider questions such as

"Was your partner's affair an isolated event or, instead, part of a long
    series of betrayals?"
"Has your partner demonstrated the ability to make difficult changes
    in the past?"
"Has he or she addressed outside factors that increased vulnerability
    to an affair—for example, limiting time with others who under-
    mined your relationship?"

Frank consideration of such questions may lead the injured partner to an
informed decision to end the relationship with the participating partner
and to take constructive steps to move on separately.

Various characteristics of the outside person involved in the affair may
also complicate treatment. When the outside person is a coworker with
whom some degree of continued interaction is required, partners should
agree on constraints regarding those interactions (e.g., not engaging in personal discussions, minimizing interactions when others are not around,
and potentially considering reassignment of responsibilities to reduce or
eliminate need for continued exchanges). The relationship with the outside
person may be further complicated if that person is in a position of trust or
power (e.g., a supervisor or superior officer)—in which case other individuals may need to be informed of the situation in order to redress issues of
power inequity. Finally, treatment may be rendered more difficult when the
outside person persists in pursuing the participating partner. In such cases,
treatment involves designing clear messages to the outside person to define
and to impose barriers to further interactions, and potentially to consider
additional administrative or legal remedies to enforce boundaries.

TAILORING TREATMENT TO ACTIVE DUTY
OR VETERAN COUPLES

Adapting the Protocol to Abbreviated Interventions

There may be circumstances that require adapting the general treatment
strategies and specific components described earlier to a highly structured,
abbreviated protocol. Especially for military couples for whom consideration of the deployment cycle precludes treatment lasting several months
or longer, an abbreviated intervention protocol may be essential. Snyder
et al. (2011) articulated an eight-session intervention protocol for military
couples recovering from infidelity based on the full-length treatment previously demonstrated to be efficacious. This abbreviated protocol, outlined
in Table 6.1, is designed to be administered in 12 hours, with Sessions 1–3
and 7 lasting 2 hours each. An intervention procedures manual outlines the
basic tasks of each session, along with handouts and reference to the self-

TABLE 6.1. Structure of an Eight-Session Abbreviated Affair-Specific Intervention

- Stage 1: Dealing with the Initial Impact
  - Session 1: Understanding What's Happened and Preventing Further Damage
  - Session 2: Reaching Good Decisions to Manage the Crisis and Contain Its Impact
  - Session 3: Dealing with Painful Feelings and Engaging in Self-Care
- Stage 2: Exploring Context and Finding Meaning
  - Session 4: Factors in and around Your Relationship That Contributed to the Affair
  - Session 5: Characteristics of Partners that Contributed to Vulnerability
  - Session 6: Putting the Pieces Together—Developing a Shared Formulation
- Stage 3: Moving On
  - Session 7: Understanding Forgiveness—Exploring Personal Perspectives
  - Session 8: Reaching and Implementing an Informed Decision about How to Move On

Note. Listed "sessions" may be conceptualized as therapeutic tasks to be accomplished in one or more actual sessions, or in extended sessions lasting 90–120 minutes.

help resource guide developed for affair couples. Preliminary implementation and evaluation of this abbreviated protocol suggest that master's-level providers can be trained to administer the intervention with modest levels of ongoing supervision or consultation, and that providers with less experience in couple counseling (e.g., unit-level military chaplains) can be trained to implement crisis containment interventions comprising Stage 1 of the protocol.

Tailoring Treatment to Separated or Deployed Couples

Rebuilding trust and intimacy following an affair generally requires effort from both partners, but sometimes one partner or the other is either unable or unwilling to participate. Even when both are able, one partner may decline—leaving the other to work at recovery unilaterally. Individual partners (typically the injured partner) can still benefit from working through the three stages of recovery outlined here. For example, learning how to withdraw from destructive escalating conflicts and to engage in self-care, learning what to disclose to others, identifying contributing risk factors for infidelity, and reaching an informed decision about how to move on are all tasks that individuals can pursue on their own. We assist individuals engaged unilaterally in recovery with ways of approaching their partner and sharing their insights, encouraging participation in a softened manner, and we frequently observe reluctant partners eventually joining in the recovery process along the way.

Sometimes, as with the earlier case of Steve and Julie, deployment or other factors initially preclude conjoint sessions. However, both technological advances (e.g., videoconferencing) and coordination of interventions (e.g., by two separate counselors adopting the same basic protocol) can facilitate couple-based interventions enhancing recovery. For example, the self-help resource book for affair couples guides partners through specific exercises aimed at promoting understanding of individual and relationship processes impacted by an affair and specific steps essential to restoring a healthy relationship. Partners separated geographically can be provided with readings that target a given stage of recovery, handouts that summarize key points, and exercises for partners to complete separately or to share and work through together. Both partners and therapists separated geographically can more readily coordinate interventions and recovery efforts by drawing upon these common resources.

Managing Issues Related to Confidentiality

Managing issues of confidentiality in couple therapy can be difficult under any circumstances, but they become increasingly complex when related to infidelity (cf. Snyder & Doss, 2005). Ongoing infidelities known by the therapist but not disclosed to the nonparticipating partner undermine a clinician's ability to conduct couple therapy. A common stance is to inform participants in the initial session that anything revealed outside of conjoint sessions becomes a part of the couple therapy and, *at the discretion of the therapist*, may be disclosed in subsequent sessions involving both partners. The qualifier regarding the therapist's discretion permits clinical judgments concerning the potential consequences for all participants of sharing or withholding specific information on either an interim or permanent basis.

Issues of confidentiality are further complicated for military couples because infidelity remains a punishable offense under Article 134 of the UCMJ. This general article of the UCMJ permits nonspecified "conduct of a nature to bring discredit upon the armed forces" to be subject to court-martial and "punished at the discretion of that court." Although not routinely pursued, military participants may still be at risk if their participation in an affair is deemed prejudicial to good order or discipline, or is "service discrediting"—with consideration given to marital status and military rank of the participating or injured partner, as well as the outside person, in addition to the affair's impact on the respective parties' ability to perform any relevant military responsibilities. Some providers within the military may *not* have the option of keeping the nature or basis of couple counseling separate from medical records available to command personnel, and any such limits to confidentiality should clearly be explained to partners at the outset of any individual or conjoint sessions.

Extension to Other Relationship Betrayals

Although sexual infidelity comprises one of the most salient examples of relationship betrayal, there are other ways in which partners' trust and emotional security can be violated with significant and enduring impact. Additional examples include (but are not restricted to) couples for whom (1) following a single episode of significant physical aggression, safety has been reliably restored but emotional injury persists; (2) one partner engages in substance abuse or relapses after rehabilitation and pledges of maintaining sobriety; or (3) one partner or the other engages in significant financial irresponsibility, bringing about enduring monetary hardship and mistrust. In each of these cases, interventions guided by the three stages outlined here (containing initial impact, examining contributing factors, and reaching an informed decision about how to move on) may complement additional interventions targeting the specific behaviors or disorder underlying the betrayal (e.g., physical aggression or substance abuse). For example, by integrating the concept of relationship trauma, partners may be better able to understand and manage reexperiencing of betrayal-related events as flashback-like phenomena. Similarly, adopting the contextual model underlying Stage 2 interventions may promote a more comprehensive, systemic understanding of contributing influences and efforts to reduce a broader range of risk factors.

Primary and Secondary Prevention:
Up-Armoring At-Risk Relationships

Surveys of soldiers returning from tours abroad confirm the adverse impact of extended deployments on military marriages. In a survey of more than 2,200 Operation Enduring Freedom (OEF) soldiers assessed during a 2-month period, about 6% of noncommissioned officers were planning separation or divorce at the beginning of their deployment, but by 15 months the percentage tripled to over 20%. Among enlisted ranks, the percentage planning separation or divorce also tripled over 15 months—from 10 to over 30%. Among soldiers deployed to Iraq, reports of marital problems increased during each year of annual surveys. Moreover, the most frequently cited cause of suicides among soldiers—reaching an all-time high in 2009—involved relationship problems, with suspected infidelity by spouses back home a leading concern.

Against this backdrop, what steps can be undertaken to strengthen at-risk relationships across the deployment cycle? Universal prevention programs typically include psychoeducational components highlighting general risk factors and interventions aimed at promoting basic communication skills and strategies for remaining connected during deployment.

However, such programs may have limited effectiveness for couples having elevated risk for infidelity, because their generality precludes individualizing components that target specific mechanisms underlying vulnerability factors and promoting resilience. Hence, predeployment assessment of relationship, as well as individual, functioning may identify those couples having moderate or higher distress, for whom more intensive support could mitigate adverse impacts of deployment. Such support might include structuring specific methods for communication during deployment, developing plans to address crises or deal with feelings of loneliness, cultivating support networks that value fidelity, and promoting a sense of shared commitment to the military lifestyle.

Case Illustration: Continued Interventions Following Deployment

Following Steve's return from his second deployment, he and Julie maintained a strained civility. Efforts at physical intimacy seemed awkward. Under persistent questioning from Steve, Julie confessed that she and Alex had engaged in various forms of sexual intimacy but had stopped short of intercourse. At that moment their marriage nearly collapsed. Steve debated whether to move out and prepare for divorce, but at the last instant called Chaplain Taylor instead, who agreed to meet with the couple later that afternoon.

Steve and Julie both described strained interactions but preferred not to separate. With Chaplain Taylor's assistance, they negotiated ways of creating separate space in their home to which either partner could retreat to regain control of his or her thoughts and feelings. Julie acknowledged Steve's lingering mistrust and agreed to provide more consistent information regarding her whereabouts when she and Steve were not together. Steve initially was reluctant to examine the impact of his own emotions on their interactions at home. However, when his alternating emotional reactivity and retreat became apparent in their counseling sessions, he agreed to address this with Chaplain Taylor and to seek further individual help if he couldn't bring this pattern under better control.

The chaplain helped the couple explore ways their marriage had become vulnerable. Steve and Julie had met during their senior year in high school. They began dating exclusively in the Fall, and the following Spring, Julie became pregnant. Although both extended families offered modest support for the couple's marriage early that Summer, Julie's parents remained embittered toward Steve and distant toward their daughter.

After Steve enlisted in the Army a few months following their marriage, the young couple struggled financially because Julie could find only sporadic part-time unskilled positions. Their baby also suffered from colic the first 6 months. Most of Steve's buddies in the service were single. Julie found it difficult to make new friends, and Steve's first deployment had been very difficult for her as a single-parent far removed from her family and friends from high school. Steve sensed Julie's unhappiness and was frequently frustrated by the limited fun they now had as a couple, his inability to resolve their financial struggles, and the decline in their emotional and physical intimacy. It seemed to him that, no matter what he did, Julie was never happy with him.

As Chaplain Taylor helped the partners to understand each other's experience, their bitterness diminished. They crafted realistic plans for spending more time together and developing healthier support systems—both separately and as a couple. Steve's intermittent emotional reactivity persisted, and each incident provoked Julie's extended retreat. Their counselor confronted this enduring pattern in one of their sessions.

COUNSELOR: I'm concerned about these flare-ups that continue and the effects they have on each of you.

JULIE: I'm just tired of it. I can never tell when some trigger's going to get Steve riled up. Maybe he can't help it, but I'm tired of feeling like the victim.

COUNSELOR: Steve, do you recognize the times when you're upset at home?

STEVE: Sometimes, not always. And sometimes she says I'm upset when I'm not.

JULIE: If you could only see and hear yourself . . .

COUNSELOR: When you do recognize that you're upset, what are the usual triggers?

STEVE: It could be anything. Sometimes it's Julie, sometimes it's something from work; other times it's something minor I can't even remember.

COUNSELOR: What happens?

STEVE: I just feel like a wave is washing over me, like I'm drowning or something, and I can't catch my breath.

COUNSELOR: Could you let Julie know those times? Could you tell her when you first start feeling that way, before your emotions take over, so the two of you could handle it differently?

STEVE: Like how?

COUNSELOR: Well, you could tell her when you are starting to feel really tense again—and whether you need to slow things down or take a break from the action until you feel more in control of your thoughts and feelings.

STEVE: Well, I'm not the *only* one who gets upset . . .

JULIE: No, Steve, you're not. I get worked up, too, and I'd be willing to do the same thing—to tell you if I start to feel like I'm losing it. But when you lose it, you get *so* worked up it frightens me. I used to be able to reassure you or talk you down, but not any more. So I just clam up or get away from you, and that seems to upset you even more.

STEVE: Because I don't know where you're going or whether you'll come back . . .

JULIE: I'm not leaving you, Steve. But you need to stop pushing me away—because that's how it feels. Listen, I know that you saw bad stuff over there, and I know you usually don't want to talk about it with me. And that's okay, although I'm also ready to listen if you want that. But mostly I just need you to know I'm on your side, I'm not the enemy, and I can give you hugs or I can give you space—whichever you need—when you start feeling that way.

COUNSELOR: Can you do that, Steve? Let Julie know what you're feeling and what you need?

STEVE: It's not always about what happened over there. Sometimes I start thinking about what was going on back here while I was gone.

JULIE: About me and Alex? That's over, Steve. I've been hoping you could see me trying hard to reassure you and show my commitment.

STEVE: I know, I see it. Sometimes I just still worry . . .

JULIE: Well, I'm willing to talk about that more, too, if that's what you want.

Over the ensuing weeks, both partners worked at handling their respective fears and stresses more effectively. However, when Steve worked late or was gone for several days during military exercises, he experienced a resurgence of anxiety and some resentment for what they'd been through the past year. Although he professed his trust of Julie, he found it difficult to manage his self-doubts and fears that she could again stray if their situation worsened as before. When Julie sensed Steve's distance or apprehensions, she feared they would never be able to recover.

Chaplain Taylor reassured the couple that trust is sometimes the last important quality to return after an affair. He helped Steve to consider evidence Julie had demonstrated regarding her commitment, and gains they had achieved in their mutual understanding and efforts to strengthen their marriage. He encouraged Steve to talk with Julie about his fears in softened ways that enabled her to respond with reassurances. They discussed ways of staying better connected when separated. Julie also came to accept some of Steve's feelings as natural consequences of all they had experienced in the last year and to trust that these could diminish with time, rather than viewing his anxieties as accusations of continued unfaithfulness. Both partners regained confidence in their marriage and after a few months, suspended their work with their counselor. A year later, both Steve and Julie felt stronger individually and as a couple, and better equipped as Steve prepared for his next deployment.

SUMMARY

Evidence abounds that stresses of the deployment cycle place military couples at increased risk for a broad range of relationship difficulties, including an affair by either the service member or civilian partner. Effective treatment requires an integrative approach that (1) recognizes the traumatic impact of an affair, (2) builds relationship skills essential to initial containment of trauma and effective decision making, (3) promotes partners' greater understanding of factors within and outside themselves that increased their vulnerability to an affair and influence their recovery, and (4) addresses emotional, cognitive, and behavioral processes essential to forgiveness and moving on—either together or separately. The integrative treatment approach described here is the first treatment designed specifically to assist couples' recovery from an affair to garner empirical evidence of its efficacy. Additional evidence is emerging in support of abbreviated adaptations of the intervention tailored to contextual constraints of the military environment and implementation by a broad range of service providers.

RESOURCES

Allen, E. S., Atkins, D. C., Baucom, D. H., Snyder, D. K., Gordon, K. C., & Glass, S. P. (2005). Intrapersonal, interpersonal, and contextual factors in engaging in and responding to extramarital involvement. *Clinical Psychology: Science and Practice, 12,* 101–130.

Atkins, D. C., Eldridge, K. A., Baucom, D. H., & Christensen, A. (2005). Infidelity and behavioral couple therapy: Optimism in the face of betrayal. *Journal of Consulting and Clinical Psychology, 73,* 144–150.

Baucom, D. H., Snyder, D. K., & Gordon, K. C. (2009). *Helping couples get past the affair: A clinician's guide.* New York: Guilford Press.

Epstein, N. B., & Baucom, D. H. (2002). *Enhanced cognitive-behavioral therapy for couples: A contextual approach.* Washington, DC: American Psychological Association.

Gordon, K. C., Baucom, D. H., & Snyder, D. K. (2004). An integrative intervention for promoting recovery from extramarital affairs. *Journal of Marital and Family Therapy, 30,* 213–231.

Gordon, K. C., Baucom, D. H., & Snyder, D. K. (2005). Forgiveness in couples: Divorce, affairs, and couples therapy. In E. Worthington (Ed.), *Handbook of forgiveness* (pp. 407–421). New York: Routledge.

London, A. S., Allen, E., & Wilmoth, J. M. (2011, August). *Veteran status, marital infidelity, and divorce.* Paper presented at the meeting of the American Sociological Association, Las Vegas, NV.

Snyder, D. K., Baucom, D. H., & Gordon, K. C. (2007). *Getting past the affair: A program to help you cope, heal, and move on—together or apart.* New York: Guilford Press.

Snyder, D. K., & Doss, B. D. (2005). Treating infidelity: Clinical and ethical directions. *Journal of Clinical Psychology: In Session, 61,* 1453–1465.

Snyder, D. K., Gasbarrini, M. F., Doss, B. D., & Schneider, D. M. (2011). Intervening with military couples struggling with issues of infidelity. *Journal of Contemporary Psychotherapy, 41,* 201–208.

Snyder, D. K., & Mitchell, A. E. (2008). Affective reconstructive couple therapy: A pluralistic, developmental approach. In A. S. Gurman (Ed.), *Clinical handbook of couple therapy* (4th ed., pp. 353–382). New York: Guilford Press.

Snyder, D. K., & Whisman, M. A. (Eds.). (2003). *Treating difficult couples: Helping clients with coexisting mental and relationship disorders.* New York: Guilford Press.

Talking about the Affair

Instructions: Use this handout during initial discussions about the affair to focus on the most important information. It's usually better to have a series of brief discussions (20–30 minutes each) focusing on a specific issue than one long discussion that tries to cover too much. Save extended discussions about "Why did you do it?" for later. If your discussion becomes too heated to handle constructively, take a 30-minute break and try again, or come back the next day.

"What Happened?"

- "When did the affair begin? Is this person someone you've known for a while? When did it become sexual, if it was sexual?"
- "Is the other person married or in a committed relationship? Does that person's partner know?"
- "How much emotional involvement was there? What else did you do together?"
- "What kinds of contraception or protection against sexually transmitted disease (STD) were used? Did you sometimes not use protection?"
- "Has the affair ended? If the affair has ended, is this just for now or permanently? What steps, if any, have you taken to ensure that no further contact takes place?"
- "Who else knows about the affair? What do others know, and how did they find out?"
- "Are there any other consequences we need to consider? Could there be any complications at work or other legal problems?"

"Why Did You Do It?"

- "Why do you think this happened? What was going on with you? What else was going on in your life? What was going on between us?"
- "Why didn't you tell me? (Or why did you wait to tell me?)"

(continued)

"Where Does This Leave Us?"

- "What about us? Should we continue to live together? Do you know what you want?"
- "Have you considered divorce? What steps, if any, have you already taken?"
- "How do we deal with the basic tasks of managing the relationship and our household?"
- "How do we make sure that we talk about the things that need to be talked about?"
- "What acts of caring feel okay right now? What other expressions of intimacy do we want?"
- "How should we handle it when our discussions start to get out of control?"
- "What commitments, if any, do either of us feel prepared to make at this time? About how to work toward moving on? About our own relationships with our children?"

Potential Contributing Factors to Vulnerability to an Affair

Instructions: Use this handout when discussing various factors that potentially contributed to vulnerability to an affair. Some possible factors suggested below probably had more influence than others. It's unlikely that the affair resulted from only two to three factors. Use this handout to keep a "broad perspective" in considering factors you may have missed.

Aspects of Your Relationship

- Frequent arguing or unresolved conflicts
- Low levels of emotional closeness
- Too little time devoted to shared fun activities
- Low levels of physical intimacy
- Unmet relationship expectations
- Difficulty balancing both relationship and individual goals

Influences Outside Your Relationship

- High demands from work or family responsibilities
- Too much time devoted to activities or persons, excluding your partner
- Stress from illness, money concerns, extended family, or other sources
- Too much time spent with individuals who failed to support your relationship
- Too little time spent with individuals supporting your relationship
- Frequent exposure to situations providing opportunity for outside emotional or sexual involvement

Aspects of the Participating Partner

- Self-doubts and vulnerability to affirmation from an outsider
- High levels of attractiveness to outsiders
- Own behaviors that contributed to or maintained relationship difficulties

(continued)

- Beliefs about affairs emphasizing positive aspects and minimizing negative consequences
- Difficulties in honoring long-term commitments

Aspects of the Injured Partner

- Self-doubts interfering with emotional or physical intimacy
- Own behaviors that contributed to or maintained relationship difficulties
- Difficulties in coping with relationship disappointments or injuries

Factors to Consider in Reaching a Decision about Your Relationship

Instructions: Use this handout to help you think through your decision about how to move forward. Consider information you have about your partner, yourself, and your relationship. Consider information from the past as well as the present. You might want to make two lists of "positive" and "negative" factors— and weight each factor for how important it is to you (e.g., 3 for *very important*, 2 for *somewhat important*, and 1 for *least important*).

Evaluating Your Partner

- Is the participating partner's affair an isolated event or part of a long-term pattern of betrayals?
- Has the participating partner been able to make and continue difficult changes in the past?
- Has the participating partner made appropriate responses to the affair by:
  - Taking responsibility and expressing remorse for his or her actions?
  - Addressing aspects of his or her own that contributed to vulnerability to an affair?
  - Addressing outside factors contributing to risk of an affair?

Evaluating Your Relationship

- Have you and your partner been able to address important relationship factors that contributed to risk of an affair?
- Have you and your partner restored a positive relationship? If not, do you believe you will be able to do so in the future?

Evaluating Yourself (for the Injured Partner)

- Have you addressed any aspects of yourself or your behavior that might have contributed to a risky situation for you and your partner?
- Have you reached a decision to move on?

(continued)

- Are you able and willing to take gradual, appropriate risks in restoring trust in your partner and your relationship?

Additional Considerations

- Implications of your decision for others (e.g., your children)
- Personal or religious values

CHAPTER 7

Intimate Partner Violence

Richard E. Heyman, Casey T. Taft,
Jamie M. Howard, Alexandra Macdonald,
and Pamela S. Collins

Compared with the first session, Mark and Kathy appeared to feel more comfortable when they entered the group therapy room this week. Kathy casually mentioned to the therapist, "I wasn't sure what to expect, but I feel like this group gets me." The therapist validated how reassuring it can feel to be with others facing similar difficulties. At the start of group, Kathy volunteered to share her practice assignment with the other group members. She explained, "This assignment was a little tough because I feel like we have *so* much to work on. But we decided that our main goals for group are to communicate better and make decisions together more often." Mark further explained, "We're not good at talking to each other; it seems like we always end up getting mad and then leaving the house, so nothing ever gets resolved." Kathy added, "We were much better before he went to Iraq, but since he's gotten back and I lost my job, things have been so hard." The rest of the group nodded to indicate that they could relate to what Kathy and Mark were saying. The therapist thanked Kathy and Mark for sharing, and instilled hope by informing the group that they were going to learn skills in the group to get their relationships back on track.

"Intimate partner violence" (IPV) comprises physical, emotional, and sexual abuse within intimate relationships. Because acts of physical and emotional IPV are common in both civilian and military populations, and because about two-thirds of couples presenting for relationship therapy report such acts in the past year, anyone involved in couple-based interventions for military and veteran families should be informed about IPV.

This chapter (1) reviews the definitions, prevalences, causes, and consequences of the various forms of IPV; (2) describes the conceptual and empirical foundations for IPV interventions; (3) provides detailed guidelines for IPV assessment and intervention with military and veteran couples; and (4) provides case studies to illustrate IPV assessment and intervention strategies.

THE PREVALENCE AND IMPACT OF IPV

Definition of IPV

The military is at the vanguard of creating and testing IPV criteria that are usable by field sites with extremely high levels of reliability and validity. Briefly, "physical IPV" is defined as at least one nonaccidental act of physical force (e.g., push/shove, scratch, slap, throw something that could hurt, punch, bite) that causes (or exacerbates) at least one of the following significant impacts: (1) any physical injury; (2) significant fear; or (3) reasonable potential for significant physical injury. "Emotional IPV" is defined as nonaccidental verbal or symbolic acts that cause (or exacerbate) at least one of the following significant impacts: (1) significant fear; (2) significant psychological distress; (3) somatic symptoms that interfere with normal functioning; or (4) fear of recurrence of emotionally abusive act(s) that causes victim to significantly limit any of these five major life activities: (1) work; (2) education; (3) religion; (4) medical or mental health services; or (5) contact with family/friends. "Sexual IPV" is the only type that does not require an impact (i.e., substantial impact is inferred). It is defined as any of the following acts: (1) the use of physical force to compel participation in a sex act against the partner's will or when partner is incapable of consent (whether or not the act is completed) or (2) the use of a physical force or an emotionally abusive act to coerce the partner to participate in a sex act. These criteria have now been adopted in the U.S. Army, Navy, Air Force, and Marines. The full criteria are available at *http://dx.doi.org/10.1037/a0017011.supp.*

Prevalence of IPV

The Air Force conducted anonymous community surveys in 2006 and 2008 (with over 50,000 respondents each) that included self-reports matching the clinically significant physical and emotional IPV criteria (i.e., act plus impact or high potential for impact) discussed earlier. About 3% of the relationships of active duty members met criteria for clinically significant physical IPV (and an additional 22% reported nonimpactful physical IPV); surprisingly, female-to-male clinically significant physical IPV was more prevalent by a small but statistically significant margin. Between 6 and 8% of the relationships of active duty members had clinically significant emotional IPV; women were more likely to be victimized by a small but statistically significant margin. IPV rates in the Army are estimated to be about one-third higher than those in the Air Force.

Different Types of Aggressive Couples?

Over the past decade, IPV clinicians and researchers have been increasingly swayed by Johnson's (2008) hypothesis that IPV comprises two distinct populations that exhibit largely different behaviors for largely different motivations and have different risk factors. "Situational couple violence"—likely the most common type seen by couples therapists—is a typically less severe form committed by both men and women. Although these couples may have conflicts that occasionally escalate to IPV (and sometimes even clinically significant IPV, involving injury or fear), their IPV, in Johnson's framework, represents the outer bounds of an otherwise "typical" couple conflict escalation pattern.

Conjoint approaches to treating "situational violent" IPV have gained more acceptability with the increasing recognition that the "situationally violent" couples (1) report that communication problems are the most common precipitant of IPV (e.g., Babcock, Costa, Green, & Eckhardt, 2004); (2) tend to report relatively low-level IPV and only within their relationships; (3) have female and male partners who are equally aggressive and who both use physical IPV for reasons other than self-defense in the vast majority of incidents; (4) have behaviors, attitudes, and personality characteristics in *both* partners that are predictive of violence; and (5) do not fit the classic patriarchal, power and control-based "intimate terrorism" profile.

In contrast, Johnson (2008) hypothesized that IPV reported by those in shelters and court-mandated treatment settings is more likely to be "intimate terrorism," a severe form caused by men's need to exert power and control over women through fear and intimidation. Individuals in these relationships are most commonly seen in shelters, the legal system, by individual mental health practitioners, and by physicians. Although Johnson's theory has not been rigorously tested, there are some preliminary supporting data and the concept is clinically compelling.

Risk Factors for Intimate Partner Violence

Alcohol Abuse

Alcohol abuse is strongly associated with IPV. This is of special note for military members, who—partly due to the higher prevalence of young people—report higher frequency and quantity of drinking than the general population, with over 10% of Air Force active duty members reporting probable DSM-level alcohol abuse or dependence. These rates are higher in the Army and Marines. Among veterans, heavy drinking was slightly more prevalent (7.5%) than it was among comparable nonveterans (6.5%).

Posttraumatic Stress Disorder

Most work investigating PTSD and IPV has focused on victims, although a growing literature indicates that PTSD is a robust risk factor for the perpetration of IPV in military populations (see Taft, Watkins, Stafford, Street, & Monson, 2011). This research has further shown that it is the symptoms of increased physiological arousal that drive the association between PTSD and IPV. Information-processing-based models of general aggression and IPV following military trauma have been proposed to help explain such research findings, and clinical observations that traumatized returning military members tend to exhibit an exaggerated perception of threat and to misread social situations in an overly hostile and negative way.

Depression

Depressive symptoms have been associated with IPV in military and veteran samples (see Marshall, Panuzio, & Taft, 2005). Seminal theories of aggression emphasize the role of dysphoric affect in connection to anger-related feelings, thoughts, memories, and aggressive inclinations.

Considering that the aforementioned risk factors exhibit high levels of co-occurrence in addition to their direct effects on IPV, it is also important to consider the possibility that the presence of more than one risk factor poses particularly heightened risk. Some preliminary evidence suggests that comorbid difficulties increase risk in a multiplicative manner. For example, separate investigations indicate that PTSD interacts with depression and alcohol use problems to increase IPV risk (see Marshall et al., 2005). The presence of traumatic brain injury likely further disinhibits aggressive behavior among those who suffer from alcohol use problems, PTSD, or depression, and may already be at heightened risk for IPV.

Relationship Conflict

Relationship conflict is the strongest risk factor for IPV, especially among situationally violent couples. As noted earlier, communication problems are the primary proximal predictor of IPV, and the vast majority of couples presenting for general couples therapy report IPV when asked but do not list it as a presenting problem.

Schema Changes

When working with military couples, it is also important to consider the possible role of alterations in core schemas that may underlie trauma reactions and relationship difficulties. For example, problems with intimacy and trust may develop if military members were betrayed or let down by others in the war zone, or perhaps did not know whom to trust during their deployment. Low self-esteem may also be common, particularly if the military member or veteran experiences guilt over acts committed during a deployment. Difficulties related to power and control may also be evident, as service members may feel powerless during traumatic events and may be more likely to attempt to exhibit control over the environment after returning from deployment. All of these changes in core schemas may lead to more hostile and controlling behaviors, and more conflict in relationships, and thus may represent important intervention targets when working on issues related to IPV.

Consequences

IPV is associated with increased risk for physical injury and seeking medical attention, increased risk for current poor health and having a chronic disease that developed after the IPV started. Being physically assaulted (especially by more severe acts such as hitting) is associated with higher rates of depressive symptoms, PTSD, substance dependence, and fear. Studies among specifically military or veteran samples have shown IPV effects similar to those shown in civilian samples, with links between IPV and injury, health problems, and depression and anxiety-related difficulties (see Marshall et al., 2005).

Exposure to IPV also affects children in the household, three-fourths of whom are exposed to it directly (i.e., witnessing or hearing it). A meta-analysis of 118 studies found that on a host of outcomes (internalizing problems, externalizing problems, social problems, academic problems, negative affect/distress, negative cognitions), children exposed to IPV fared significantly worse than nonexposed children. Research in military samples also indicates that IPV is associated with higher child abuse potential; lower parenting satisfaction; and increased aggression, hostility, and behavioral problems among the children exposed to the IPV (see Marshall et al., 2005).

Military Context and IPV

There is a belief, common among IPV advocates and the popular press, that military service increases risk for IPV. Clinicians working with military and veteran families should be aware that there are no well-conducted studies that demonstrate such an increase in risk. The only study to (1) use comparable measures and (2) control for age and ethnic/racial composition (Heyman & Neidig, 1999) found that representative Army and civilian samples had equivalent rates of mild to moderate violence. However, soldiers had higher rates of male-to-female severe violence (e.g., 2.5% severe physical IPV reported by male soldiers vs. 0.7% reported by male civilians). It should be noted that the Army data were collected during relative peace in the early to mid-1990s; the aftermath of repeated deployments for Operation Enduring Freedom (OEF)/Operation Iraqi Freedom (OIF)/Operation New Dawn (OND) and changes to recruiting standards may produce different results if a similar study were conducted now.

The intense interest in military–civilian comparisons is often distracting and misplaced. First, because the military population is predominantly young and more ethnically/racially diverse than the general population (both risk factors for IPV), base rates in the military will likely always be higher. Second, because the military is predominantly male, male-to-female IPV will be predominately military member (or veteran)-to-civilian partner. Third, because the military recruits and accepts its members from the U.S. population, individuals bring the problems and risks found in varying degrees in the general population. Many young individuals from underprivileged, chaotic, or violent environments are attracted to the military to achieve a better life, yet are at higher risk for IPV. However, all military members are, by definition, employed, have completed high school (or a general equivalency degree [GED]); and are screened for drug use and psychological health, all of which lower the risk for IPV. Thus, it is impossible to infer from any existing research that military training and service increase risk for IPV; careful control of the myriad factors that may render the military population and the civilian population different would be necessary.

CONCEPTUAL AND EMPIRICAL UNDERPINNINGS

Treating IPV conjointly is often an appropriate match both for the interactional dynamics that put couples at risk for escalation to physical or emotional IPV and for how intact, distressed couples conceptualize their problems. Studies of intact couples presenting for relationship therapy indicate that physical IPV is underreported as a presenting problem because it is not considered by them to be as important, as frequent, or as negative as the communication problems, psychological IPV, or lack of love in the relationship. Therefore, separating dyads into individual, gender-specific treatment that focuses solely on IPV reduction would likely decrease motivation or compliance more than would conjoint treatment that focuses on the couple but prioritizes the reduction of IPV. Indeed, couples report that conjoint therapy allows them to see things from a new perspective, renew togetherness, and underscore teamwork in a way that individual treatment would be unlikely to accomplish.

An additional benefit of treating IPV conjointly is that if, as indicated earlier, the key determinants of situational IPV are tied to couples' interactions, having direct access to observing and modifying these determinants is advantageous for clinicians. For example, most incidents of IPV occur during an argument between partners in which conflict escalates until one or both partners strike the other (e.g., Babcock et al., 2004). Furthermore, destructive couple conflict and mutual verbal aggression have been found through observational studies to be strongly associated with physical IPV. In other words, the majority of IPV occurs within a particular context (i.e., problematic communication), not in the context of patriarchal "power and control," and approaching this problematic communication directly (as in most forms of couple treatment) is efficacious for both the couple's distress and for IPV.

Because each person's behavior is not only a response to the partner's behavior but also a stimulus for the partner's subsequent response (the systems theory concept known as "circular causality"), both partners frequently contribute to conflict escalation; thus, each can work to reduce escalation (and in turn the risk for IPV), although each individual is ultimately responsible for his or her own use of physical IPV. In fact, men's IPV is least likely when *both* partners adopt a nonviolent philosophy. Therefore, having the system within which the IPV takes place (i.e., the couple) in the therapy room allows this circular causality to reveal itself and allows multiple points of intervention. Furthermore, because each person's actions elicit certain thoughts, emotions, and behaviors in the partner, having both people present in conjoint sessions allows for such problematic cognitions and affect to be used therapeutically.

Another major advantage of treating IPV in conjoint therapy is the possibility of a shared, transparent treatment plan. Because partners often are already working at cross-purposes and have separate goals and strategies, their attempts at relationship change are typically ineffective and often misattributed as provocation. Thus, it is advantageous for both partners to be cognizant of what each is attempting to do to better the situation. Furthermore, because *both* individuals are encouraged in conjoint treatment to accept personal responsibility for their behavior, the therapist is less likely to be met with the persistent resistance and partner blaming that is typical in gender-specific treatment, in which the sole focus on the individual and the omission of discussion of the partner's responsibility can foster defensiveness.

One final benefit of conjoint treatment is that monitoring of IPV is more easily accomplished when both partners are asked to report it. In conjoint therapy, both partners are typically forthcoming about IPV that occurs, and any discrepant reports can be clarified and thoroughly examined. More accurate tracking of IPV allows for better assessment of progress, sharper conceptualizations, and more appropriate treatment adjustments.

However, conjoint treatment is contraindicated under certain circumstances, such as severe victimization (marked by significant injuries, fear, or assessment that IPV is used to intimidate or control) and extremely volatile and poorly controlled affect and behavior. Finally, substance abuse (including alcohol) by either partner is a contraindication for conjoint therapy to eliminate IPV; specialized therapy for the substance problem, followed by conjoint treatment, has showed promise as an efficacious approach to reducing not only substance use and relationship distress but also IPV.

In summary, randomized treatment efficacy trials clearly indicate that conjoint therapy is often suitable and even desirable for treating IPV. Furthermore, few women in intact relationships presenting for couple therapy are fearful of remaining with their partners or of participating in a treatment with them. Thus, research indicates that concerns about inappropriateness of conjoint treatment are unfounded for most intact couples presenting for relationship therapy and even for the majority of intact couples who are identified through formal reports of IPV. This is especially true among active duty military members, whose IPV tends to be of the mild, situational type. Furthermore, direct involvement of command in setting expectations for nonviolent relationships has been shown to decrease recidivism for both IPV and child maltreatment by 50%.

GUIDELINES FOR IPV ASSESSMENT AND INTERVENTION WITH MILITARY MEMBERS OR VETERANS

Emotional and physical IPV are ubiquitous but rarely are the problems for which couples present. Thus, thorough assessment of the couple and potential function of IPV is crucial, both for proper treatment and for determination of whether conjoint treatment is appropriate. Questionnaires provide an easy and efficient manner of obtaining information about relationship and individual variables of interest. As discussed in other chapters in this volume, a model brief assessment packet for couples with a military member/veteran would include—in addition to an IPV measure—questionnaires assessing relationship satisfaction, areas of desired change, steps toward divorce, alcohol and other substance use/abuse, PTSD symptoms, and depression symptoms.

Questionnaires can also be used to begin the assessment of IPV and offer certain advantages: they provide higher detection than interviews, provide behaviorally specific definitions of abuse, offer a common language for the clinician and client, can be completed outside of session (if doing so does not compromise victim safety), and make it easier to broach the topic for both clinician and clients. Although the Revised Conflict Tactics Scale (CTS2; Straus, Hamby, Boney-McCoy, & Sugarman, 1996) is the most widely used measure of IPV in relationships, it is long. Richard E. Heyman and colleagues have recently used the large Air Force community assessments (that included detailed IPV measures) to create short screeners with extremely high (over 90%, and typically above 95%) sensitivity and specificity. To screen for male-to-female physical IPV, four questions still result in excellent detection (pushing/slapping, grabbing, biting, and punching). To also screen for female-to-male violence, three acts should be added (slapping, scratching, and throwing objects that could hurt). To screen for emotional abuse, only one item is needed: "During the past 12 months, were you ever so stressed by things your partner did/said that it affected you almost every day for 2 weeks?"

Although the questionnaires are a good starting point for assessment, individual interviews provide richer clinical information. In separate sessions, individuals who screened positive for possible physical or emotional IPV should receive a detailed assessment. Structured clinical interview modules for physical, emotional, and sexual abuse are available (Foran, Beach, Slep, Heyman, & Wamboldt, in press). Furthermore, individuals should be asked to estimate the overall frequency of aggressive episodes in the past year and to discuss the most severe and several recent episodes of IPV in the past year. Individuals should be asked to describe these incidents from beginning to end, as if narrating a video, and should be asked to rate, on a scale of 1 to 10, how hard each act of force was. The clinician should ask for additional detail until he or she can visualize the incident as if watching a movie. Clients may try to resist reporting such in-depth descriptions of the incident, opting to minimize the severity with comments such as "We just started pushing and shoving" or "There was only some slapping and grabbing." However, when pressed to describe those incidents in detail, they frequently reveal more serious abuse than initially indicated.

In addition, individuals often describe the other's behavior as more severe than do their partners, who frequently minimize their own acts or impacts and try to portray themselves in a positive light. Obtaining both sides of the story increases the likelihood of an accurate (or at least plausible) account and allows the clinician to weigh credibility. Factors such as severity, chronicity, injury or potential for injury, need for medical attention, fear, police involvement, context, and the inferred function of the IPV should be directly assessed.

A key aim of the initial assessment is to determine whether a conjoint format is appropriate—that is, if the IPV is not extreme in frequency or severity, if neither partner has sustained injuries serious enough to merit medical care, if the aggressor(s) admits to and takes responsibility for the use of IPV and wants to stop, and if neither partner reports fear of participating in conjoint sessions or of increased IPV as a result of participating (Mitnick & Heyman, 2008). If conjoint treatment is indeed appropriate, the therapist might also have the couple discuss a problematic topic, to observe the strengths and weaknesses of communication patterns during conflict.

Table 7.1 contains risk factors identified in the research literature, tested in military samples, and used daily by Air Force assessors. When such risk factors are present, the clinician should discuss the dangerousness of the situation with the victim and make the victim aware of resources to increase safety should he or she choose to leave the partner. The clinician's discussions with high-risk IPV perpetrators should identify the risky behaviors (e.g., stalking, forced sex, injuring victim, threats to kill) and make referrals for gender-specific IPV group treatment (or at least individual treatment focused on IPV). It is not until the gender-specific IPV treatment is successfully complete, and IPV and coercive control tactics have stopped, that conjoint therapy should be reconsidered.

Finally, even if conjoint treatment appears appropriate based on these guidelines, the clinician should assess the speed and explosiveness of the couple's emotionally or physically aggressive situations. If physical or emotional IPV occurs in the context of high emotional liability, it may be difficult to ensure that conjoint sessions would be productive and safe. Individual sessions for the partners are desirable until there is demonstrable improvement in anger control.

COUPLE-BASED IPV INTERVENTIONS WITH MILITARY MEMBERS OR VETERANS

There are currently no empirically validated couple-based or gender-specific IPV interventions for civilian or military populations. Casey T. Taft and

TABLE 7.1. Risk Factors for IPV Perpetration and Victimization

Risk factors for repeated IPV perpetration	Risk factors for repeated IPV victimization	Relationship risk factors
1. Is, or has been, physically abusive toward a child	1. Fears for self or children or pets	1. Ongoing pattern of relationship discord
2. Used weapons in any relationship conflict	2. Was injured in alleged incident	2. Conflict over children
3. Strangled or attempted to strangle partner in any relationship conflict	3. Used weapons in any relationship conflict	3. Financial problems
4. Violence toward partner has escalated in frequency or intensity	4. Has access to firearms	
5. Forced or coerced sex in the past	5. Physically aggressive toward current partner	
6. History of harming or threatening to harm pets	6. Has current problem with substance use	
7. Current problem with substance use	7. Used substances during incident	
8. Caused severe injury that required medical attention in alleged incident	8. Overlooks or easily forgives IPV	
9. Expresses ideas or opinions that justify violence toward a partner	9. Believes that physical violence by partner/spouse is acceptable within the relationship	
10. Threatened harm to partner/spouse, especially a threat to kill partner/spouse	10. Has unrealistic perceptions of nature and severity of incident	
11. Problem with significant jealousy	11. Currently has anger/hostility toward partner	
12. Attempts to control partner/spouse's access to friends/family/resources	12. Exhibits current symptoms of depression	
13. Violation of order of protection	13. Does not have, or is unwilling to use, informal support system (family/friends)	
14. Has access to firearms	14. Is unwilling to use formal support system (hotlines, shelters, Commander, emergency room, police)	
15. Exhibits stalking behavior in this relationship	15. Reports significant dissatisfaction with military life style	
16. Recently separated from partner against his or her wishes	16. Witnessed/experienced violence as a child	
17. Physically aggressive toward a partner/spouse in the past		
18. Violent toward others in the past		
19. Witnessed/experienced violence as a child		
20. Emotionally abusive to partner		
21. Property destroyed in any relationship conflict		
22. Used substances during incident		
23. Caused minor injury that did not require medical attention in alleged incident		
24. Is uncooperative with assessment		
25. Threatened harm to self		
26. Currently feels options in relationship are exhausted		
27. Currently feels military career is over		
28. Exhibits current symptoms of depression		
29. Currently has anger/hostility toward partner		
30. Blames others for current incident		
31. Denies the incident occurred		
32. Demonstrates inability to see partner's point of view		
33. Reports significant stress		
34. Reports significant dissatisfaction with military lifestyle		
35. Unrealistic expectations of partner/spouse		
36. Has criminal history		
37. Unit/command is *not* supportive of initial safety plan, when advised IPV is occurring		
38. Expresses rigid beliefs in traditional sex roles		

Note. Data from U.S. Department of Defense Intimate Partner Violence Risk Assessment Working Group.

his colleagues, however, are in the process of evaluating the efficacy of a couple-based group intervention to prevent IPV (i.e., the couple has not engaged in recent IPV) in OEF/OIF/OND veterans who report relationship distress (Taft et al., 2010). This 10-week program, Strength at Home: Couples' Group, is funded via a cooperative agreement through the Centers for Disease Control and Prevention, and is currently being evaluated in a controlled clinical trial.

Although this program takes a prevention approach in avoiding IPV before it develops in veteran couples, the intervention strategies used are highly relevant for couples who may already be engaging in situational couple violence. Furthermore, although this intervention is currently being delivered in groups, which confers certain advantages (e.g., sense of shared experience and support from other couples, observational learning and positive role modeling among couples), it may also be delivered with individual couples. The program is cognitive-behavioral in nature and targets communication skills and social information-processing deficits that may be present in veterans with increased likelihood of having experienced trauma. The intervention includes components from empirically validated interventions for IPV and PTSD.

The initial phase (Sessions 1–3) of the Strength at Home: Couples' Group program focuses on psychoeducation about trauma, IPV, and other relationship problems. The second phase (Sessions 4 and 5) presents conflict management skills to help couples identify and effectively manage difficult issues when they arise. The third phase (Sessions 6–9) covers basic communication skills. The 10th and final session focuses on gains achieved over the course of the intervention and plans for continued change. Across all of the sessions, group members complete in-session practice exercises and are provided "practice assignments" to consolidate information learned in group. Assignments also involve intimacy-enhancing exercises (e.g., self-monitoring of positive relationship behaviors) across sessions. Following is a fuller description of each of the three primary phases of the intervention, and a discussion of process considerations in working with potentially violent couples.

Phase I: Psychoeducation

The initial group session provides the rationale and goals for the program, explains the importance of practice assignments, and begins a discussion of couples' treatment goals. Therapists also teach participants the skill of paraphrasing, which is the foundation of active listening and is a critical skill for managing conflict. In Session 2, couples continue to discuss treatment goals and their beliefs about healthy and unhealthy relationships. Therapists emphasize that IPV represents the extreme end of unhealthy relationships, and material is provided to educate couples about different forms of IPV (physical, psychological, sexual). There is particular emphasis on understanding psychological forms of IPV, because this type of IPV is often more subtle and can have devastating effects. Group discussions focus on behaviors that (1) make the partner afraid, (2) attack the partner's self-esteem, (3) limit the partner's basic rights and freedoms, and (4) punish the partner or make him or her feel insecure in the relationship. All partners are asked to sign a form indicating that they will remain nonabusive, because making such a public statement may serve to enhance motivation to refrain from IPV. Sessions 2 and 3 also discuss the link between trauma and relationship problems, and common themes related to trauma and deployments that can affect relationships (i.e., trust, intimacy, esteem, power, and control). The overarching clinical tasks of these early sessions are to enhance motivation, educate couples about IPV, and help couples gain insight into factors contributing to their relationship difficulties.

Phase II: Conflict Management

This phase of the intervention focuses on conflict management and assertive anger expression. Session 4 begins with review of a practice assignment in which partners interview each other about how they learned their current way of expressing anger and other emotions. Participants often indicate that when growing up, they were taught that "real men" do not talk about their feelings and should not discuss negative feelings. These are important areas for discussion, because in order to modify dysfunctional and coercive communication styles, couples must first understand how they initially developed them. This assignment leads to psychoeducational material describing the differences between passive, aggressive, and assertive expressions of anger. "Assertive" communication is presented as the goal for couples, and involves openly communicating thoughts and feelings as issues come up without "stuffing anger" or keeping in feelings (passive), or letting them out all at once in a hostile or violent manner (aggressive). Couples are provided "Conflict Analysis Sheets" to self-monitor their own passive, aggressive, and assertive responses to difficult situations. These sheets are used across these conflict management sessions.

In Session 5, couples are asked to generate and implement a detailed "Time-Out Plan" to use during potential conflict situations. The development of these plans is a vital crisis management tool that helps to ensure safety for the couple and provides a skill that helps to lay the groundwork for future work on communication. Several basic principles of time-outs are discussed. It is important to emphasize that the earlier a time-out is called, the better, and that time-outs should never be used to avoid one's partner. Rather, the basic principle behind a time-out is that the couple takes a "break in the action" to calm down before discussing an issue. Couples are then provided with a number of tips for what to do during time-outs, such as replacing negative thoughts with more positive thoughts, becoming aware of feelings other than anger, and using relaxation strategies. Next, therapists assist couples in developing individual, written time-out plans, including who has the right to call a time-out, how the couple signals a time-out, where each person will go and what he or she will do during a time-out, how long it will last, how the couple will signal the end of a time-out, and what the couple will do once the time-out has ended. Couples are then provided a written assignment to take their time-out plans home and practice them during a conflictual situation.

Phase III: Communication Skills

The final phase of the Strength at Home: Couples' Group program involves strengthening communication skills. Active listening skills are emphasized at the outset of this phase (Session 6), because they are the foundation of good communication and are critical for deescalating conflict. Listening skills are particularly important when significant trauma symptoms are present in one or both partners, because information-processing abilities are often compromised by emotional arousal. Specific skills covered during this session are paraphrasing, clarifying through questions, and validating. Key points therapists make during this discussion are that (1) active listening does not mean losing the argument or giving in to one's partner, and (2) listening is a difficult skill that takes practice.

Session 7 builds on the active listening skills material by assisting couples in learning how to give assertive messages. For example, partners are taught the importance of giving a clear and concise description of the behavior that they would like changed, describing their feelings about the behavior and its effects, and making suggestions or requests about what they would like their partners to do or how the problem might be resolved.

In Session 8, emotional expression skills are covered, because a variety of feelings are likely to underlie expressions of anger. Military members and veterans often have difficulties recognizing and expressing their emotions due to either symptoms of emotional numbing or the ways in which they have been socialized to express feelings. Psychoeducation about basic emotions (anger, sadness, fear, disgust, and happiness) and identifying one's feelings is provided. Also, specific tips are given about expressing emotions (e.g., using "I statements" to express feelings underlying anger) and listening to partners' expressions of emotions (e.g., remembering to listen, being nonjudgmental).

Session 9 covers a number of ineffective communication strategies or "traps" that people commonly fall into and also provides some examples of those traps. For example, military members and veterans may be particularly likely to engage in "mind reading," in which they assume they know what their partners are thinking and often assume that their partners have negative intentions. Such negative interpretations may be particularly likely among those who have experienced extended periods of danger, especially if traumatized and exhibiting symptoms of posttraumatic stress, consistent with the notion that they may have an exaggerated perception of threat and exhibit faulty social information processing.

Across each communication session, couples practice the skills covered in session and participate in role plays. Therapists and other group members provide constructive feedback. Furthermore, couples complete "Communication Analysis Sheets" between sessions to monitor their own positive and negative communication behaviors and to troubleshoot negative communication patterns and abusive behavior. "Daily Feelings Expression" forms are also given to partners to self-monitor and practice the expression of feelings other than anger to one another each day. Military members and veterans who have long focused on control of emotions may need assistance in reconnecting with the normality of experiencing a range of emotions regularly.

Relapse Prevention

The 10th and final session focuses on exploring gains made in the group, identifying goals and strategies for future change, and identifying barriers to change and strategies to overcome these barriers. The primary clinical tasks of the session are to help group members develop a realistic appraisal of changes made and to identify areas needing continued attention and strategies for continuing this work after the group ends.

Process Considerations and Tips for Therapists

In addition to delivering the intervention protocol, it is important that group leaders promote nonabusive relationship norms, model empathy and supportive listening, provide an optimistic perspective on the ability to change, encourage self-disclosure, and identify important couple and group dynamics that may hinder treatment progress. The following strategies for working with couple conflict are also important considerations.

At times during the sessions, participants may be critical or hostile toward their partners. It is important for therapists to intervene as soon as participants begin to engage in this type of behavior, and to be straightforward and clear about labeling abusive behavior. During such situations, it is often helpful to request that partners speak to one another in "the softest, kindest way possible." For example, the therapist may say the following:

"I'm going to stop you right there. Let's bring this to the group. What skill would help [names of partners] be more effective? How can they have a different conversation together?" It is often helpful to have couples paraphrase for one another to slow the process down and to provide practice in more effective communication strategies.

Throughout the intervention, therapists may need to remind participants that hostility, criticism, and abusive behavior (including psychological abuse) is destructive to relationships. Therapists should state this directly and be compassionate but firm. By allowing participants to criticize one another, therapists are tacitly condoning this behavior. When naming participants' destructive or psychologically abusive behavior, it is helpful to pair it with the opposite behavior (i.e., a positive or assertive response). For example, a therapist might say, "I'm wondering if there's another word you could use, because *stupid* is abusive. Let's rewind and try again."

It is also important that therapists do not encourage a dynamic in which partners take turns explaining their side to the therapist. Instead, the therapist may state: "I am not the judge here. This is something that you need to work out as a couple, and we're all here to help you do that."

For individual crises, therapists may make provisions to speak with individuals or couples for 20- to 30-minute sessions to deal with emergent issues (e.g., infidelity or suicidality) prior to or following group sessions. Regarding the escalation of IPV, couples are provided safety planning information and referral and hotline information for victims of IPV. Such disclosures are kept confidential from the perpetrator to enhance safety, and dangerous escalation of IPV may lead to the determination that a couple-based approach is no longer appropriate due to safety considerations. (See Handout 7.1, *Couple's Safety Plan*, at the end of this chapter.)

Case Illustration: Couple-Based IPV Treatment

Pretreatment Assessment

Mark and Kathy presented to the clinic because of relationship distress. They had been married for 6 years and did not have children. The couple reported frequent arguments and expressed frustration that these arguments typically involve yelling and door slamming. At the first session, Mark and Kathy's therapist asked them to complete some self-report questionnaires. Their responses to these questionnaires indicated high levels of relationship dissatisfaction and physical IPV in the relationship over the past 12 months. Additionally, Mark endorsed clinically significant symptoms of PTSD and subclinical alcohol dependence, and Kathy endorsed clinically significant symptoms of depression. Mark explained that he often ended up drinking more alcohol than he planned, and occasionally this cut into time he would spend exercising or going out with Kathy; however, Mark denied increased tolerance or withdrawal symptoms, and he did not meet full symptom criteria for alcohol dependence. Upon interviewing the couple, the therapist learned that Mark and Kathy were not typically violent with one another during arguments, but they had pushed each other during one particularly heated argument about 9 months ago. During this incident, Mark grabbed Kathy, which left a bruise on her arm, and Kathy threw a drinking glass toward Mark's head. At the therapist's request, the couple described this incident in detail. Mark rated the force of Kathy's violence as a 2 on a scale of 1 to 10 (with 10 = *severe physical IPV that warrants medical care*), whereas Kathy rated Mark's as a 4. Both denied feeling fearful in the relationship. Despite significant conflict and distress in the relationship, Mark and Kathy both expressed a desire to improve the relationship and appeared motivated for treatment. Considering all of this information together, the therapist determined that conjoint therapy was appropriate. Mark and Kathy were recommended for enrollment in a group intervention for military couples experiencing relationship distress and possible low-level IPV in the past.

Background Information

Mark was an Army Reservist who saw significant combat when he served as a gunner during his second of two deployments to Iraq in 2007. During one mission, Mark's vehicle drove over an improvised explosive device (IED); the driver was killed and Mark sustained some injuries, including a mild traumatic brain injury and facial lacerations. Since returning home, Mark displayed symptoms of PTSD, including nightmares, sleep disturbances, problems with attention, and increased irritability and anger. Mark reported occasionally coping by drinking alcohol, stating that some nights he needed to have a couple of drinks to get to sleep. Mark denied any prior mental health or alcohol problems or treatment. He was currently working full-time, with notable difficulty concentrating.

Kathy had a history of depression as a teenager that remitted following a course of psychotherapy. She had noticed a resurgence of symptoms over the past year, coinciding with Mark's return home. Current symptoms included loss of interest in activities she used to enjoy (e.g., yoga, jogging, concerts, going to parks), weight gain, sleep disturbance, significant fatigue, and low energy. Kathy had been working full-time while Mark was deployed, but her hours had recently been reduced at her retail job, which caused the couple financial strain.

Both expressed frustration and sadness at the state of their relationship. They reported few shared positive activities since Mark's return home, considerable difficulty communicating with one another, and thoughts of divorce. They stated that they had come for treatment as a last resort.

Psychoeducation

In Session 1, Mark and Kathy participated in group introductions. They appeared reassured to hear that other couples like themselves were struggling with similar issues. They practiced paraphrasing with one another in session; the group laughed about how easy it was, yet noted that they rarely did this with one another at home. Mark and Kathy generated ideas about what constitutes a healthy relationship: good communication, doing things together, making decisions, and supporting each other. They agreed to practice paraphrasing the upcoming week and to talk with one another about setting mutual treatment goals using the handout on healthy relationships given in the group.

During Session 2, group leaders reviewed the practice assignments. Several group members set goals to reduce verbal and physical IPV. Mark and Kathy set two main goals for their relationship: improving communication—as evidenced by more frequent conversations that did not involve yelling, door slamming, or aggression—and increasing their shared decision making. After this group discussion, Kathy reported "a strong connection" to the other group members, because "they understand the problems I'm having with Mark." Next, group leaders presented more detailed information about what constitutes abuse, including psychological abuse. Mark initially rejected the idea that controlling whom Kathy could talk with constituted abuse; he believed that he was protecting her from getting hurt by others. The group challenged Mark's thinking about this issue, and eventually he acknowledged that limiting a spouse's ability to make and keep friends may not be part of a healthy relationship, but he maintained that this was not abuse. Group leaders used Mark's belief that controlling Kathy's friends was protection as a springboard to discuss the handout on common reactions to trauma. The group discussed the ways in which traumatic experiences had affected their lives and relationships. For the practice assignment, group members were asked to write about the ways in which trauma had affected their relationship.

The group members reviewed this assignment together in Session 3 and discovered that many of the service members thought of the world as a dangerous place, and believed that they must scan their environment for danger at all times. Mark revealed that he often felt angry with Kathy because she was too flippant about her safety. Kathy explained that she felt as though she was "walking on eggshells," because she didn't know what would "set Mark off." She realized that she had been avoiding difficult conversations, such as the couple's finances, because she did not want to elicit anger and irritability in Mark. With the new insights gleaned from psychoeducational material about trauma, the couple acknowledged that respective hyperarousal and "shorter fuses" were leading to increased conflict. They also stated that they did not realize that they were angry until they were already shouting. Other group members shared similar experiences, and all stated that they felt "on edge" in their relationships a lot of the time. Group leaders identified beliefs related to safety and control, and the feelings of hyperarousal, as typical trauma responses. As the session progressed, leaders emphasized that however the beliefs developed or patterns of IPV were established, these were learned behaviors and the intervention was designed to help them learn alternative patterns of responding to anger. By the end of the session, Mark reported that this session was "eye-opening," because he could see how his attempts to control Kathy could be abusive, and how this might be related to the IED attack in which he felt so helpless.

Conflict Management

Session 4 began the conflict management stage of therapy with a review of the different styles of anger responses and how group members learned them. Mark and Kathy both admitted that they did not believe they could get their point across, or would not be taken seriously, without shouting or threatening to leave the relationship. Mark reported that he typically had a passive anger response, with occasional aggressive explosions; Kathy characterized herself as mainly assertive, with some periods of aggressive communication, and becoming passive when she "saw rage in Mark's eyes." Both Kathy and Mark reflected that their patterns of conflict and interpersonal aggression were displayed within their families of origin. Mark said that his use of IPV was "honed" during his military service. Their realization that the way one expresses anger is *learned*, instead of an innate trait, helped to increase their sense of efficacy to change their behavior. Group leaders introduced the Conflict Analysis Forms to help group members monitor their conflict styles and increase assertive expressions of anger. In Session 5, group leaders introduced time-outs as a tool to prevent conflict in situations in which one or both members of the couple struggle to remain assertive and nonabusive. Mark said he thought this was "juvenile," but agreed to try it.

Communication Skills Training
and Consolidation of Treatment Gains

In Session 6, both Mark and Kathy reported success with calling a time-out during the prior week. Kathy said they had trouble "timing in" and returning to the conversation after they called the time-out. Other group members helped them problem-solve ways to rejoin (e.g., one couple used a timer set to 30 minutes, so they at least checked in about whether they were ready to start talking again). As the therapy moved into the communication phase, active listening skills were reviewed, including additional practice paraphrasing, clarifying with questions, and validating. During Session 7, Mark and Kathy struggled to use these skills consistently when having difficult discussions. They believed that active listening, and especially validating, meant agreeing with their partner, "giving up control" of the conversation, and losing the argument. Other couples in the group who reported greater success with the skills agreed to role-play the active listening; the first role play represented a "typical" conversation, and the second demonstrated the active listening skills. Mark and Kathy commented that the second conversation was more productive than the first, which seemed more like an argument that the couple was trying to "win." The group leaders then encouraged the group to combine these active listening skills with the new skill of giving an assertive message to one's partner. When they returned in Session 8, Mark and Kathy reported two successful conversations during which both felt supported. They stated that, as with the earlier skills, it felt unnatural at first, but they could see how this would continue to improve their communication with one another.

During Session 8, the group members discussed their struggles in expressing emotions, and group leaders reviewed handouts on identifying and expressing feelings. In this session, Mark described how anger seemed to be the primary emotion that he felt and expressed. Group discussions focusing on the range of emotions one can feel resonated with him. Group leaders explained that people often find it easiest to express anger, even if other feelings underlie their anger. Although it is painful to reflect on feelings such as sadness, fear, and guilt, it is important not to avoid these emotions, because they can prolong distress and disconnection from one's partner. Through this discussion, Mark acknowledged that he felt sad and powerless much of the time, and Kathy indicated that she did not realize this. The couple returned to Session 9 without having completed their Daily Feelings Expression practice assignments, stating that they did not share any feelings with each other during the week. Group leaders facilitated an active listening task between Mark and Kathy to identify what got in the way: Kathy admitted that she was scared to share feelings with Mark, because he always just shut down or blew up when she tried, and Mark said that he assumed Kathy knew what he felt, so there was no need to say it. Group leaders used these as examples of common communication traps into which couples can fall. Both Mark and Kathy recognized their own typical traps (generalizing, mind reading), and agreed to schedule a time to share at least one emotion each day.

By the final session, Mark and Kathy had completed their Daily Feelings Expression sheet each day and reported that the assignment had increased their sense of closeness. Group members then shared what they learned during group and their goals for continued improvement after this final session. Mark and Kathy identified the active listening and assertive communication skills as two of their "favorite things about the group." The partners reported improvements in their relationship over the course of therapy; they stated that they were able to discuss difficult topics without "flying off the handle," and they enjoyed spending time together again. Both agreed that communication about emotions would be their biggest area for growth in the future, but they felt hopeful that they would continue to progress.

Posttreatment Assessment

Mark and Kathy were again administered the same self-report questionnaires they had completed prior to treatment. Both partners reported increased relationship satisfaction and no additional incidents of physical IPV. Additionally, Mark reported a reduction in his drinking, stating that he now rarely felt like he needed a drink to get to sleep, and he noticed he was concentrating somewhat better at work. Kathy reported that her depressive symptoms had decreased. She had began to enjoy more activities and felt less fatigue. Taken together, this information indicated that the treatment had been effective in reducing presenting complaints, including some symptoms that were not directly targeted in the treatment.

SUMMARY

Like comparable civilian couples, physical IPV occurs in at least 1 in 4 homes of military families, with clinically significant physical or emotional IPV occurring in at least 1 in 10 homes of military families. If couples with a military member or veteran are similar to civilian couples, the majority will present to couple treatment having experienced physical IPV in the last year, although very few will report it spontaneously as a presenting problem. Thus, knowledge of how to assess and treat this large group of couples is necessary.

In this chapter we have distinguished between acts of physical and emotional IPV and clinically significant IPV. Nearly all cases of relationship problems that fall short of clinically significant IPV (but with physical or emotional IPV) can be treated conjointly. We discussed one approach for couples with a military member or veteran, Strength at Home. (Other recent discussions of conjoint treatment for aggressive couples can be found in LaTaillade, Epstein, & Werlinich [2006] and Stith, McCollum, Rosen, Locke, & Goldberg [2005]—both groups have forthcoming, empirically guided books—and Mitnick & Heyman [2008]). We noted factors related to military service—emotional numbing, emotional and cognitive amplification of threat cues, PTSD, strain on relationships from repeated deployments, among many others—that may make treatment of such couples distinctive.

As they do with civilian couples, therapists should be cautious when military couples report clinically significant IPV. Conjoint approaches are clearly contraindicated when assessment reveals "intimate terrorism" (Johnson, 2008). Although partners with clinically significant IPV who are in the "situationally violent" group (i.e., do not use IPV as a power and control tactic) can sometimes be seen effectively conjointly, IPV should be the primary clinical focus. Treating such partners can sometimes be conjoint, but sometimes it is best accomplished via a mixture of individual and conjoint sessions. Such considerations are covered in LaTaillade et al. (2006), Mitnick and Heyman (2008), and Stith et al. (2005).

RESOURCES

Babcock, J. C., Costa, D. M., Green, C. E., & Eckhardt, C. I. (2004). What situations induce intimate partner violence?: A reliability and validity study of the Proximal Antecedents to Violent Episodes (PAVE) Scale. *Journal of Family Psychology, 18,* 433–442.

Foran, H. F., Beach, S. R. H., Slep, A. M. S., Heyman, R. E., & Wamboldt, M. Z. (Eds.). (in press). *Family problems and family violence: Reliable assessment and the ICD-11.* New York: Springer.

Heyman, R. E., & Neidig, P. H. (1999). A comparison of partner abuse rates in U. S. Army and civilian representative samples. *Journal of Consulting and Clinical Psychology, 67,* 239–242.

Johnson, M. P. (2008). *A typology of domestic violence: Intimate terrorism, violent resistance, and situational couple violence.* Boston: Northeastern University Press.

LaTaillade, J. J., Epstein, N. B., & Werlinich, C. A. (2006). A conjoint treatment of intimate partner violence: A cognitive behavioral approach. *Journal of Cognitive Psychotherapy, 20,* 393–410.

Marshall, A. D., Panuzio, J., & Taft, C. T. (2005). Intimate partner violence among military veterans and active duty servicemen. *Clinical Psychology Review, 25,* 862–876.

Mitnick, D., & Heyman, R. E. (2008). Couples approaches to treating intimate partner violence. In J. Keeling & T. Mason (Eds.), *Domestic violence: A multi-professional approach for healthcare practioners* (pp. 157–166). Berkshire, UK: Open University Press/McGraw-Hill.

Stith, S. M., McCollum, E. E., Rosen, K. H., Locke, L., & Goldberg, P. (2005).

Domestic violence focused couples treatment. In J. Lebow (Ed.), *Handbook of clinical family therapy* (pp. 406–430). New York: Wiley.

Straus, M. A., Hamby, S. L., Boney-McCoy, S., & Sugarman, D. B. (1996). The revised Conflict Tactics Scales (CTS2): Development and preliminary psychometric data. *Journal of Family Issues, 17,* 283–316.

Taft, C. T., Monson, C. M., Murphy, C. M., Howard, J. M., Resick, P. A., & Walling, S. M. (2010). *Strength at Home: Couples' Group.* Unpublished manual. Available by emailing Casey.Taft@va.gov.

Taft, C. T., Watkins, L. E., Stafford, J., Street, A. E., & Monson, C. M. (2011). Posttraumatic stress disorder and intimate relationship functioning: A meta-analysis. *Journal of Consulting and Clinical Psychology, 79,* 22–33.

Couple's Safety Plan

The goal of this safety plan is to prevent partner maltreatment during times of potential stress and conflict by establishing rules and agreements for mutually respectful behavior.

If a situation begins to escalate:
Male partner and female partner agree to avoid all unwanted touching or physical aggression.
Male partner and female partner understand how to use time-out procedures.

Describe the time-out plan: _____

_____

_____

_____

_____

Male partner and female partner were provided emergency phone numbers.

911 _____   _____

Male partner and female partner will agree on a safety plan for the children.
Teach children emergency numbers and how to use them.
Teach children to leave the conflict area.

_____

_____

Male partner and female partner agree not to stop each other or children from leaving or using the telephone.

If conflict continues to escalate, a partner will call an emergency number and/or leave the situation and go to a safe location.

Male partner agrees to the details of this safety plan   Yes   No

Female partner agrees to the details of this safety plan   Yes   No

(continued)

Client Name (Please Print): _____

Client Signature: _____ Date: _____

Client Name (Please Print): _____

Client Signature: _____ Date: _____

Provider Signature: _____ Date: _____

Provider Title: _____

Source: U.S. Air Force Family Advocacy Program.

CHAPTER 8

Posttraumatic Stress Disorder and Its Comorbidities

Candice M. Monson, Steffany J. Fredman,
and David S. Riggs

Amber, John's wife of 5 years, contacted their family physician's office approximately 5 months after John's return from his third deployment to Iraq. She had done this without his awareness, because she knew that John would be angry with her for contacting them, but Amber was extremely distressed. Things were becoming increasingly tense in their relationship, and they had had a big confrontation the day before. In an argument about money, John cleared the contents of the kitchen table with a swipe of his arm. Since returning from Iraq this most recent time, John had been acting very differently. He vacillated between anger and sullenness. He wasn't sleeping well, and when he did sleep, it was fitful. Several times he had accidently hit Amber during nightmares about his time in Iraq. She noticed that he seemed "spacey" and preoccupied on occasion; he was unreachable. John was terse with their two young children, often seeming annoyed with them. This was a real change for John, who had previously adored his children and was very hands-on with them. In addition, John had always been a casual drinker, but since his return, his drinking had become a daily occurrence and he was drinking up to a 12-pack of beer per day. One time she thought she smelled marijuana on his clothes, but he adamantly denied it and was so belligerent with her about her asking that she didn't want to broach the topic again. She didn't tell the nurse on the phone that they had made love only twice since his return, in the immediate days after coming home; he seemed uninterested, if not disgusted, by her affection. This was a change from their prior warm and easy relationship. Amber's family and friends had told her to be patient—the transition can take time. However, she knew that things were supposed to be better by now or at least headed in a better direction.

Amber and John are not alone in their experience of the intimate relationship problems associated with individual posttraumatic stress-related problems. An alarming number of service members, veterans, and their families are experiencing these and other relational difficulties associated with traumatic stress-related symptoms. In this chapter, we describe the time-limited and manualized intervention we have been implementing with these veterans and their loved ones that has led to improvements in both veterans' mental health and their partners' well-being, and enhanced relationship satisfaction. We describe the conceptualization of these issues in an interpersonal framework and illustrate the intervention with a case study. We also discuss considerations in the delivery of the intervention with these couples and other dyads.

INCIDENCE AND IMPACT OF POSTTRAUMATIC STRESS DISORDER AND ITS COMORBIDITIES

Compared with other mental health conditions, the specific precipitant of posttraumatic stress disorder (PTSD)—a traumatic stressor—is known. Those who have served in the military are particularly at risk for exposure to a traumatic stressor, and combat trauma exposure is associated with a high likelihood of PTSD diagnosis when compared with most other types of trauma exposure. In the wake of trauma exposure, it is common for many people to reexperience the event, to feel irritable or hypervigilant, to avoid reminders of it, and to feel emotionally numb. However, for most people, these symptoms abate through a process of natural recovery over a period of weeks or months. For a minority of traumatized individuals, that natural recovery process is impeded, and PTSD results. Other conditions frequently accompany the disorder, with depression, substance use disorders, and personality disorders being among the most common.

Research on the most recent cohort of North American combat forces indicates that a substantial number of them are experiencing clinical levels of postdeployment mental health problems. PTSD symptoms, problematic substance use, and depression are common and increasing in prevalence over time. One striking finding from a landmark U.S. study of soldiers and marines over time was that interpersonal difficulties were growing at a rate outpacing that of individual mental health problems (Milliken, Auchterlonie, & Hoge, 2007). In treatment-seeking samples, more than three-fourths of married/partnered veterans of Iraq and Afghanistan have reported difficulties with partners or children. PTSD and major depression were particularly associated with difficulties in family adjustment (Sayers, Farrow, Ross, & Oslin, 2009).

Research with combat veterans from prior eras and different countries further establishes the corrosive and likely recursive effects of PTSD and family relationship problems. Across studies, veterans diagnosed with PTSD and their romantic partners report more numerous and severe relationship difficulties, more parenting troubles, and generally poorer family adjustment, and they divorce at higher rates relative to trauma-exposed veterans without PTSD (see Galovski & Lyons, 2004, and Monson, Taft, & Fredman, 2009, for reviews). The avoidance/numbing symptoms of PTSD, in particular, are associated with intimate relationship dissatisfaction, impaired intimacy, and lower parenting satisfaction, and may be at least partly attributable to diminished self-disclosure in intimate relationships. The hyperarousal symptoms, especially dysregulated anger, have been implicated in intimate partner aggression and aggression more generally. This association appears to be strengthened by frequent use of large quantities of alcohol.

CONCEPTUAL AND EMPIRICAL UNDERPINNINGS

Elsewhere we more fully describe a theory underlying our therapy, cognitive-behavioral conjoint therapy for PTSD (CBCT for PTSD), which accounts for the association between intimate relationship problems and PTSD (Monson, Fredman, & Dekel, 2010). The theory holds that individual cognitive, behavioral, and affective mechanisms reciprocally interact within each individual, then between individuals mutually in the dyad to influence their individual and relationship functioning. Here we briefly discuss how the therapist in John and Amber's case conceptualized problems in John's posttrauma recovery and their associated relationship problems.

The therapist observed that John's learning at the time of the traumatic event had caused certain people, places, and things in his postdeployment life to provoke the fight-or-flight response that occurred at the time of his most distressing trauma. A suicide bomber had killed a soldier under John's command, whom John had sent on the operation. The sight of backpacks and the smell of petroleum and heat triggered his distress. To deal with this distress, John began avoiding these reminders by staying away from situations such as his children's day care and family barbecues, among other

things. Like other PTSD sufferers, his avoidance expanded beyond specific trauma-related reminders to include avoidance of emotions, a term
known as "experiential avoidance." Experiential avoidance can include
avoidance of not only negative emotions (e.g., fear, anger, and sadness)
but also positive emotions, which contributed to Amber and John's diminished emotional connection and intimacy. John's substance use served as an
additional way for him to avoid unwanted memories and feelings, which,
like other methods of avoidance (e.g., self-injury, aggression, overeating),
interfered with John learning new associations in his postdeployment life
and his successful trauma recovery.

At the dyadic level, Amber's well-intended caretaking behaviors, such
as running interference between John and extended family, taking over
more child care responsibilities, and not challenging John's substance use,
served to promote or maintain John's avoidant behavior. In this way, Amber
inadvertently colluded to "accommodate" or make space for the symptoms
of PTSD in John's life and their relationship. This accommodation of the
avoidance so characteristic of PTSD also diminished John and Amber's
intimate relationship satisfaction through decreased engagement in mutually enjoyable activities (e.g., going out to eat), restricted emotional expression, and diminished self-disclosure, including trauma-related disclosure.
The therapist also conceptualized that the couple's poor communication
and conflict management skills, in concert with this avoidance, decreased
effective trauma disclosure for John's recovery and the couple's relationship
enhancement.

The therapist also noticed that there were thoughts held by John and
Amber that might be maintaining John's posttraumatic stress-related
problems and their relationship struggles. The therapist ascertained in the
assessment of John's trauma history that the soldier under John's command
was killed in the course of what sounded like routine operations following the current rules of engagement. Yet, when describing this event, John
commented, "I should have prevented [his soldier's] death," attributing the
death to his own poor judgment. And, as a result, he concluded in his
current-day life, "I can't trust myself to make decisions in my own life or
my marriage because when I choose wrong, people die." Amber expressed
thoughts relevant to their recovery as well, including, "I just want things to
be back the way they were. I don't want us to do *anything* to further upset
John." Discussing the ways in which traumatized individuals and their
loved ones make sense of traumatic experiences, and addressing beliefs that
might get in the way of trauma recovery, allows for trauma processing and
resulting individual and relationship improvements.

Consistent with the theory that underlies CBCT for PTSD, the therapist was keen to the range of emotional disturbances beyond anxiety that
accompany traumatization, including John's guilt, shame, anger, grief, and

sadness. She conceptualized that John, in particular, was struggling with the identification and expression of these emotions, which is common in those who have PTSD. These challenges were contributing to diminished emotional communication and self-disclosure, and decrements in the couple's emotional and physical intimacy. Amber was reticent to express her positive or negative emotions, or to do anything that might cause John to experience his feelings.

Evidence of Treatment Efficacy

Our recent review of the literature on couple and family therapy for PTSD reveals only one published randomized controlled trial of couple or family therapy for PTSD with veterans (see Riggs, Monson, Glynn, & Canterino, 2009). In that study, researchers tested the addition of a more general behavioral family therapy (BFT) to individual evidence-based PTSD therapy (Glynn et al., 1999). Veterans who received trauma exposure therapy followed by BFT exhibited decreases in the positive symptoms of PTSD (e.g., reexperiencing and hyperarousal symptoms) that were roughly twice as large as those observed in the group that received individual exposure therapy alone. Veterans who completed BFT also showed more improvements in interpersonal problem solving than those who did not receive BFT.

CBCT for PTSD is a 15-session conjoint treatment that is disorder-specific, meaning that it is a conjoint therapy specifically designed to treat individual PTSD and its comorbid conditions, as well as relationship problems (Monson & Fredman, 2012). Monson, Schnurr, Guthrie, and Stevens (2004; Monson, Stevens, & Schnurr, 2005) published the results of an earlier version of the treatment with Vietnam veterans and their wives. From pre- to posttreatment, there were large and statistically significant improvements in clinicians' and partners' ratings of the veterans' PTSD symptoms. The veterans reported moderate improvements in PTSD and large statistically significant effect size improvements in their depression, anxiety, and social functioning. Wives also reported large effect size improvements in their relationship satisfaction, general anxiety, and social functioning.

The current treatment described here is more trauma-focused in nature, has a greater emphasis on decreasing couple-level avoidance, and externalizes the disorder to have a greater dyadic and systemic orientation. Results of the current version of the therapy, using a sample of both Iraq war combat veterans and nonveterans who were diverse with respect to their index traumatic event, sexual orientation, and sex of the identified patient, have revealed statistically significant and large effect size improvements in clinicians', patients', and partners' ratings of patients' PTSD symptoms from pre- to posttreatment. Partners also reported large effect size improvements in their relationship adjustment (Monson et al., 2011). A randomized controlled trial of the therapy with a community sample is in process, and another randomized controlled trial comparing CBCT for PTSD to prolonged exposure, a well-validated individual therapy for PTSD, in an active duty population has been funded by the U.S. Department of Defense.

GUIDELINES FOR ASSESSMENT AND INTERVENTION

CBCT for PTSD is organized into three phases. The phases of the therapy are represented by the acronym R.E.S.U.M.E. Living, which is consistent with our belief that all individuals with PTSD can experience a natural recovery from traumatization as the impediments of avoidance and problematic ways of thinking are removed (see Table 8.1):

1. *Rationale and Education (R.E.)*: psychoeducation about the reciprocal influences of PTSD symptoms and relationship adjustment, and instruction in conflict management skills.
2. *Satisfaction enhancement and Undermining avoidance (S.U.)*: behavioral interventions that improve dyadic communication and increase couple-level approach behavior.
3. *Meaning making and End of therapy (M.E.)*: cognitive interventions designed to address maladaptive ways of thinking that maintain both PTSD symptoms and relationship difficulties.

Psychoeducation and conflict management strategies are introduced first to provide a rationale for the conjoint approach, and to enhance the physical and emotional safety of both members of the couple prior to beginning the communication skills training and joint *in vivo* exposure exercises that characterize Phase 2. The behavioral interventions in Phase 2 precede the dyadic cognitive restructuring in Phase 3, so that couples can draw upon their improved communication skills and new tendency to approach rather than avoid when asked to do the trauma-focused work that forms the basis of the third phase of treatment.

The sessions of CBCT for PTSD are designed to be 75 minutes long and to conclude with out-of-session assignments designed to promote the couple's skills use in their everyday lives between sessions. In contrast to individually delivered exposure-based therapies for PTSD, in which patients are encouraged to review repeatedly events in detail until habituation of anxiety related to feared memories occurs, CBCT for PTSD is trauma-focused but not imaginal exposure-based. In other words, traumatic events are discussed in enough detail for those involved in CBCT for PTSD (patient, partner, and therapist) to have a shared sense of what occurred, so

TABLE 8.1. Overview of CBCT for PTSD

R.E.S.U.M.E. LIVING

Phase 1: Rationale for Treatment and Education about PTSD and Relationships
Session 1:   Introduction to Treatment
Session 2:   Safety Building

Phase 2: Satisfaction Enhancement and Undermining Avoidance
Session 3:   Listening and Approaching
Session 4:   Sharing Thoughts and Feelings—Emphasis on Feelings
Session 5:   Sharing Thoughts and Feelings—Emphasis on Thoughts
Session 6:   Getting U.N.S.T.U.C.K.
Session 7:   Problem Solving/Decision Making

Phase 3: Meaning Making of the Trauma(s) and End of Therapy
Session 8:   Acceptance
Session 9:   Blame
Session 10:   Trust
Session 11:   Control
Session 12:   Emotional Closeness
Session 13:   Physical Intimacy
Session 14:   Posttraumatic Growth
Session 15:   Review and Reinforcement of Treatment Gains

that problematic interpretations of the event(s) may be addressed. Explicit renditions of the events to include sights, sounds, smells, and so forth experienced at the time are discouraged. We have found that the strategy of discussing the trauma(s) as if from a "10,000-foot view" rather than in "nitty-gritty" detail facilitates new ways of thinking about the event and its consequences, but without patients and their partners becoming unduly emotionally distressed in response to disclosure of trauma-related material. Our experience is consistent with recent research on individual trauma-focused cognitive therapy for PTSD.

CBCT for PTSD is systemic in its conceptualization of posttraumatic stress and intimate relationship problems. At the outset, we tell couples that even though one or both partners have been diagnosed with PTSD, we consider their *relationship* to be the "patient" or "client" and, hence, focus simultaneously on improving both posttraumatic stress symptoms and their relationship problems. The language used in the treatment is designed to externalize the posttraumatic stress problems outside of the individual(s), so that it exists within their shared relationship and they can work on it together. To maintain the PTSD focus throughout treatment, communication skills practice is oriented toward how partners together will address the role of PTSD in their relationship. If, for example, they present to a session arguing about topics that are not specific to PTSD and it does not appear that they can resolve it quickly and successfully, we redirect them to focus on PTSD-relevant content, and encourage them to use their conflict management and communication skills to do so. We tell them that the focus for now is the PTSD and how it intersects with their relationship, and that we expect that they will be able to negotiate these other topics successfully as the role of PTSD in their relationship shrinks further and they have greater mastery of the communication skills.

Pretherapy Engagement and Assessment

It is our experience that veterans' couple and family relationship problems or their loved ones' difficulties are often the precipitants for veterans' treatment for mental health problems. Thus, using these relationships as a conduit to treatment and delivering the therapy in a conjoint format can be important ingredients to successful engagement of service members and veterans, who are reticent to seek treatment for a variety of personal and professional reasons. A full discussion of engagement strategies is beyond the scope of this chapter. However, we have been successful in engaging veterans in treatment by acting quickly on requests for help and getting an initial agreement to at least meet with a therapist who can provide feedback about couple functioning.

We encourage therapists in clinical practice to meet with the partners together for one session, then to schedule a second assessment session in which the therapist meets with each member of the couple individually. Fully informing the couple that this will be done one time to collect each individual's history, and sharing with the couple that anything discussed in an individual meeting with the therapist *can* be brought to the couple therapy, is imperative to maintaining the conjoint frame. At the second assessment meeting, one partner's history is taken while the other partner completes brief objective measures of mental health and relationship difficulties; then the two partners exchange places. A third assessment session is then scheduled, in which the therapist provides feedback to the couple regarding diagnostic impressions and the couple's functioning. This is used as a foundation for the rationale for pursuing a course of CBCT for PTSD. In the spirit of fully informed consent, we urge therapists to describe explicitly the nature of the intervention (e.g., time-limited, trauma-focused after requisite skills are built), the expectations of the couple (e.g., participating in in-session practice of skills, out-of-session assignments), and the expectations of the therapist (e.g., to guide and structure sessions). A clear outline of the course of therapy is important for the successful initiation of all therapies, but especially when working with traumatized individuals who have experienced unpredictable situations in which they were helpless. In this approach, the fourth session with the couple is the first session of the intervention protocol.

In conducting the individual assessments, it is important for the therapist to establish whether the veteran or partner meet DSM criteria for PTSD. A careful assessment of the traumatic event(s) not only informs diagnosis but also helps the therapist to anticipate things that the couple likely avoids, and the nature of the trauma-focused cognitive work that will ensue in the third phase of the therapy. A "gold standard" method of assessing the presence and severity of PTSD is the Clinician-Administered PTSD Scale (CAPS). The CAPS provides both ratings for the frequency and severity of each of the 17 DSM symptoms of PTSD, which can then be used to make a diagnosis of PTSD, and a quantitative measure of overall severity. In clinical practice, it may not be possible to administer the CAPS to establish the *severity* of PTSD symptoms, in which case the PTSD Checklist (PCL), might be used as a substitute. The PCL is a brief (i.e., less than 5 minutes to complete) self-report measure that allows respondents to rate the severity of each of the DSM PTSD symptoms. We have created and routinely use a Partner Version of the PTSD Checklist (PCL-P) that asks intimate partners to rate their perception of their loved one's PTSD symptoms. The partner's perception of the patient's PTSD symptoms can provide invaluable clinical information in general, especially in light of research and our own clinical experiences that veterans of the current conflicts tend to minimize their posttraumatic stress symptomatology. Discrepancies in the multimodal assessment of PTSD can provide important clinical information regarding the case conceptualization and possible barriers to maximal treatment benefit.

It is also important to assess for the presence of comorbid conditions with which veterans commonly present, such as major depression and substance use disorders (see Whisman & Sayers, Chapters 9, and Schumm & O'Farrell, Chapter 10, this volume, for suggested assessment strategies). In addition, research indicates that veterans' intimate partners will likely present with their own mental health symptoms, with symptoms of depression, substance abuse, or general anxiety as the most likely suspected types of problems. This is, in part, why we encourage clinicians to meet with each partner individually and to have each complete a brief battery of self-report assessment instruments.

We recommend that each partner complete objective, self-report assessments of relationship satisfaction and intimate aggression as part of the initial assessment. In our research and clinical practice, we treat couples who have engaged in minor acts of aggression, according to objective assessment, and include cessation of physical aggression as a treatment goal (see Heyman, Taft, Howard, Macdonald, & Collins, Chapter 7, this volume, for more information regarding assessment and treatment). We provide referrals for individual or group treatment for clients or couples who are engaging in more severe forms of aggression.

Over the course of therapy, we recommend that at least the Veteran and Partner versions of the PCL (anchored for the past week) and some brief assessment of relationship satisfaction (can be as simple as an overall rating of relationship satisfaction in the past week) be administered to evaluate ongoing functioning. We recommend that these across-treatment assessments be done prior to every other or every third session because of their brevity. Other relevant comorbid conditions in the veteran or partner should also be monitored. This assessment information should be conveyed to the couple to reinforce progress or to determine impediments to a successful course of therapy.

Phase 1: Rationale and Education

Treatment Challenges and Strategies

In our experience, the modal partners presenting for CBCT for PTSD include a PTSD-identified individual with at least one comorbid condition and a partner with some mental health symptoms, who, as a couple, experience clinical levels of relationship distress. Thus, the first phase of the therapy is designed to provide greater understanding of the symptoms of PTSD and its association with relationship problems. It also involves laying out a clear rationale of why the therapy should help the veteran with PTSD, the couple's relationship, and the distress that the veteran's partner is likely experiencing. Hope is infused by providing a recovery-oriented model of posttraumatic problems and by conceptualizing the couple's relationship as a major vehicle for healing after a traumatic event(s).

Instilling safety within the couple's relationship is also a major goal of Phase 1. Trauma victims were not safe at the time of the trauma and continue to live as though others and the world pose threats to their emotional and physical safety. Also, high levels of relationship conflict, including intimate aggression, can disrupt safety in the couple's relationship. The therapist should assume a compassionate but strong stance in creating a safer environment, in which partners work on their relationship, by teaching and incorporating conflict management strategies into the relationship. In some cases, these couples avoid conflict at all costs by chronically disengaging from one another. The goal is to create safety and skills to regulate anger and other distressing emotions, so that partners can safely reengage, or engage for the first time, in a more authentic and intimate relationship with one another.

Therapeutic Components of Phase 1

In the first session following assessment, the therapist provides psychoeducation about PTSD and a rationale for PTSD-focused conjoint treatment, an explanation of how avoidance and problematic thoughts maintain PTSD, and ways that PTSD can contribute to and maintain relationship problems. The session concludes with the couple collaboratively identifying treatment goals in the areas of their relationship and PTSD. Couples are encouraged to be as specific as possible, so that progress can be easily monitored and assessed over the course of treatment. For instance, a therapist helps partners who identify improved intimacy as a relationship goal to make this more tangible by saying, "That's a great goal. Now, let's figure out how we'll know that you're being more intimate." In response, the partners might identify hand holding, daily hugging and kissing, cuddling, or having sex as behavioral signs that their intimacy is improving. Similarly, with regard to PTSD-related goals, couples who identify decreased irritability as a goal are encouraged to generate behavioral markers of decreased irritability (e.g., less yelling at the children, fewer arguments with the partner).

The second session of this phase focuses on enhancing physical and emotional safety in the relationship for both partners. Couples are provided with psychoeducation about the role of PTSD in relationship functioning as it relates to dysregulation in the fight-or-flight system and are taught primary and secondary prevention strategies for managing conflict. An example of a primary prevention strategy includes slowed breathing when one notices escalating anger; an example of a secondary prevention strategy is time-out, which can be used once couples are involved in a heated exchange and one or both partners want to prevent the situation from escalating further. To increase the likelihood that each of these skills will be practiced outside of the session, the couple is asked to practice both skills during the session. This also provides the therapist with the opportunity to clarify any aspects of the skills that are unclear and to reinforce the couple's efforts.

Phase 2: Satisfaction Enhancement and Undermining Avoidance

Treatment Challenges and Strategies

In Phase 2 (Sessions 3 through 7), the overall goals are to improve relationship satisfaction and to decrease behavioral and experiential avoidance. Communication skills are presented and practiced in each session sequentially to help the partners label and share their emotions and then notice the way thoughts influence their feelings and behaviors. Communication skills are practiced with discussion of PTSD-related content, which is presented as a method to "shrink" the PTSD that exists in their relationship. This simultaneously facilitates communication skills building and a collaborative approach to addressing trauma-related behavioral and experiential avoidance.

Another major treatment intervention to address trauma-related

avoidance that begins in this phase of the therapy and continues throughout is tailoring "approach assignments" for each couple. These dyadically
focused *in vivo* approach assignments have the dual goals of (1) having the
traumatized partner approach the avoided here-and-now people, places,
things, and feelings that maintain posttraumatic problems, and (2) increasing mutually pleasurable activities for the partners to enhance their relationship satisfaction (e.g., going to movies and restaurants). It is important
to note that for the purposes of CBCT for PTSD, the couple relationship,
rather than the individual with PTSD, is the unit of intervention in these
approach assignments. Thus, the partners are encouraged to complete these
exercises as a team rather than seeing them as a task to be completed by the
PTSD-identified individual, with the partner serving as "coach" to encourage the completion of the approach assignments.

Therapeutic Components of Phase 2

In Session 3, the role of avoidance in maintaining PTSD and relationship
problems is introduced (see Handout 8.1, *PTSD and Avoidance*, at the
end of this chapter), and improved communication is conceptualized as an
antidote to both PTSD and relationship distress. The couple is taught the
communication skill of reflective listening and then given the opportunity
to practice this skill while discussing PTSD-specific content. In keeping
with the idea of externalizing the PTSD, partners are first asked to discuss
people, places, feelings, and situations that PTSD makes them avoid as a
couple; they are then asked to use their reflective listening skills to discuss
the things that they, as a couple, would be doing if they avoided less.

Starting in Session 4, a list of avoided stimuli serves as the basis for
assigning out-of-session couple-level approach activities at the end of each
session throughout the remainder of the treatment. Session 4 also introduces
the notion that couples typically have one of two types of conversations at
any given point in time: sharing thoughts and feelings ("sharing") or problem solving ("solving"). The therapist explains that the next several sessions
will focus on sharing, starting with emphasis in Session 4 on identifying
and sharing feelings. The ability to identify and share feelings is believed
to be important in combating both PTSD-related "alexithymia" (i.e., difficulty identifying and naming one's emotions) and relationship distress.
In this session, partners practice reflective listening and emotional sharing
skills by simultaneously labeling and sharing their feelings in response to
the discussion topic of how they each feel about the role of PTSD in their
relationship, and how they each feel when they imagine shrinking the role
of PTSD in their relationship. This exercise also serves as a powerful way
to teach couples about the intimacy-building role of sharing feelings in that
most couples report feeling closer after the exercise compared to before,

even if partners share negative feelings (e.g., sadness, disappointment). Session 5 focuses on sharing thoughts and associated feelings.

Session 6 introduces a process for teaching couples how to identify and potentially modify thoughts that may be contributing to distress in one or both partners. The process is summarized in the acronym U.N.S.T.U.C.K.:

- Unified and curious as a couple as partners join together in collaborative empiricism.
- Notice and share thoughts and feelings.
- (Brain)Storm alternative thoughts or interpretations, even if they seem implausible.
- Test the thoughts (i.e., consider the evidence for each alternative thought).
- Use the most balanced thought(s).
- Changes in emotions and behaviors that result from the balanced thought(s).
- Keep practicing (i.e., recognition that it requires effort to change one's mind when there have been entrenched patterns of thinking).

The *Big Picture Worksheet* is used to facilitate this process (see Handout 8.2 at the end of this chapter).

Session 7 reviews recommended steps for problem solving and decision making. As with the previous sessions, skills instruction in Sessions 5 through 7 is followed by in-session practice of the skills using PTSD-related content. For example, in Session 7, partners are asked to apply their problem-solving skills to plan their next *in vivo* approach assignment.

Phase 3: Meaning Making and End of Therapy

Treatment Challenges and Strategies

Building on the couple's increased satisfaction, improved communication, and decreased behavioral and experiential avoidance, Phase 3 addresses trauma-relevant thoughts that maintain PTSD and associated relationship problems. The partners use the U.N.S.T.U.C.K. process to discuss and consider alternative methods of understanding traumatic events, present-day events, and relationship issues. There is an initial focus on historical appraisals specific to the traumatic event(s); present-day beliefs commonly disrupted by trauma are then addressed. This sequence is chosen because changes in the ways in which a traumatized person and the partner make sense of the specifics of the trauma(s) can have cascading effects on beliefs operating in the here and now. For instance, a veteran who blames herself for being raped in the military may have trouble trusting her judgment in the here and now. Reappraisal of the event as the result of contextual factors that may have been beyond her control at the time (e.g., the rapist had the element of surprise, fighting back may have resulted in further injury or even death), helps the traumatized individual develop different views of her judgment and ability to trust herself in the present.

Therapeutic Components of Phase 3

Sessions 8 and 9 are historical in nature and target maladaptive thinking patterns that interfere with acceptance of the traumatic event and appropriate placement of blame, respectively. Examples of problematic thinking that can impede acceptance of traumatic events include hindsight bias, the tendency to assume that one had the knowledge at the time of the event that one has now, and "undoing," the tendency to play out the event with alternative courses of actions that could have prevented it (e.g., "I should have done this instead of that . . ."). To facilitate a more accurate and balanced reappraisal of the traumatic event(s), the couple uses the U.N.S.T.U.C.K. process.

Sessions 10 through 13 focus on historical appraisals until more balanced thoughts are achieved, as well as here-and now interpersonal beliefs in the areas of trust, control, emotional intimacy, and physical closeness that may have been disrupted by the trauma (e.g., "I can't trust people; they will hurt me," "I have to retain control at all times in order to stay safe"). Couples continue to use the U.N.S.T.U.C.K. process to address these PTSD-related thoughts, as well as any thoughts held by either partner that may maintain relationship discord ("I cannot accept a compliment from my partner because then she will try to manipulate me").

Session 14 focuses on benefit finding and the potential for posttraumatic growth as a result of traumatic events. Finally, Session 15 includes a review of skills learned and improvements made over the course of treatment, and a discussion to help couples anticipate and address fluctuations in their individual and relationship functioning over time.

FACTORS INFLUENCING TREATMENT

There are a variety of factors that can influence a course of CBCT for PTSD. We categorize these factors here according to individual, interpersonal, and institutional factors. With regard to individual factors, as the number and severity of mental health conditions in either partner increase, the challenges in delivering the treatment generally increase. For example, the partner of a veteran struggling with his or her own symptoms of PTSD may be reluctant to engage in *in vivo* approach activities with the veteran due to his or her own anxiety, may have difficulties labeling and sharing his or her own emotions, and may tend to engage in more rigid, black-and-white thinking. Similarly, a partner experiencing major depression may find it difficult to marshal the energy and motivation needed to engage in and complete the approach assignments with the veteran. Additionally, a partner with a substance use disorder may rely on alcohol or other substances as an overlearned coping strategy, potentially interfering with the couple's adoption of newer, more adaptive ways of coping with stressful situations or managing negative emotions.

Most of our research on CBCT for PTSD has excluded couples in which both partners meet criteria for current PTSD. However, we recently received funding to investigate the treatment of such couples by adapting the protocol so as to target both members' PTSD-related cognitions. We currently exclude couples in which one or both members have met criteria for substance dependence within the previous 3 months in both our research and clinical practice. The rationale for this is that the medical risks of untreated substance dependence, such as death due to overdose or seizures secondary to withdrawal, require swift and targeted treatment that is beyond the scope of the CBCT for PTSD protocol. However, we have successfully treated couples in which one or both of the partners were diagnosed with substance abuse disorders. For example, the partner of one veteran we treated met criteria for cannabis abuse and was initially quite reluctant to use less, because it helped him to relax. Over the course of therapy, he agreed to smoke less as an "experiment" to see if he could learn other ways to cope with stress and to show support to the partner with PTSD, who was being asked to confront numerous anxiety-provoking situations without relying on her typical avoidant coping strategies. By the end of treatment, he had successfully reduced his marijuana use, and the couple reported feeling closer as a result of "being in this together." Efforts are also under way to modify the protocol to target couples in which one member meets criteria for both PTSD and substance dependence.

We have seen improvements in partners' moods over the course of treatment, which may be partly attributable to less conflict and an overall improved emotional tone in the relationship. However, we have also observed that asking both partners to complete the U.N.S.T.U.C.K. process on their respective thoughts during Phase 3 helps partners adopt a more balanced way of thinking in general, which can help them to examine and modify more general maladaptive negative thoughts.

In this vein, "cognitive flexibility," or the ability to consider a range of possible interpretations for events, is another individual factor that may influence the delivery of the intervention. There is variability among individuals in their ability to brainstorm a range of possible interpretations about traumatic events and other events. In general, greater cognitive flexibility is a positive prognostic indicator. Partners' ability to adopt a "big picture" view of events can help in reappraisals of historical and current events. In addition, this strength can help the partner to make healthier attributions for the patient's PTSD-related behavior and to build empathy. For instance, reconceptualizing a veteran's "controlling" behavior, such as discouraging the partner from leaving the home after dark, as the result of a desire to keep one's family safe after having been in a life-threatening situation rather than a desire to take away another person's freedom, can help to maintain good will on the part of the partner and a commitment to work on the relationship. This latter consideration is particularly relevant in light of the finding that when service members endorse high levels of PTSD symptoms, but their female spouses perceive that they experienced low levels of combat exposure, female spouses report lower levels of relationship satisfaction (Renshaw, Rodrigues, & Jones, 2008).

An interpersonal factor that may be of concern to some clinicians is the possibility of partners' vicarious or secondary traumatization, or the possibility of loved ones developing their own case of PTSD as a result of hearing about veterans' traumatic experiences. Consistent with research, our clinical experience is that most problems experienced by partners are due to the difficulties of living with someone with untreated symptoms of PTSD rather than hearing about traumatic events per se. In the case of CBCT for PTSD specifically, the risk of secondary traumatization is extremely low. As noted earlier, the treatment is trauma-focused, but it is not imaginal exposure-based; that is, events are not reviewed in minute detail. Rather, traumatic events are discussed from a "big picture" perspective to assist both members of the couple in forming a more cogent trauma narrative. This, in turn, facilitates the patient's recovery from PTSD through greater acceptance of the event and a more accurate appraisal of it. We have also observed that many partners are quite skilled in promoting patients' adoption of a different perspective on the event in response to this "big picture" trauma disclosure. For instance, we worked with a couple in which the veteran's traumatic event involved killing enemy combatants at close range. He harbored intense self-blame for these actions, believing that he somehow could have chosen not to fire on them even while he was being fired upon. His wife helped him appreciate that he actually had no choice but to fire, given that this is what his training had prepared him to do, and that if he had not fired back, he would have been court-martialed or, worse, killed. She also allayed his concerns that she would think of him as a "bad person" for having killed other people by explaining to him that he was doing the job he had been trained to do, and that she understood how these actions had occurred in the context of war.

An institutional factor that may influence delivery of the treatment relates to concerns about secondary gain motives involving getting medically discharged from the military, receiving financial compensation for mental health problems, or fulfilling the "sick role" in the case of discharged veterans. It is important to note that the literature supporting these notions is scant and equivocal. Nevertheless, we have seen cases in which the PTSD diagnosis interacted in this context, with some veterans reporting that the diagnosis served as validation of their military service or trauma exposure (especially in cases in which they were originally disbelieved) or was a burden that they carried because of their survivor guilt. Some have transparently expressed concern that profiting from an evidence-based therapy could threaten their disability rating and ultimately the compensation that accompanies it. There are advantages and potential limitations of pursuing an evidence-based treatment that must be discussed upfront and be ongoing as part of a fully informed consent process. We encourage clinicians to consider the timing of delivering evidence-based interventions. When someone is being evaluated to establish a mental health disability, it is not likely the best time to pursue a treatment that can work. Other supportive therapy may be indicated.

TAILORING TREATMENT TO ACTIVE DUTY AND VETERAN COUPLES

Adapting the Protocol to Abbreviated Interventions

There are occasions when veterans may have the opportunity to receive evidence-based individual PTSD treatment, CBCT for PTSD, or both. CBCT for PTSD is designed to serve as a stand-alone treatment for PTSD. Nonetheless, there may be situations in which veterans and clinicians may elect to deliver elements of CBCT for PTSD in concert with individual evidence-based PTSD treatment. For couples in which the patient wishes to pursue individual treatment but would like his or her partner to learn more about PTSD and why it has affected their relationship, Phase 1 of CBCT for PTSD could be offered. Alternatively, Phases 1 and 2 could be delivered if the patient elects to receive a course of individual treatment and the couple would like to address relationship issues. We recommend against offering the full 15-session CBCT for PTSD protocol simultaneously with other trauma-focused PTSD treatment, not only to avoid overwhelming the patient with multiple intensive treatments but also to avoid confusing the patient regarding how to approach review of the traumatic event. More specifically, some evidence-based individual treatments for PTSD (e.g., prolonged exposure, cognitive processing therapy) encourage patients to review a trauma account in detail, and sometimes over and over again, until their anxiety is habituated, whereas CBCT for PTSD encourages taking a "big picture" perspective.

We are currently evaluating an abbreviated version of the intervention delivered in groups that comprise romantic and nonromantic dyads and include an active duty or discharged Iraq/Afghanistan veteran with posttraumatic stress problems. This eight-session protocol includes the sessions of Phases 1 and 2 of the intervention but substituting the U.N.S.T.U.C.K. session with a session focused on generalization of the communication skills to a range of relationships. The final session focuses on consolidation of skills and review of treatment gains. Clinicians delivering this group intervention have commented on the advantages of the multidyad format in facilitating social support among veterans and their loved ones and the vicarious learning and feedback across dyads. They have also commented that the dyads appreciated that the treatment was shorter in duration given the multiple demands impinging on these veterans and their loved ones.

Tailoring Treatment to Separated or Deployed Couples

We are sometimes asked whether cohabitation is required for a couple to participate in and benefit from CBCT for PTSD. Our perspective is that cohabitation is not necessary, provided that the couple can complete the out-of-session assignments. For instance, we have treated couples who did not live together and where one or both partners travel frequently for work. These couples have successfully navigated this potential barrier by speaking on the phone and e-mailing each other daily, and making sure to see each other in person during the week to do their assigned *in vivo* approach activities.

Many of the returning veteran couples whom we have treated work, go to school, or have young children, making it difficult for them to attend regularly scheduled appointments during daytime hours. To facilitate their session attendance, we have found it helpful to be as flexible as possible when scheduling appointments by offering evening appointments and the option to schedule appointments around work, school, or child care responsibilities. As a result, we have generally had excellent session attendance, and couples routinely express appreciation for this accommodation given all the other demands that they are juggling.

Some military members have expressed concern that treating PTSD during active duty status will result in a less able and prepared fighting force. Specifically, the concern is that recovery from PTSD will lead to service members being less vigilant to threat cues and less responsive to true danger. We and others submit that treating PTSD actually makes for a more able and prepared fighting force, because service members can more accurately appraise real versus imagined threat. Research does not support the notion that a human's hardwired fight-or-flight response to legitimately life-threatening situations is extinguished with psychotherapy. The goal is to decrease hypervigilance and other hyperarousal symptoms that can contribute to "hair-trigger" reactions, as well as reexperiencing symptoms that can interfere with attention and mental acuity. Chronic irritability can also make PTSD-affected service members less able to work as a team with fellow service members, all of which may place themselves and others at increased risk of harm.

We are exploring the delivery of CBCT for PTSD via telephone and videoconference to meet the needs of veterans and loved ones who do not have ready access to the treatment due to geography or therapist availability. We have not yet had a case in which a deployed service member was receiving mental health services and had a partner at home who was aware of such. In those circumstances, we suggest that a therapist consider using technology (i.e., phone, Internet) to deliver some of the interventions from Phase 1 of the therapy alongside an evidence-based treatment for PTSD. More specifically, therapists can e-mail information regarding psychoeducation about trauma and the recovery-oriented model of posttraumatic problems, and also discuss the rationale for the PTSD intervention. The couple could also be asked to notice and exchange positive characteristics or behaviors via technology every day. These interventions could also be used with other adult loved ones who support the service member and the intervention from a distance. In those cases in which there is ongoing relationship conflict, the individual and interpersonal conflict management strategies in Session 2 could be delivered via telephone to the service member and his or her partner to decrease the ambient stress that could interfere with the service member's treatment and compromise the partner who continues to manage the many demands at home.

Case Illustration: CBCT for PTSD

Below we describe the course of treatment for Amber and John by the phases of CBCT for PTSD.

Phases 1 and 2

The implementation of Phases 1 and 2 of CBCT for PTSD were largely uneventful for Amber and John, with the exception of some initial difficulties with their out-of-session assignment adherence, addressing John's alcohol abuse, and programming approach assignments specific to the couple's physical intimacy. The partners came to the second session of therapy having completed most of their out-of-session assignments, but John did not complete his version of the Trauma Impact Questions, admitting that he did not want to think in any way about what had happened to him in Iraq.

The therapist had him answer the questions verbally and, prior to the end of the session, engaged him in a discussion about his understanding of the role of avoidance in preventing his completion of the assignment. She also problem-solved with the couple about how John would record what he had shared in session regarding the Trauma Impact Questions to complete fully this out-of-session assignment before the next session. John came to the third session having completed his Trauma Impact Questions. The therapist applauded his efforts and reviewed John's responses briefly in the third session.

In the first intervention session, in which the couple engaged in goal setting, Amber mentioned John's alcohol use. John was initially defensive about this topic but acquiesced a bit after Amber pointed out his tendency to pass out each night on the basement couch and disclosed that their eldest child had asked her, "Why is Daddy so sleepy all of the time?" John agreed to a goal of decreasing the amount of alcohol he consumed each day. The therapist monitored John's alcohol use at each session, reinforcing his decreased consumption and prompting Amber to reinforce his decreased use. However, Amber began Session 5 expressing her concern that John had driven home after drinking at a bar. The therapist reassured Amber that they would discuss the issue within the session and redirected them to review the out-of-session work that they had done. During the in-session practice, the therapist posed the questions identified in the protocol about the various thoughts that PTSD had made them have (e.g., John's thought, "If I get close to someone, one of us will get hurt," and Amber's thought, "If I try to get close to John, he will lash out at me") and added that they each may have thoughts about the role of alcohol as an avoidance strategy of PTSD in their relationship. Amber was able to express her thoughts and related feelings in response to John's alcohol use. More specifically, she expressed, "I'm concerned that you might die because of drinking, and I'm scared for me and our kids." This softened John, and he disclosed the trauma-related precipitant for his alcohol use that particular day—his coworker's injury at work. After highlighting the couple's use of the skill of identifying thoughts and feelings impacted by posttraumatic stress symptoms, the therapist commended the partners for their increased self-disclosure and approach of important emotions that each of them was experiencing. She noted the increase in their intimacy scores from the beginning to the end of the in-session practice. The therapist also introduced the notion of John taking a "break" from drinking as an experiment to combat the avoidance that drives PTSD and "pushes him and their relationship around" (externalizing the disorder). This seemed to appeal to John's competitive spirit; Amber was relieved.

The couple came to Session 6 reporting that since the last session John drank alcohol only once at a holiday gathering, and only two beers at that event. The therapist had assigned progressively more challenging *in vivo* approach assignments related not only to John's index trauma, the death of his comrade by suicide bomber (i.e., sitting in less comfortable positions in public places, going to a funeral of a family friend), but also approach assignments related to physical intimacy. Specifically, the therapist assigned increasingly intimate relationship encounters (e.g., holding hands, snuggling on the couch), but discouraged the partners from focusing on achieving sexual intercourse so that they did not necessarily become outcome-focused in their physical intimacy efforts. They came to Session 6 reporting that they had engaged in sexual intercourse twice since the last session, which the therapist and the couple celebrated as a major treatment accomplishment. She also wondered out loud with the couple, "I wonder if John's decreased alcohol consumption and your commitment to address the presence of PTSD in your relationship have in any way contributed to your increased physical intimacy?"

Phase 3: Getting U.N.S.T.U.C.K.

With a foundation of improved relationship satisfaction and communication skills, the course of therapy transitioned to focus on Amber and John's trauma-specific ways of thinking. Amber knew almost nothing about John's experiences in Iraq. She wanted to know, but she avoided asking about it because she didn't want to "rattle his cage." John's index traumatic event that was determined during the individual assessment was the death of one of his men, Chris, by a suicide bomber. As his commanding officer, John had ordered Chris to go on the mission in place of another soldier who was ill that day. John saw Chris approaching the bomber just before the bomb went off. John's reexperiencing symptoms were riddled with images of the explosion.

The therapist, knowing that Amber knew little of what had happened, asked John to give Amber and the therapist a "brief overview" of what had happened in Iraq that was most distressing to him. John reluctantly provided the details, and Amber seemed relieved, as if her imagination had created a worse image. To target John's difficulty accepting the reality of what happened, the therapist then asked John, "What do you want to change the most about what happened?" To which John said, "The fact that I sent Chris to his death." The therapist recognized this as the Noticed thought (stuck point) for the U.N.S.T.U.C.K. process, and John agreed to write down their work on the Big Picture Worksheet (see Figure 8.1). The therapist asked Amber if she had any questions for John, now that she knew more about John's experience and what he was thinking about it. Amber responded, "I'm not sure what to ask." The therapist role-modeled asking questions and being curious for Amber.

THERAPIST: I guess I'm wondering what you mean, John, when you say "I sent him to his death?"

JOHN: He was under my command, was supposed to be off that day, and I sent him in there to die.

AMBER: You didn't send him to die. It's not your fault.

JOHN: Well, then whose fault is it (*sarcastically*)?

THERAPIST: (*softly*) That's a really good question for all of us, because it sounds like right now you think it is 100% your fault. Am I right?

JOHN: Of course, it's all my fault. I sent him there.

THERAPIST: You did send him there as his commander, but let me ask the two of you something in the spirit of the brainStorming step of the U.N.S.T.U.C.K. Did you know when you sent Chris on the mission that he was going to get bombed by an insurgent?

JOHN: Of course not.

AMBER: Oh, yeah, like that something-sight bias you mentioned.

THERAPIST: Yes, hindsight bias—knowing information now that you didn't know at the time.

JOHN: I should have known.

AMBER: How could you have known that he was going to get blown up?

THERAPIST: That's a good question, Amber.

JOHN: It was a dangerous area.

THERAPIST: Before we keep going, let's get down on our sheet the idea that John couldn't see into the future when he sent Chris into the area. John is not a fortune teller. It is an idea that we want to put on the table. John, can you get that thought down? (*Pause for writing.*)

AMBER: I just thought of something: Wouldn't someone have had to go on the mission no matter what?

JOHN: Yes, and I let Chris go.

THERAPIST: You let Chris go? What do you mean?

AMBER: Did he want to go?

JOHN: I wouldn't say he wanted to go, but he was trying to advance up the ranks, which meant that he was always more willing and "good-to-go."

THERAPIST: Let's get that idea down. Amber, can you paraphrase what you heard John say about Chris's "good-to-go-ness"?

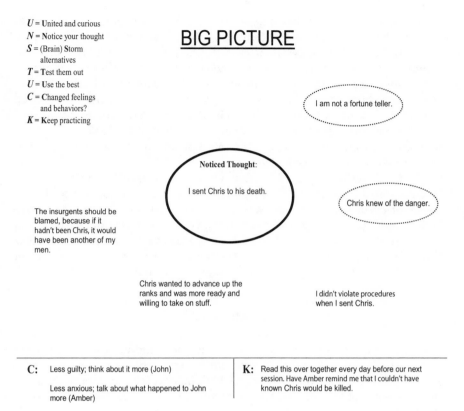

FIGURE 8.1. Big Picture Worksheet for John.

AMBER: I heard you say, "Chris wanted to advance up the ranks and was more ready and willing to take on stuff." It sounds like he was even willing to take on potentially dangerous assignments.

JOHN: He was. We knew it was dangerous.

THERAPIST: Are you saying that Chris, like you, knew of the potential danger?

JOHN: Yeah, he wasn't stupid.

THERAPIST: Okay. Let's get that down. . . .

John indicated that the two most compelling alternatives to the thought he initially noticed were the notions that Chris knew of the danger and "proceeded in spite of it, like a good soldier," and that John didn't know at the time that anyone would be bombed. In a subsequent session the couple added to the Big Picture Worksheet that "the insurgent should be blamed, because if it hadn't been Chris, it would have been another of my men." The therapist also paired an *in vivo* approach assignment with a Big Picture Worksheet about control in Session 11. More specifically, the couple used U.N.S.T.U.C.K. on John's thought, "The shopping mall is dangerous," and agreed to read the sheet before going to the mall at a nonpeak time. At the next session, they agreed to go to the mall on a Saturday afternoon, when it was likely to be more crowded.

They came to the final session with their respective posttreatment Trauma Impact Questions. In response to the question about why John's traumatic event occurred, John wrote "Stupid dumb luck. Chris was a good soldier and agreed to go on the mission. We knew it was dangerous, and he served his country when I asked him. It wasn't my fault that Chris was killed. It was the bomber's fault. If it wasn't Chris, it would have been someone else. I wish people didn't die in war, but that is a reality."

SUMMARY

A large portion of our returning service members and veterans come home from their deployments with posttraumatic stress problems. Fortunately, our knowledge about how to treat PTSD has grown exponentially since previous wars of this scope. This is accompanied by greater awareness in the clinical, layperson, defense, and veteran health communities of the effects of military-related PTSD on couple and family functioning, and vice versa. The time-limited and trauma-focused treatment presented here, CBCT for PTSD, is the first of its kind in its simultaneous treatment of the origins of PTSD and the intimate relationship problems associated with it. The therapy is also designed to be flexible in its phased format to incorporate veterans' loved ones in an overall treatment plan to address PTSD. Though PTSD and its frequently comorbid conditions can wreak havoc on couples' relationships, intimate relationships hold great promise in helping our veterans heal from the physical and mental scars of war and improving the lives and well-being of those who surround them.

RESOURCES

Galovski, T., & Lyons, J. A. (2004). Psychological sequelae of combat violence: A review of the impact of PTSD on the veteran's family and possible interventions. *Aggression and Violent Behavior, 9,* 477–501.

Glynn, S. M., Eth, S., Randolph, E. T., Foy, D. W., Urbaitis, M., Boxer, L., et al.

(1999). A test of behavioral family therapy to augment exposure for combat-related posttraumatic stress disorder. *Journal of Consulting and Clinical Psychology, 67,* 243–251.

Milliken, C. S., Auchterlonie, J. L., & Hoge, C. W. (2007). Longitudinal assessment of mental health problems among active and reserve component soldiers returning from the Iraq war. *Journal of the American Medical Association, 298,* 2141–2148.

Monson, C. M., & Fredman, S. J. (2012). *Cognitive-behavioral conjoint therapy for posttraumatic stress disorder: Harnessing the healing power of relationships.* New York: Guilford Press.

Monson, C. M., Fredman, S. J., Adair, K. C., Stevens, S. P., Resick, P. A., Schnurr, P. P., et al. (2011). Cognitive-behavioral conjoint therapy for PTSD: Pilot results from a community sample. *Journal of Traumatic Stress, 24,* 97–101.

Monson, C. M., Fredman, S. J., & Dekel, R. (2010). Posttraumatic stress disorder in an interpersonal context. In J. Gayle Beck (Ed.), *Interpersonal processes in the anxiety disorders* (pp. 179–208). Washington, DC: American Psychological Association.

Monson, C. M., Schnurr, P. P., Guthrie, K. A., & Stevens, S. P. (2004). Cognitive-behavioral couple's treatment for posttraumatic stress disorder: Initial findings. *Journal of Traumatic Stress, 17,* 341–344.

Monson, C. M., Stevens, S. P., & Schnurr, P. P. (2005). Cognitive-behavioral couple's treatment for posttraumatic stress disorder. In T. A. Corales (Ed.), *Trends in posttraumatic stress disorder research* (pp. 245–274). Hauppague, NY: Nova Science.

Monson, C. M., Taft, C. T., & Fredman, S. J. (2009). Military-related PTSD and intimate relationships: From description to theory-driven research and intervention development. *Clinical Psychology Review, 29,* 707–714.

Renshaw, K. D., Rodrigues, C. S., & Jones, D. H. (2008). Psychological symptoms and marital satisfaction in spouses of Operation Iraqi Freedom veterans: Relationships with spouses' perceptions of veterans' experiences and symptoms. *Journal of Family Psychology, 22,* 586–594.

Riggs, D. S., Monson, C. M., Glynn, S., & Canterino, J. (2009). Couples and family therapy. In E. B. Foa, T. M. Keane, M. J. Friedman & J. A. Cohen (Eds.), *Effective treatments for PTSD: Practice guidelines from the International Society for Traumatic Stress Studies* (2nd ed., pp. 458–478). New York: Guilford Press.

Sayers, S. L., Farrow, V., Ross, J., & Oslin, D. W. (2009). Family problems among recently returned military veterans. *Journal of Clinical Psychiatry, 70,* 163–170.

PTSD and Avoidance

Instructions: Use this handout to reinforce psychoeducation presented to the dyad in the session about the role of avoidance in maintaining PTSD and relationship problems and to develop a list of avoided places, people, situations, and feelings that the couple will begin to approach systematically during therapy.

As we discussed in the session, many people who have experienced trauma try to avoid thoughts and feelings associated with that event. Similarly, many people also avoid situations, places, and activities that remind them of the trauma or because they just feel scary. People with PTSD can also become frightened of the thoughts, feelings, and physical sensations associated with anxiety itself. This tendency has been described as a "fear of fear." Although avoiding can make you feel more comfortable in the short run, it actually can make the problem worse in the long run, because it prevents you from overcoming your fears.

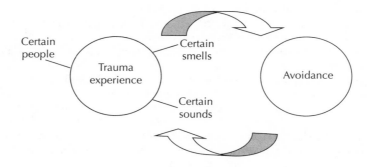

Like avoiding situations, places, and activities that remind them of traumas, people with PTSD come to avoid their own internal experience, such as their thoughts, feelings, and physical sensations. We sometimes describe this as a "fear of feeling." Techniques to avoid your inner experience might include obsessive thinking, emotional numbing, overcontrolling your emotions for fear of being out of control, or injuring yourself to distract from painful emotions.

When you confront feared conversations, memories, situations, or feelings several things begin to happen:

- Facing these situations helps you make sense of them (e.g., "Why am I afraid to talk to my spouse about our children?" → "She might figure out that I don't feel like I'm an adequate parent").
- You learn that thinking about these experiences is not dangerous and that being upset or anxious is not dangerous (e.g., "I won't go crazy if I'm sad after talking about these situations. In fact, my partner and I feel closer").
- You become less fearful of other situations that remind you of these situations (e.g., "Now that I've faced this and had a positive experience, why wouldn't that be the case in the future?").
- You learn that you can handle your fear and anxiety; therefore, you feel better about yourself (e.g., "I'm strong enough to handle being sad or angry without acting on these feelings. I don't have to feel *good* all of the time, but rather be *good* at feeling").
- You learn that when you repeatedly confront memories or situations you have avoided, the fear and distress gradually decrease. In other words, you again become relatively comfortable in these situations (e.g., "I don't get nearly as upset as I used to discussing these things with my partner").

Choosing to more directly address difficult issues for yourself and your relationship is hard work, but will lead to long-term payoff.

List below as many things as possible that, as a couple, you "help" avoid.

Places	**Situations**
_____	_____
_____	_____
_____	_____
_____	_____
_____	_____

People	**Feelings**
_____	_____
_____	_____
_____	_____
_____	_____

Big Picture Worksheet

Instructions: The Big Picture Worksheet is used to facilitate the dyadic cognitive intervention process. The noticed thought is written in the center of the page; alternative thoughts are written around the noticed thought. The best balanced thought(s) are circled. At the bottom of the form in the "C(hanged feelings and behaviors?)" section the dyad notices the changed feelings and related behaviors and identifies ways that they will practice these changes in the "K(eep practicing)" section.

U = **U**nited and curious

N = **N**otice your thought

S = (Brain) **S**torm
  alternatives

T = **T**est them out

U = **U**se the best

C = **C**hanged feelings
  and behaviors?

K = **K**eep practicing

BIG PICTURE

Noticed Thought:

C:

K:

CHAPTER 9

Depression

Mark A. Whisman and Steven L. Sayers

Paul and Jennifer felt like they "just did not get along" and disagreed "about everything." Their struggles as individuals and challenges as a couple preceded Paul's deployment to Iraq as a communications specialist. Paul had experienced several previous episodes of depression, and within the year after his return from Iraq to his Army Reserve unit, he had begun to feel anhedonic and experienced irritable mood, as well as poor sleep, hopelessness, self-criticism, and lack of motivation. Jennifer had a history of generalized anxiety disorder, but she was managing her symptoms well with the help of her psychiatrist. They struggled financially in the period after Paul's combat deployment, having to live with Jennifer's mother. The spouses battled over money and child discipline, the latter being complicated by long-standing conflict over Jennifer's 12-year-old son and Paul's 8-year-old son from their previous relationships. The couple entered therapy with some positive experiences with individual treatment but remained locked in a pattern of frequent loud verbal conflict and convinced that the other spouse was the guilty party.

INCIDENCE AND IMPACT OF DEPRESSION
AND COMORBID CONDITIONS

Depression is a common and debilitating mental disorder. The National Comorbidity Survey—Replication (NCS-R), which is a population-based survey of 9,282 English-speaking adult household residents of the continental United States, provides prevalence estimates of major depressive disorder (MDD) of 16.2% for lifetime and 6.6% for the 12 months preceding the interview (Kessler, Merikangas, & Wang, 2007).

Depressed persons are also likely to meet criteria for other disorders in addition to their depression. In the NCS-R, nearly three-fourths (72%) of people with lifetime MDD also met criteria for at least one other disorder assessed in the NCS-R, including 59% who met criteria for at least one lifetime comorbid anxiety disorder, 32% with at least one lifetime comorbid impulse control disorder, and 24% with at least one lifetime comorbid substance use disorder. Similarly, approximately two-thirds (65%) of people with 12-month MDD met criteria for at least one other 12-month disorder, including 58% with comorbid anxiety disorder, 21% with comorbid impulse control disorder, and 9% with comorbid substance use disorder. Therefore, the majority of people with 12-month or lifetime histories of MDD are likely to meet criteria for at least one comorbid disorder. With respect to clinical severity, 38% of respondents with 12-month MDD were classified as being seriously or severely depressed, based on a self-report measure of depressive symptoms.

It is important to note that military populations may be more vulnerable to MDD following exposure to combat, with the prevalence rates of military personnel returning from combat in a mostly male combat population as high as 14%. As with the broader population, a large percentage (78%) of combat veterans with posttraumatic stress disorder (PTSD) are likely to experience depression within their lifetime. Couples in which the service member has served in combat may be more likely than civilian couples to face multiple medical and mental health comorbidities due to the traumatic nature of combat (Sayers, 2011).

Combat veterans may be particularly less likely to seek or receive treatment for depression. In one survey of service members who had just returned from combat and met screening criteria for a mental disorder, about 60% were concerned that their fellow soldiers or commanding officers would lose trust in them or treat them differently if they sought treatment, and 65% stated that seeking treatment made them appear "weak" (Hoge et al., 2004). Thus, there are likely special challenges related to stigma for combat veterans.

Depression is also associated with role impairment, such as impairments in the areas of work and social life (Kessler et al., 2007). One area that has generated a considerable body of research is the association between depression and quality of intimate relationships such as marriage, as reviewed by Whisman and Kaiser (2008). Much of the research on intimate relationship functioning has focused on global relationship adjustment, measured by self-report, and described in terms of "distress" or "discord." Specifically, prior research has shown that relationship distress is associated with concurrent depressive symptoms and depressive disorders (i.e., major depression, dysthymia). Furthermore, results from longitudinal studies indicate not only that relationship distress is predicted by earlier depression, but also that baseline relationship distress predicts change in depressive symptoms and incidence of depressive disorders; the prospective association between relationship distress and MDD has been found in several large-scale studies, supporting the generalizability of these associations. Finally, research has shown that relationship distress is associated with poorer outcomes in individual-based treatments for depression, such as individual psychotherapy, and that relationship distress does not generally improve following individual-based treatments for depression. In summary, there is a growing literature indicating that relationship distress is important for understanding the etiology, severity, course, and treatment of depression.

CONCEPTUAL AND EMPIRICAL UNDERPINNINGS

Several theoretical models have been advanced to account for the association between relationship functioning and depression. In this section, we discuss three of the most popular of these models.

First, according to the *marital discord model of depression* (Beach, Sandeen, & O'Leary, 1990), relationship distress decreases available support from the partner and increases the level of stress in the relationship. For example, relationship distress may result in decreased couple cohesion, coping assistance, and intimacy, and increased verbal and physical aggression, threats of separation, and criticism and blame. These processes, in turn, increase the likelihood of the onset and maintenance of depression. Although often cited as a model that focuses on the role of relationship distress as a precursor of depression, this model also proposes that depression can contribute to the onset and maintenance of relationship distress, resulting in a perpetuating cycle of greater depression and greater relationship distress. Thus, the service member who is experiencing severe conflict in his or her marriage is more vulnerable to depressive episodes due to the stress associated with this conflict and more limited in the ability to work with the partner over time to decrease this significant source of stress.

Second, according to the *interactional perspective of depression* (Coyne, 1976), depressed individuals seek reassurance from other people to alleviate their doubts concerning their own worth and whether others care about them. Although other people often provide reassurance, depressed individuals often doubt what they are told, leading to further reassurance seeking. Because this pattern is repetitive and resistant to change, significant others become frustrated and irritated with the depressed person, and become increasingly likely to reject the depressed person and become distressed themselves. In the context of military couples, the service member who is excessively focused on reassurance from a spouse regarding his or her military career may produce an ongoing irritant to the spouse within the relationship. As seen from this perspective, relationship distress is likely to be a consequence of the excessive reassurance seeking of the depressed partner.

Third, according to the *stress generation model of depression* (Davila, Bradbury, Cohan, & Tochluk, 1997), depressed people inadvertently contribute to the occurrence of stress in their lives and thereby contribute to the maintenance and recurrence of depression. In particular, this theory focuses on interpersonal events and stressors that may be contributed to by the depressed person's characteristics, situations, or behaviors. By creating contexts that are stressful, the person increases the likelihood of recurrent or chronic depression. As applied to close relationships, this theory suggests that depressed people make an unwitting contribution to the generation of stress in their relationship, which in turn leads to further depression. For example, a service member with recurrent depression may have chronic low mood, and a pessimistic view focused on the struggles associated with military life. This service member may distance the partner and have a more difficult time obtaining support from him or her.

In summary, there are at least three theoretical models for understanding how relationship distress and depression may be associated with one another. Although differing in their emphasis, each model allows for bidirectional pathways of influence. Consequently, relationship distress and depression are likely to influence one another in a recursive and reciprocal fashion. As applied to treatment, these models suggest that interventions targeting better relationship functioning should not only improve the quality of relationships but also reduce depression. In support of this perspective, research has shown that couple-based interventions are effective in reducing relationship distress and decreasing depression. Most of the clinical trials to date have focused on couples who are experiencing relationship distress and one partner is depressed, although some trials focus on couples who do not have distressed relationships. A recent meta-analysis of eight controlled trials provided evidence for the effectiveness of couple-based interventions in the treatment of depression (Barbato & D'Avanzo, 2008). Couple therapy appears to be comparable to individually oriented treatment in reducing depressive symptoms and more effective than individually oriented treatment in improving relationship distress. Although meta-analytic studies are helpful in providing an overall estimate of the effectiveness of couple-based interventions for depression, it is important to note that treatments included in this meta-analysis differ in important ways, including differences in interventions and underlying models of change. For example, couple-based interventions that have been shown to be effective in reducing depression include cognitive and cognitive-behavioral couple therapy, emotion-focused couple therapy, systemic couple therapy, and coping-oriented couple therapy.

GUIDELINES FOR ASSESSMENT AND INTERVENTION

In this section, we provide clinical guidelines for assessment and intervention with couples in which at least one partner is depressed and the relationship is distressed. We rely heavily on the cognitive-behavioral framework of assessment and intervention (Beach et al., 1990; Epstein & Baucom, 2002), as this is the most thoroughly studied couple-based approach to treating depression, although we discuss other interventions that have also been developed for use with couples in which one or both partners is depressed.

Assessment

Therapy typically begins with an assessment of the couple. Following is a brief overview of common assessment domains and methods; readers are referred to Snyder, Heyman, and Haynes (2005) for a more detailed review of evidence-based assessment of couples. As with most couple-based therapy, the initial assessment includes an interview of the couple. During this interview, the therapist asks each partner for his or her perceptions of the ongoing problems in the relationship. In addition to their own statement of the problems occurring in the relationship, it is generally helpful to ask partners about the frequency and intensity of conflicts in their relationship, the common sources of conflicts in their relationship, and how these conflicts are typically resolved in their relationship. In asking about conflicts, it is important to find out if either partner is currently engaging in verbal or physical abuse and, if not, whether they have a history of partner violence. (See Heyman, Taft, Howard, Macdonald, & Collins, Chapter 7, this volume, for guidelines for treating domestic violence if the initial assessment reveals that this is occurring.) Other common areas for assessment in the initial interview include partners' beliefs and thoughts about each other and about their relationship (e.g., the attributions they make about their partner's behavior, their unmet expectations and unfulfilled standards they have for each other and the relationship), and to what extent and under what circumstances they experience positive and negative feelings about each other and their relationship. Finally, partners are asked about their goals for therapy, focusing on specific examples of how they would know that each goal had been reached. Following the interview, partners can be asked to complete one or more self-report questionnaires to provide additional information on their perceptions of specific domains of the relationship, as well as their global evaluation of their relationship; the reader is referred to Snyder et al. (2005) for a review of specific measures.

In addition to assessing relationship functioning, it is important for the therapist also to assess for depression. There are a variety of interview and self-report methods of assessment, and these assessment techniques can be further categorized into those that assess for the presence of depression (diagnostic assessments that focus on specific inclusion and exclusion criteria) and those that assess the severity of depression; the interested reader is referred to Joiner, Walker, Pettit, Perez, and Cukrowicz (2005) for a review of evidence-based measures for assessing depression in adults. In interviewing a partner about his or her depression, the therapist seeks to obtain a relevant and complete history, including information about the current episode, past episodes, medical history, and family history. In addition to these verbal reports, a partner's nonverbal behavior (e.g., crying, psychomotor retardation or agitation) can provide useful information about the level of depression. Furthermore, therapists should assess for possible suicide ideation or behavior when assessing a partner's depression. It is important for therapists to assess for depression not only in the "identified patient" but also in the other partner, as research has shown that partners of depressed individuals are also often distressed.

Clinicians will also want to familiarize themselves with military culture sufficiently to assess the relevant aspects of military life and military deployments (see Martin & Sherman, Chapter 2, this volume). Key aspects include the length and location of assignments, the specific jobs or Military Occupational Specialty (MOS) of the service member, exposure to combat, and experiences with the military and veteran health systems. Relationship- and family-related aspects of military life include the arrangements made during extended training and deployments of the service member for managing their household, the nature and source of supports for the service member's partner during these times, and their perceptions of their functioning prior to and following deployments.

Although relationship functioning and depression are often the primary foci of an initial assessment, the previously reviewed research on psychiatric comorbidity suggests that a thorough evaluation also includes an assessment of other possible mental health problems that might not otherwise be identified by the couple. Readers are referred to other chapters in this volume for methods for evaluating other forms of emotional or behavioral disorders.

In addition to a thorough assessment at the onset of treatment, we recommend that therapists conduct brief, ongoing assessments throughout the course of treatment. At a minimum, this would involve regular (e.g., weekly) assessment of depressive symptoms and relationship distress. There are a variety of brief self-report measures of depression, and partners can complete these measures in a waiting area prior to the session. Measures that are commonly used to monitor change in treatment include the 21-item Beck Depression Inventory—Second Edition (BDI-II) and the 9-item Depression scale of the Patient Health Questionnaire (PHQ-9). Ongoing assessment allows the clinician to monitor symptom levels, thereby evaluating whether interventions are having their intended effects. Furthermore, because most symptom-based measures of depression include questions about suicide, regular ongoing assessment provides therapists with information to make informed judgments about potential suicide risk.

Intervention

Based on the information gathered during the assessment, couple therapists develop a treatment plan that is tailored to the needs and treatment goals of each couple. Couple therapy for depression is usually time-limited (usually 20 or fewer sessions) and focuses on the current relationship. Each session typically involves (1) setting the agenda for the session, in collaboration with the couple; (2) reviewing the homework (or "assignment" or "task") that the couple has done during the week; (3) addressing a problem, learning new skills, or practicing new ways of relating to one another to tackle problems or issues in the relationship; (4) deciding upon a new homework assignment to do before the next session; and (5) summarizing what was covered in the session and eliciting feedback about the session.

Couple therapy for depression generally follows three stages (Beach et al., 1990). The first stage involves eliminating major stressors and reestablishing positive activities in the relationship. The second stage involves improving communication and problem solving in the relationship. The third stage involves preparing for termination, with a focus on maintenance of gains and preventing relapse. In the following sections, each of these three stages is described in greater detail.

Stage 1

The goal of the first stage of therapy is to eliminate major stressors and to reestablish positive activities in the relationship. This stage begins with the initial therapy session, during which the therapist discusses the treatment plan and the goals of therapy. In discussing couple therapy for depression, it is important that the therapist convey to a couple that although they are being seen together in therapy because relationship problems and depression often influence each other, neither is more important nor necessarily the cause of the other. Rather, the therapist can suggest that both members of the couple are caught up in a difficult situation, and that by working together they can better hope to improve the quality of their relationship and their individual well-being. In the first session, it is also usually helpful to provide information to the couple about depression, particularly if neither partner has been treated for depression in the past. For example, it is helpful for couples to learn about the symptoms of depression, which sometimes helps the partner of the depressed person understand that behaviors such as loss of interest in general, and loss of libido in particular, are symptoms of depression and not signs of rejection or indicators of how the person feels about the relationship. It is also useful to note that after experiencing the intensity of combat, many of those who served may appear to "not care." It may take some time before the combat veteran's emotional reactions readjust to everyday family life. Furthermore, it is often helpful for partners to learn that depression can be a chronic or recurring problem, and that the depressed person cannot just "snap out of" or overcome the depression by sheer willpower. In general, partners evaluate depressed individuals more negatively than nondepressed individuals; therefore, educating couples about the symptoms and course of depression may help to change some of the negative thoughts and feelings a partner may have about the depressed person. The guidelines offered in Handout 9.1, *Do's and Don'ts of Supporting a Partner with Depression*, at the end of this chapter, can help partners know how to respond to the depressed individual early in treatment.

If the assessment indicates the presence of severe negative behaviors in the relationship, such as verbal or physical abuse, threats to leave the relationship, or extramarital affairs, then stopping these behaviors become the first goal of therapy. Therapists discuss the consequences of these behaviors for the relationship and for the individual well-being of the partner, and treatment is directed at stopping these behaviors. (See Snyder, Baucom, Gordon, & Doss, Chapter 6, and Heyman, et al., Chapter 7, for interventions for infidelity and domestic violence, respectively.) These clinical problems might be revealed privately to the therapist during the assessment or during treatment sessions after the treatment has begun. It is important that they become the focus of clinical intervention. Depending on the severity, scope, and clinical context of these issues, the therapist may refer one or both partners to additional or alternative treatments, according to the guidelines discussed in the chapters referenced earlier.

In addition to eliminating major relationship stressors, the other objective of the first part of therapy is to increase the frequency of positive activities in the relationship. Partners are taught the importance of "caring behaviors"—behaviors that show interest, respect, concern, or affection—that can be offered several times a week and demonstrate that the partner is valued and that the relationship is important. In session, partners are encouraged to pinpoint specific behaviors they could do that could increase the happiness of the partner (e.g., compliment the partner, ask the partner about his or her day, fix the partner a special meal). They are encouraged to write down but not share a list of such behaviors with the partner. For homework, they are then asked to increase the frequency during the coming week of these "unexpected" behaviors that demonstrate caring. Each person is also asked to watch for positive behaviors from their partner, and to acknowledge and thank the partner when they notice the partner engaging in a caring behavior; thanking the other person for specific acts of caring should help to increase the likelihood that the behaviors will occur again in the future. Both depression and relationship distress are associated with the tendency to attend to and remember negative experiences; encouraging people to focus on the positive helps to reduce these tendencies and promote hopefulness. In the following session, therapists ask each person what he or she noticed the partner doing during the week and check to make sure that both partners acknowledged these behaviors when they occurred. Subsequent sessions can include having each person make specific requests for behaviors they would like the partner to add to his or her list of caring behaviors ("I would like you to X" or "Please do X").

There are several types of difficulties to be expected when increasing positive interaction in military couples. In some couples in which the service member is preparing for deployment, the service member may be withdrawing emotionally because of the need to prepare for this deployment. In addition, the increased rate and frequency of training in the weeks or months prior to deployment decrease the opportunity and focus for activities meant to increase positive interaction. Acknowledging these constraints and openly discussing them may help the couple put forth the needed effort to increase positive interaction. Service members who are deployed for an extended time to a combat zone often struggle with challenges of redeveloping routine ways of interacting with their spouse in the months following their return (Sayers, 2011). Thus, it may be helpful to discuss this task in the context of reestablishing patterns of leisure interaction after the extended separation.

A second method for increasing positive exchanges in the relationship is for the couple to increase the frequency of pleasurable shared activities ("companionship activities"). During the session, partners are encouraged to think of activities they can do together that they find enjoyable, such as going for a walk, to a movie, or out to dinner. They can then pick one or two of these fun, shared activities to do during the week as part of their goals for the week. Sometimes, depressed individuals are reluctant to engage in this exercise, stating that nothing they do brings them pleasure or enjoyment. In such cases, it may be helpful for therapists to engage in "pleasure predicting" with depressed individuals, asking them to predict in advance how much pleasure or enjoyment they anticipate from the activity, and comparing their expected pleasure with the actual pleasure they experienced during the activity. Many depressed individuals will find that the actual degree of pleasure they experience during the shared activity is higher than what they had anticipated. Again, as noted earlier, some consideration to adjusting to civilian life, and discussion of the contrast of everyday interaction to the adrenaline generated in combat deployment can be useful in order to help the partners adjust their expectations about their emotional reactions.

Models of both relationship distress and depression suggest that the respective problem may be due in part to high levels of negative exchanges or low levels of positive exchanges. By reducing the frequency of severe negative behaviors and increasing the frequency of positive behaviors, relationship distress and depression should begin to be reduced by the end of the first stage of treatment.

Stage 2

The goal of the second stage of therapy is to improve communication and the couple's ability to solve problems in the relationship. Improving communication in general, and communication regarding solving problems in the relationship in particular, is a central focus of many couple-based treatments for depression.

Couples are first taught nonverbal and verbal skills for empathic listening and speaking. With respect to listening skills, partners are encouraged to demonstrate understanding and acceptance through tone of voice, facial expression, and posture, as well as through paraphrasing or reflecting what they hear their partner say. Regarding speaking skills, partners are encouraged to use "I" statements ("I feel X when you do Y in situation Z"); to speak in a clear and direct fashion; to limit themselves to speaking only a few sentences at a time so as to not overwhelm the listener; and to express their subjective view through sharing their thoughts, ideas, and feelings. In session, therapists typically begin by providing instruction and modeling of positive listening and speaking skills. Couples then practice these skills talking about positive or neutral topics, with the therapist supervising them and providing feedback on their performance. Couples can then continue practicing communication skills during the week as part of their between-session task or assignment. In subsequent sessions, therapists review the homework, troubleshoot any difficulties the couple may have had in completing the assignment, and continue practicing effective communication. As in any population of couples, partners in military couples vary greatly regarding their expression skills and inclination to value emotional expression. Therapists might find, for example, that some combat veterans value emotional expression less in the immediate postdeployment period. This is due to the expectation that service members in the combat situation suppress their emotions, which may persist into the postdeployment period. Some discussion of the needs of service members in these different contexts can be useful in facilitating emotional expression training.

Once couples master general communication skills when talking about positive or neutral topics, the focus can shift to more emotionally laden or conflict topics. In this stage, the goal is to teach couples how to discuss and solve problems in their relationship. Couples are taught the basic steps in problem solving—problem definition, brainstorming, decision making, implementing solutions—and are encouraged to use their constructive communication as they work on solving ongoing problems in the relationship. They start with solving smaller problems in the relationship, with the goal of solving larger problems in later sessions. As with communication training, problem solving begins in the session, with the therapist instructing the couple about effective problem solving, then providing feedback on the couple's performance of these skills. Couples can then continue these kinds of problem-solving assignments on their own during the week.

Observational research on problem-solving interactions of couples with a depressed partner has shown that these couples engage in many of the same negative patterns of communication observed with distressed couples in general. Therefore, general communication and problem-solving training should prove to be useful for many distressed couples with a depressed partner. However, it has also been shown that a poorer course of depression is predicted by (1) criticism expressed by the partners of depressed individuals and (2) "perceived criticism," which refers to the degree to which depressed individuals think their partner is critical of them. Therefore, in addition to general communication and problem-solving training, therapists working with couples in which a partner is depressed seek to educate couples about the importance that criticism has for depression, and focus on reducing the occurrence of criticism. Furthermore, because perceived criticism is incrementally associated with depression above and beyond the effects of observed criticism, therapists also focus on reducing perceptions of criticism.

One way of working with perceived criticism is to focus on potential differences between a speaker's intent of a particular message and the impact the message has on the partner. Consistent with the interactional perspective of depression (Coyne, 1976), depressed individuals may have doubts concerning their own worth and whether others care about them, which may impact how they interpret the partner's behavior; specifically, they may be more likely to perceive criticism in situations in which the partner does not intend to be critical. Consequently, it may be useful for the depressed person to tell the partner when he or she thinks the partner is being critical and "check out" whether the partner intended to be critical at the time. By encouraging people to check with their partners regarding the intent of messages they perceive as critical, partners may learn to pinpoint behaviors in which they may unwittingly engage that the depressed partner perceives as critical; partners can then focus on changing these behaviors. Furthermore, the depressed individual may learn that the partner did not intend to be critical, which can result in a change in his or her interpretation of the partner's behavior and a general reduction in the perceptions of criticism. The therapist can encourage the spouse to "check out" assumptions in the manner illustrated below:

> "Paul, let me ask you to check out Jennifer's intentions with that statement. I know it is easy to assume you know what is in her mind, but as we've been discussing, you can take the opportunity to challenge your assumptions. Can you ask her the following: 'I am feeling criticized here; can you say more about what you are thinking?' "

Stage 3

The goal of this final stage of therapy is to help couples solidify the gains they have made in the earlier stages of therapy, to prepare for termination, and to prevent relapse. One strategy for solidifying gains and preparing for termination that can be implemented in one of the final sessions is for a therapist to review the main topics covered in therapy, then have each partner write about what he or she learned and found most helpful in therapy for homework. These summaries can then be kept together with therapy materials (e.g., handouts and worksheets) as part of a "therapy toolkit" to which the couple can refer as a refresher of the skills learned in therapy and a resource of things to do if the partners encounter problems again in the future.

In the final sessions leading up to termination, therapists can also work to identify "high-risk" situations that the couple might anticipate encountering in the future that could pose a challenge to their relationship or relapse of depression. For example, a prolonged deployment, a change in residence, or a change in military assignments might all result in changes in the way the couple handles family responsibilities and time together, which could increase the likelihood of conflict and relapse. The couple would then be encouraged to develop strategies for coping with these situations before they occur. For example, partners anticipating a change in military assignments and resulting decrease in amount of time together during the week may choose to set aside additional time on the weekend to engage in activities together.

Because depression is a recurrent disorder, it is also important in the final stages of therapy to discuss the recurrent nature of depression, to talk about how to recognize the early warning signs of depression, and to identify steps each partner can take to identify or prevent a recurrence of depression. For example, a person who recognizes that social withdrawal is an early warning sign of becoming depressed might agree to schedule time with friends and extra joint activities with the partner to reverse this pattern of withdrawal.

A final strategy for preventing relapse for people with co-occurring depression and relationship distress involves treatment "fading" and booster sessions. With respect to treatment fading, weekly sessions could be followed by biweekly and then monthly sessions. Such a schedule would allow couples greater opportunity to practice and master the skills learned in therapy on their own while still being able to check in periodically with their therapist to get feedback and guidance in areas in which they are experiencing difficulties. With respect to booster (or maintenance) sessions, treatment is seen as consisting of two phases: an active treatment phase and a maintenance or continuation phase. Once a couple has completed active treatment and is no longer experiencing depression or relationship distress, the partners then enter a maintenance phase involving periodic (e.g., monthly) scheduled sessions; these sessions are commonly described as "checkup" sessions, similar to a dental checkup or automobile maintenance checkup. For some couples, booster sessions are used to review skills learned in treatment, whereas other couples use booster sessions to solve problems that emerge during the passage of time or that were not anticipated during the course of therapy.

FACTORS INFLUENCING TREATMENT

Although many couples respond to couple-based interventions for depression, other factors may prove to be important in conceptualizing depression that occurs in a couple's relationship and tailoring treatment accordingly. In this section, we review some common factors that may influence the process or outcome of treatment and offer guidelines for adapting treatment to these factors.

Suicide

One factor that may influence treatment for people with depression and co-occurring relationship distress is the risk of suicide. In most clinical trials, active risk of suicide is an exclusion criterion for participation in the trial, so little is known about the impact of couple-based interventions for suicidal individuals. However, there are reasons to believe that couple therapy may be helpful. For example, hopelessness has been identified as a risk factor for suicidal ideation and behavior, and helping couples improve their relationship may help to transform hopelessness into hopefulness. Suicidal individuals are also often conceptualized as poor problem-solvers, because suicide is seen as the only "solution" to their problems. Problem-solving training, therefore, may provide suicidal individuals with a framework for solving problems that extends beyond their relationship and helps them to be better problem-solvers in general, thereby reducing their risk of suicide.

Because little is known about the impact of couple-based treatments for suicidal individuals, therapists working with suicidal individuals are encouraged to use other treatments that have been shown to be effective in treating suicidality prior to engaging in couple-based treatment for depression. In addition, it may be helpful to have an individual therapist work with the person with active suicidality, and to ensure that both partners consent to the couple therapist having communication and a good working alliance with that clinician. For some therapists, individual treatment for the person with depression and suicidality may be an important prerequisite for entering or continuing in couple therapy. Without separate, individual treatment, a great deal of attention and session resources would need to be devoted to treating suicidality.

A plan for handling suicidal thoughts and behaviors in couple-based treatment can be delivered in a matter-of-fact way. First, arrangements for crisis care to facilitate safety are discussed. For example, service members and veterans, as well as their partners, can be given the Veterans Department of Affairs (VA) Veterans Crisis Line number (1-800-273-8255, press 1 for veterans) for emergencies. Second, a plan for managing suicidal thoughts and behaviors is developed in concert with the depressed person's individual therapist, and a role for the partner can be negotiated that is consistent with this plan. For example, when a person is experiencing suicidal thoughts, a prearranged plan for increased self-care (i.e., becoming active, or listening to music to reduce suicidal thoughts) can be enacted and supported verbally by the partner. In this way, the partner can support a higher level of functioning in the most appropriate way. A check-in each session helps determine whether the plans have been used and to track the depressed person's current level of depressive symptoms, including suicidality. This can be accomplished using a weekly brief self-report measure of depression completed before the session, as described earlier in the section on *assessment*, and discussion during the appointment about any relevant findings.

Depression in Both Partners

Research has shown that partners of depressed individuals are at risk for distress and increased depressive symptoms themselves. Partners report that the depressed person's lack of energy, feelings of worthlessness, lack of interest, and constant worrying are a source of burden, and that the burdens of living with a depressed person can increase their own level of distress. This raises an interesting question regarding the treatment of couples in which both partners are depressed. In most clinical trials to date, depression in the partner is an exclusionary criterion. Therefore, little is known regarding the impact of couple-based treatment on couples in which both partners are depressed. However, it seems likely that the interventions described in this chapter could also be helpful for couples in which both partners are depressed. In such cases, the therapist may want to consider the impact that depression in both partners may have on the treatment process. For example, because of diminished levels of motivation and energy in both partners, it may be more challenging to engage such couples in homework assignments. In such cases, therapists may want to make use of graded task assignments, starting with small assignments and building to larger assignments.

Engaging Reluctant Military Service Members and Their Partners

Several factors associated with the active military and veteran populations may lead to greater reluctance to participate in individual or, especially, couple therapy for depression. Older, Vietnam-era veterans are more used to engaging in treatment without the participation of their partners due to less active outreach and inclusion of family members by VA in previous decades. Cultural factors among both older and younger active military and veteran cohorts likely lead to greater concern about the stigma of mental health treatment, even in the presence of a close family member. Family members are not used to being included in VA treatment modalities due to all these factors. Following up on new federal law (Public Law 110-387: Veterans' Mental Health and Other Care Improvements Act of 2008), the VA has begun to ensure that couple- and family-based services are provided to veterans for conditions related to their military service. In addition, family member involvement in treatment is being encouraged more actively in order to support treatment efforts for the overall goal of improving clinical care.

Emphasis on early assessment sessions as a time-limited way to hear about the difficulties each partner is having is usually sufficient to elicit initial participation, with no extended commitment of participation in treatment implied or required. In some situations with very reluctant partners, the initial contact can be defined as "for the veteran's benefit," without requiring initial buy-in of the partner in a dyadic approach. Asking both partners to describe how they each reacted to the initial session and addressing any concerns or uncertainties often helps the reluctant partner feel more comfortable through an initial three- to four-session assessment period.

The Impact of Military Life on Relationships and Couple Therapy

Military life demands accommodations in lifestyle and related limitations not common to nonmilitary families. Relationship separations and reunions are frequent due to deployment for training purposes and to combat deployments to the recent conflicts in Iraq and Afghanistan. Periodic family relocations are also common, leading to disruptions in children's schooling and potentially disruption of ongoing mental health treatment. Partners of military service members also may become frustrated with disruptions in their work life, leading to less career advancement for the partner or the decision of the partner not to enter the workforce. Thus, the common theme of sacrifice for military service borne by the entire family may have an impact on the dynamics of couple interaction and sense of burden on the service member. It is useful for the couple therapist to normalize these feelings.

As noted earlier, military life is marked by intermittent marital separation for a range of reasons. Thus, for many military couples there is greater risk of treatment being temporarily interrupted or shortened than that for their civilian counterparts. In many cases the therapist may not know whether treatment will be resumed when the service member again becomes available. Thus, it is important to provide the couple the most straightforward and helpful aspects of the couple intervention, which are likely to be interventions to increase positive exchanges (Stage 1). If a therapist knows that discontinuation of treatment will occur, then it may be helpful to integrate previously described aspects of the treatment from Stage 2 earlier in Stage 1. This can be accomplished by focusing more formal communication training on the positive feelings associated with the positive exchanges. In that way, the couple could potentially obtain some benefit from a briefer form of couple treatment and, when possible, feel encouraged to resume treatment to focus on more intractable problems using a problem-solving approach.

Age-Related Comorbidities

Military veterans who served in the Vietnam era form the largest single group of current or former U.S. military service members, and remain the predominant group of veterans receiving VA services. These veterans, who are usually at least 60 years old, bring with them the medical concerns of older adults, including diabetes, cardiovascular disease, and related difficulties. The therapist is encouraged to consider the following factors associated with age-related physical disability: (1) an increased degree of dependence or mutual dependence between partners; (2) an additional source of burden on one or both partners providing assistance to the disabled individual; and (3) limitations in the range of activities available to the couple to address depression (i.e., difficulty in ambulating, fewer social outlets). The therapist can consider addressing directly these normative problems in formal or informal problem-solving training.

TAILORING TREATMENT TO ACTIVE DUTY OR VETERAN COUPLES

Couple Complexity

A distinguishing feature of military and veteran couples is the greater likelihood of high clinical complexity (Sayers, 2011). This is particularly true for couples experiencing reintegration after the service member was deployed to a combat zone. As noted earlier, PTSD and depression are common comorbid disorders. Additionally, there is a range of other social and family reintegration stressors associated with the service member being out of the household for training assignments and combat deployment for weeks or months. Concerns about infidelity during deployment and the discovery of actual infidelity lead to additional relationship problems. Prioritizing among these problems can be a highly complex process. In many cases, this requires individual and couple-based treatments simultaneously, sequenced interventions for the service member or veteran, or multiple foci within the couple-based intervention sessions. The overall impact on the couple is a greater burden of time and effort devoted to treatment, and a longer commitment to treatment on the part of the clinician.

Adjunctive Treatments

Additional treatments for depression and other disorders such as PTSD or substance use might also be necessary when addressing depressive symptoms using couple therapy. This is particularly likely for military service members and veterans who have experienced combat exposure and also report significant relationship problems (Sayers, Farrow, Ross, & Oslin, 2009). There are several ways of addressing this issue, depending on the clinical circumstances and the degree of clinical impairment. In the case of substance abuse and comorbid depression, a period of sobriety is usually recommended for participation in couple therapy. If sobriety has been achieved prior to couple treatment, ongoing individual or group support for this sobriety is a useful adjunctive treatment because of the disruptive nature of relapse. In cases in which comorbid depression and PTSD are significant problems, then significant session time would be needed to focus on alleviating the PTSD symptoms. Thus, individual treatment for PTSD and depression prior to couple therapy could be indicated. In other cases, partners with depression can benefit from the adjunctive individual treatment of depression, especially in cases involving suicidality, as noted earlier. Readers might also consider the feasibility of other couple-based treatments of PTSD or substance abuse (see Monson, Fredman, & Riggs, Chapter 8, and Schumm & O'Farrell, Chapter 10, this volume).

Reintegration Issues

Even aside from dealing with depression, an important factor for many military couples concerns the impact of separation due to training and deployment to combat zones (Sayers, 2011). The experience of reintegration upon the return of the service member leads to several potential areas of concern that can be addressed using a psychoeducational approach as part of the couple therapy. Specifically, during the separation, the partner of the service member usually develops the ability to manage a household without the service member's presence. Thus, the partner may experience a reduction of autonomy after the service member's return. In addition, the service member and partner may not have similar expectations and desires about the pace of renewing emotional and sexual intimacy. The remaining partner may have lingering resentment about feeling "abandoned," and the service member may have difficulty accepting changes in his or her partner and family routines, or changes in discipline or privileges granted the children in his or her absence. Basic household chores and routines need to be renegotiated and reestablished, and the couple needs to reestablish or strengthen joint problem-solving and decision-making abilities, and reestablish support networks inside and outside the nuclear family. It is necessary for both partners to accept changes that have occurred in the relationship and in each other during the deployment. Addressing these concerns as normative experiences using a psychoeducational approach is often useful.

In addition, combat veterans often return from deployment exhibiting behaviors that are adaptive in the context of a military combat deployment and general military environment but maladaptive or inappropriate in civilian and family life. Military service members are trained to operate in the combat situation using deadly force, to function in tight-knit units, and to follow high operational security, often under severe conditions, with the daily threat of injury or death. Aside from the high risk of specific traumatic events, military training and the combat situation call for specific behaviors, including increased aggression, that are adaptive in this very specialized context but problematic at home. As shown in Handout 9.2, at the end of this chapter, these attitudes and behaviors have been given the acronym *BATTLEMIND*, which presents these behaviors as normative for combat but problematic in civilian and family life. The *BATTLEMIND* program has now been developed into a broader resilience training program (U.S. Army Medical Command, 2011), but these core concepts as originally defined can be useful as a teaching aid to help the couple understand the impact of military training and combat on relationship functioning. The clinician can use this information in a psychoeducational intervention and integrate it into the couple therapy.

Case Illustration

Paul, age 30, and Jennifer, age 31, entered evaluation for couple therapy at a large urban VA medical center with complaints that they experienced frequent loud disagreements. Their status as a blended family became more complicated in that Jennifer became pregnant with a daughter during the first year of their marriage, who was born during the army reservist's yearlong deployment to Iraq. The couple had not planned to become pregnant that soon after marriage, and the combat deployment was an important factor that increased the level of unpredictability in their lives, an experience common to military families.

Both Paul and Jennifer described acrimonious family upbringings, with Paul having witnessing domestic violence from his father, and Jennifer reporting extended conflict with her mother during her teen years. Jennifer also had significant contact with the mental health system during these years for generalized anxiety disorder, and since then had managed these symptoms well. Jennifer had developed a psychotherapy relationship with a psychiatrist and had been functional in the retail workforce for approximately 8 years, except for several months' maternity leave after the birth of their daughter. Paul described several previous depressive episodes that led to treatment in the public mental health system, in which he received both medication and individual psychotherapy. He reported very little exposure to trauma in his yearlong combat deployment and significant depression during the year before presenting for couple therapy. He had engaged in inconsistent individual psychotherapy and pharmacotherapy at his VA

Medical Center in the year after returning from his deployment prior to starting couple therapy. Paul met diagnostic criteria for depression, and described being anhedonic and experiencing irritable mood, in addition to poor sleep, hopelessness, self-criticism, and lack of motivation. He was working as a security guard at a local public high school, except during the summer, when he was primarily responsible for care of the children.

Paul had been persistent in pursuing Jennifer after they met, and although she felt positive about the attention that he paid to her and her son, he often exhibited jealousy and concern at the prospect of other men's attention. Over time this behavior grew into a pattern of internal desperation wherein he pursued closeness when feeling that their bond was threatened, and Jennifer withdrew emotionally because of feeling confined and controlled. Paul's tendency to pursue closeness also occurred during marital arguments, which would frustrate Jennifer. One partially successful solution was for Jennifer to demand that Paul go to another part of the house because of his desire to continue to engage in verbal arguments with her. The couple reported recently having loud and escalating fights, often over differences in their communication style, child rearing, and Jennifer's parental role in their marital relationship. Paul had reported some mild reciprocal violence during his first marriage, but both spouses indicated that they had never engaged in any physically violent or threatening behavior with one another.

Starting in the first evaluation session, suggestions were offered to the couple to reduce the level of verbal conflict, including "time-out" from arguments. As the evaluation proceeded, the couple found some success in reducing their overall level of conflict. They were very engaged in the evaluation, and readily accepted the therapist's suggestion to focus on reducing their rapidly escalating conflict, and their recent avoidance of positive interaction. Early in treatment, however, both individuals maintained a consistent pattern of focusing on changing their partner's unpleasant behavior. Refocusing partners on their internal experience when they were in conflict was helpful in recasting the problem and softening their reactions to each other. For Paul, this involved noting his urgency for closeness, whereas for Jennifer, discomfort with Paul's emotional intensity was important. It was possible then to ask each partner to consider solutions to these problems other than demanding that the partner change.

Early treatment interventions focused on collaboratively developing opportunities for the spouses to enjoy positive time together. Paul was resistant and pessimistic about many potential activities ("We hate each other's movies"), although an initial positive shift in treatment came from Paul's developing a family outing that included the children. Jennifer facilitated this shift by going along with the activity, even though this particular outing, a water park, was an activity Paul and the older children enjoyed more than she. This helped Paul develop a more positive attitude toward selecting activities that might suit them both.

After some increase in couple satisfaction and decrease in the conflict at home, Paul was able to visit his psychiatrist more consistently. He subsequently became more consistent and accepting of medication for his depressive symptoms. He also reported both an increase in motivation and a decrease in irritability and worry about contacts that Jennifer had with other men at work, all changes that were consistent with improvements in depression. Jennifer corroborated the degree to which his behavior was less negative toward her and more consistent with their children. She reported a range of positive interactions they had, even while they continued to deal with the relatively difficult situation of living with her mother.

With this momentum, treatment focused on helping the couple use informal brainstorming and more systematic problem-solving strategies to generate additional ideas for positive activities. Communication guidelines for focusing on solutions and avoidance of blaming were helpful, although the spouses often reverted to complaints about the other without support from the therapist. The couple began to talk about developing resources to move out of their current living situation to a place of their own. That had continuing difficulty, however, with conflict between Jennifer's 12-year-old son and Paul, in part because of difficulties inherent in the son's current developmental stage, as well as the disruption in their relationship due to Paul's military deployment.

Discussion of the multiple ways the veteran's deployment affected his role in the family and the impact on his relationship with Jennifer's son was a critical step. The spouses were coached to use more positive communication strategies, revealing the sense of displacement Paul felt after his return from deployment, and Jennifer's feeling of being abandoned during this time, with her mother as her only support. The couple continued to face many individual and family challenges. After 12 treatment sessions, however, the spouses showed significant improvement in their satisfaction, and Paul's depressive symptoms continued to improve.

SUMMARY

Depression is a common and disabling condition, and relationship distress has been shown to predict the onset, severity, and course of depression. Couple therapy has been shown to be effective in reducing depression and improving relationship quality. The most thoroughly researched approach to couple therapy for depression is cognitive-behavioral couple therapy, using the structure and many of the same interventions used for treating general relationship distress. In treating co-occurring depression, however, there is a greater emphasis on education about depression; rapid reduction of destructive conflict, including the reduction of criticism and perceived criticism; and redevelopment of social support and intimacy that may have been lost due to the impact of depression on the relationship. Military service members and combat veterans often present with greater clinical complexity than nonmilitary/veteran couples, with problems ranging from multiple comorbidities, reintegration stresses of the service member returning from a combat deployment, and the behavioral sequelae of combat training and combat experiences. Therapists need to consider the impact of additional treatments and the sequence of treatments in order to care for the multiple problems experienced by these couples. Therefore, couple therapy may be longer and may need to be more flexible to address the clinical needs of military couples. The couple-based strategy described here provides a useful strategy for treating depression in this population.

RESOURCES

Barbato, A., & D'Avanzo, B. (2008). Efficacy of couple therapy as a treatment for depression: A meta-analysis. *Psychiatric Quarterly, 79,* 121–132.

Beach, S. R. H., Sandeen, E. E., & O'Leary, K. D. (1990). *Depression in marriage: A model for etiology and treatment.* New York: Guilford Press.

Coyne, J. C. (1976). Toward an interactional description of depression. *Psychiatry, 39,* 28–40.

Davila, J., Bradbury, T. N., Cohan, C. L., & Tochluk, S. (1997). Marital functioning and depressive symptoms: Evidence for a stress generation model. *Journal of Personality and Social Psychology, 73,* 849–861.

Epstein, N. B., & Baucom, D. H. (2002). *Enhanced cognitive-behavioral therapy for couples: A contextual approach.* Washington, DC: American Psychological Association.

Hoge, C. W., Castro, C. A., Messer, S. C., McGurk, D., Cotting, D. I., & Koffman, R. L. (2004). Combat duty in Iraq and Afghanistan, mental health problems, and barriers to care. *New England Journal Of Medicine, 351,* 13–22.

Joiner, T. E., Walker, R. L., Pettit, J. W., Perez, M., & Cukrowicz, K. C. (2005). Evidence-based assessment of depression in adults. *Psychological Assessment, 17,* 267–277.

Kessler, R. C., Merikangas, K. R., & Wang, P. S. (2007). Prevalence, comorbidity, and service utilization for mood disorders in the United States at the beginning of the twenty-first century. *Annual Review of Clinical Psychology, 3,* 137–158.

Sayers, S. L. (2011). Family reintegration difficulties and couples therapy for military veterans and their spouses. *Cognitive and Behavioral Practice, 18*(1), 108–119.

Sayers, S. L., Farrow, V. A., Ross, J., & Oslin, D. W. (2009). Family problems among recently returned military veterans referred for a mental health evaluation. *Journal of Clinical Psychiatry, 70,* 163–170.

Snyder, D. K., Heyman, R. E., & Haynes, S. N. (2005). Evidence-based approaches to assessing couple distress. *Psychological Assessment, 17,* 288–307.

U.S. Army Medical Command. (2011). Resilience training. Retrieved November 1, 2011, from *www.resilience.army.mil.*

Whisman, M. A., & Kaiser, R. (2008). Marriage and relationship issues. In K. S. Dobson & D. J. A. Dozois (Eds.), *Risk factors in depression* (pp. 363–384). San Diego: Academic Press.

Do's and Don'ts of Supporting a Partner with Depression

Instructions: Partners of depressed individuals want to demonstrate their care and support but are often unsure about how to go about doing this in an effective manner. Following are several general guidelines for you to consider in supporting your partner.

- Do learn about depression.
- Do provide support and encouragement.
- Do acknowledge your partner's feelings and express your willingness to try to understand his or her experiences.
- Do provide opportunities for fun activities, but don't pressure your partner to participate.
- Do keep your expectations realistic.
- Do be patient and recognize progress, even small steps.
- Do try to remain active and healthy, maintaining your normal routine and activities as much as possible.
- Do take care of yourself.
- Don't expect your partner to "snap out of" his or her depression.
- Don't ignore your partner's depression, hoping it will go away.
- Don't offer unsolicited advice about what your partner "should" do to overcome his or her depression. Instead, support your partner's efforts to overcome the depression.
- Don't tell your partner why he or she should feel better.
- Don't say you know what your partner is going through, even if you have been depressed.
- Don't take your partner's behavior personally.
- Don't criticize or be negative.
- Don't threaten to leave the relationship.
- Don't avoid the subject of suicide out of fear of giving your partner "ideas."

BATTLEMIND

Instructions: Please review the table below. You'll note that each item describes an important objective that helps service members perform their duties when deployed. It may helpful for you *(the service member)* to describe the value of each item, such as why it is important to have "tactical awareness." Then it will be helpful for you *(the nonmilitary spouse)* to tell your partner when you notice that he or she is "relaxing" from these strict job requirements back home. An example: "Honey, I noticed that you appeared much more open and relaxed when we were out last night."

Behaviors	Consequences for home and relationship behavior
Buddies (cohesion) versus Withdrawal	Bonds built in combat lead to sometimes showing a preference for time with military buddies over family members.
Accountability versus Controlling	Accountability for control of weapon/gear and one's behavior leads to the need to control access to one's "stuff" and irritability toward family members about this.
Targeted Aggression versus Inappropriate Aggression	Use of anger and aggression in combat leads to a short temper at home.
Tactical Awareness versus Hypervigilance	A high degree of situational awareness results in appearing jumpy at home.
Lethally Armed versus "Locked and Loaded" at Home	The need for a weapon for survival in combat leads to feeling like one needs to have a weapon at home, in the car.
Emotional Control versus Anger/Detachment	Keeping a necessary lid on one's emotions becomes second nature and leads to being seen as "uncaring" by spouse.

(continued)

Mission Operational Security (OPSEC) versus Secretiveness	Keeping secrets in war may lead to not telling one's whereabouts to one's spouse and discussing very few deployment-related details.
Individual Responsibility versus Guilt	Survivors' guilt about combat events may lead to feelings that the spouse "just can't understand."
Nondefensive (combat) Driving versus Aggressive Driving	Unpredictable combat driving survival skills are risky at home—driving down the middle, not stopping, fast lane changes.
Discipline and Ordering versus Conflict	Giving and following orders in the military carries over to conflicts with spouse or children.

Source: Adapted from education material developed by the Walter Reed Army Institute of Research.

CHAPTER 10

Substance Use Disorders

Jeremiah A. Schumm and Timothy J. O'Farrell

Jason and Cassie had been together a year before Jason was deployed to Afghanistan. Prior to Jason's deployment, the couple would occasionally go out on the weekends to have drinks with friends or have friends over to drink and watch sports. Although Jason would sometimes have as many as five or six beers, neither partner regularly drank to intoxication or had recurrent negative consequences from their drinking. However, since Jason's return from Afghanistan 4 years ago, his drinking steadily increased to the point that he was drinking at least 12 beers nearly every day and began smoking marijuana at least once per week. This led to Jason missing work often, and there were times when he was driving home intoxicated. Jason began frequently to isolate from Cassie, spending much of his time drinking in their basement, and the couple rarely spent time together in activities that they used to enjoy. When they were together, Jason and Cassie also began to argue more frequently, particularly when Jason had been drinking. On several occasions, these arguments led to Jason pushing Cassie, and there were also times when Cassie slapped Jason. These arguments were frightening to the couple's 3-year-old daughter Sarah, and Jason had begun to withdraw from his daughter and instead spent most of his time drinking. It was obvious to Cassie that Jason's substance use had become out of control, but it was not until he was arrested for his second offense for driving under the influence that Jason agreed to seek help.

Couples such as Jason and Cassie experience firsthand the damaging effects of substance use disorders, which, unfortunately occur among a significant proportion of active service members and veterans. This chapter describes behavioral couples therapy for substance use disorders (BCT-SUD), which has been well-studied among various populations, including individuals who have served in the military. BCT-SUD is a manualized, 12-session treatment that concurrently targets promoting alcohol and drug sobriety, while improving the couple relationship. We describe the application of this model in the treatment of substance use disorders, along with a case example.

THE INCIDENCE AND IMPACT OF SUBSTANCE USE DISORDERS AND THEIR COMORBIDITIES

Large-scale samples from the U.S. population and members of the military suggest that substance use disorders affect a substantial number of individuals. The National Longitudinal Alcohol Epidemiologic Survey (NLAES) utilized face-to-face interviews of 42,862 individuals in the United States who were age 18 and older and assessed current (past 12 month) and lifetime substance use disorder diagnosis according to the DSM. According to the NLAES, approximately 7.4% of individuals met criteria for a current alcohol use disorder. This rate of current alcohol use disorders found in the general U.S. population may be slightly lower than what is found in military samples. Milliken, Auchterloine, and Hoge (2007) examined data from a sample of 88,235 Army soldiers completing the Post-Deployment Health Reassessment after returning from Iraq. This study showed that 11.8% of active duty and 15% of reservist soldiers endorsed experiencing alcohol problems during the 6 months after returning from Iraq. These apparent higher rates of alcohol use disorders in the military may be, in part, related to demographic factors; that is, military members are generally younger, with a higher proportion of males, and the NLAES indicates that in the general U.S. population approximately 1 out of 5 men ages 18–24 exhibit a past-year alcohol use disorder diagnosis.

Although there are not large-scale, representative studies of military members to provide estimates of drug use disorder prevalence, drug use disorders are found to be less common than alcohol use disorders in the general U.S. population. NLAES estimates suggest that approximately 1.5% of individuals meet past 12-month diagnosis for drug use disorders. The NLAES also found that many of those with a current drug use disorder are likely to also have a current alcohol use disorder. Specifically, results showed that having a past-year drug use disorder increased the risk for a past-year alcohol use disorder by 2,500%. Hence, those with current drug use disorders are highly likely to also experience current problems with alcohol use.

Studies clearly show that substance use disorders are associated with worse couple relationship functioning. In a review of the literature, Marshal (2003) concluded that couples in which at least one member has an alcohol use disorder have worse self-reported relationship functioning than those in which neither partner has an alcohol use disorder. In addition, couples in which one member has an alcohol problem demonstrate poorer communication skills compared to couples without an alcohol use disorder. Also, substance use disorders are related to elevated rates of intimate partner violence.

Psychiatric comorbidities are also fairly common in substance use disorders. Representative community sample studies find that individuals with substance use disorders are at elevated risk for experiencing other mental health disorders, with variations in the rates of comorbidity according to demographic factors and whether alcohol or drug use disorders are being considered. In the National Vietnam Veterans Readjustment Study (Kulka et al., 1990), 73% of Vietnam veterans with combat-related posttraumatic stress disorder (PTSD) were found to have lifetime prevalence of an alcohol use disorder. There is a lack of research to understand the rates of psychiatric comorbidity among female veterans and or service members. However, data from U.S. representative samples suggest that various mood and anxiety disorders are likely to co-occur among a significant subset of women in the military and female veterans who exhibit substance use disorders. Although the direct treatment of comorbid psychiatric disorders is outside of the realm of the protocol described here, it is important for clinicians to be aware of the likelihood of psychiatric comorbidity so that they can work directly with other treatment providers to provide appropriate referrals. Awareness of these co-occurring conditions is also important, so that clinicians can adapt the sequencing of the treatment to fit with a couple's current treatment needs.

CONCEPTUAL AND EMPIRICAL UNDERPINNINGS

The theoretical rationale underlying this treatment is more fully described in a book by O'Farrell and Fals-Stewart (2006). In contrast to most other substance use treatment approaches, BCT-SUD focuses on disrupting the reciprocal cycle between substance abuse and relationship functioning by directly addressing each domain.

In this model, a four-stage approach addresses the bidirectional relationship between substance abuse and relationship functioning. Abstinence from alcohol and drugs is emphasized as the primary goal, since it is assumed that abstinence must first occur before the couple is able to work through relationship problems effectively. Improvements in relationship functioning are viewed as an important secondary goal. It is important to point out that the various stages do overlap to a certain degree. For example, interventions to support abstinence are heavily emphasized in earlier sessions, although these sessions also provide the opportunity for couples to work initially toward the secondary goal of improving the relationship. The four stages are as follows:

- *Stage 1: Engaging the couple.* The couple is assessed, introduced to treatment rationale, and engaged in the initial commitment and expectations.
- *Stage 2: Supporting abstinence from alcohol and drugs.* The couple works on building support for abstinence within the couple domain and addressing issues that are likely to impact sobriety.
- *Stage 3: Improving the relationship.* The partners engage in positive couple behaviors that support sobriety and help to improve relationship satisfaction. The partners also learn effective communication strategies to improve chances of achieving sobriety and remaining sober, and improving relationship quality.
- *Stage 4: Continuing recovery.* The couple develops a plan for continuing recovery and for addressing the possibility of relapses to alcohol or drugs following the completion of therapy.

Evidence of Treatment Efficacy

Multiple randomized controlled trials demonstrate that family-based interventions for substance use disorders are associated with higher substance use abstinence rates in comparison to individual-based treatments. Behavioral couples therapy for these disorders has particularly strong empirical support, with several randomized clinical trials from various independent researchers demonstrating its superiority to individual-based substance use treatment approaches. These studies have shown that this approach is equal to or more effective than individual-based substance abuse treatments in producing abstinence from alcohol or drugs, fewer days of heavy drinking, and fewer problems related to substance use. In addition, these studies have typically found that this treatment is associated with better relationship outcomes than are individual-based approaches.

Although we are unaware of any studies of this protocol among active duty service members, several studies of this approach have been conducted among veterans. O'Farrell, Cutter, and Floyd (1985) describe results from a randomized clinical trial among 36 male veterans with alcohol use disorders and their female partners. In this study, heterosexual couples in which the male veteran had an alcohol use disorder were randomly assigned to receive (1) BCT-SUD delivered in group format plus individual alcoholism counseling, (2) interactional marital therapy group plus individual counseling, or (3) individual counseling with no marital therapy. Results showed that those receiving BCT-SUD had a lower number of days drinking during treatment than the treatment comparison conditions. Also, those who received BCT-SUD had a larger improvement in marital adjustment over the course of treatment. During the 2-year follow-up period (O'Farrell, Cutter, Choquette, Floyd & Bayog, 1992), the three treatments did not differ on days abstinent, although those receiving BCT-SUD had better marital adjustment than the two comparison treatments. In addition, those receiving BCT-SUD showed a trend ($p = .056$) toward fewer drinking-related problems than those receiving individual counseling only.

Along with the positive effects on the primary outcomes of substance use and overall marital adjustment, this treatment is also associated with significant reductions in partner aggression. Among a sample of 88 male veterans with alcohol use disorders and their female partners, O'Farrell, Van Hutton, and Murphy (1999) found significant reductions in partner aggression from the year prior to treatment to the 2 years following treatment. Results further showed that those who remitted from alcohol problems following treatment had similar levels of partner aggression to that of a demographically case-matched, nonalcoholic sample. However, those who relapsed to exhibit alcohol problems following treatment had elevated rates of partner aggression. These data suggest that the treatment may promote a reduction in substance use, which, in turn, is a key to reducing partner aggression.

Finally, O'Farrell and colleagues (1996) demonstrated that this approach is a cost-effective addition to veteran outpatient substance abuse treatment. In analyzing data from the previously described randomized clinical trial ($N = 36$), O'Farrell et al. showed that BCT-SUD was associated with significant reductions in health care and legal costs during the 2 years following treatment. In addition, results showed a positive benefit-to-cost ratio, indicating that the health care and legal cost savings offset the treatment delivery cost. In contrast, interactional couples group therapy failed to provide a positive cost–benefit following treatment. This suggests that among veterans with alcohol use disorders this approach appears to provide a unique advantage to reducing health care and legal costs over interactional marital therapy.

Although results from these and other studies support the efficacy of BCT-SUD for male veterans with alcohol use disorders, more research is needed to investigate the effects of this treatment for other populations. There exist no randomized clinical trials to examine the efficacy of this treatment among active duty service members or among female veterans or service members. In addition, there is a lack of research to determine whether this treatment is effective when used with couples in which both members exhibit a substance use disorder.

GUIDELINES FOR ASSESSMENT AND INTERVENTION

Stage 1: Engaging the Couple

The overarching goal of Stage 1 is to get the couple invested in engaging and returning for therapy appointments. Within this overarching goal, there are four primary therapeutic tasks: (1) initial engagement and contact, (2) initial interview, (3) assessment, and (4) gaining commitment and starting treatment.

Treatment Challenges and Strategies

One of the most frequently asked questions at our training workshops is how to engage the patient and his or her partner who did not seek out treatment. Often BCT-SUD is delivered in the context of a larger addiction treatment program, in which the patient may have sought help for the addiction but did not necessarily request couples-based treatment, nor did his or her partner necessarily request to be directly involved. In this scenario, there may be several specific challenges and strategies for dealing with these issues.

One challenge is overcoming patient concerns that may arise from the therapist contacting the patient's partner. Patients may fear that the intention of the therapist is to encourage the partner to leave the relationship or use "tough love" in dealing with the patient. They may also be concerned that the therapist is going to reveal information about the severity of the patient's substance use of which the spouse is currently unaware. Substance abusing patients may also have a tendency to avoid dealing with problems directly and may find the idea of addressing their partners' anger in a direct manner to be aversive.

To address these concerns, there are several suggested steps. Therapists should state that their intention is to help the patient to gain positive support toward achieving sobriety and that spouses typically respond in a positive manner when they are asked to be included. We have found it to be effective in engendering patient cooperation in contacting the spouse when we explain that we want to support the patient by explaining to the patient's spouse what a positive step he or she has taken by seeking help. We also explain to the patient that contacting the partner is a routine part of substance abuse treatment planning and invite the patient to sit in while we make initial contact with the partner. Patients sometimes suggest that they speak with their partners first and then the therapist can contact the partner afterward. Our anecdotal evidence suggests that this approach is often less effective, particularly among male veterans, and that contacting the patient's partner directly is usually more effective in eliciting initial partner involvement.

During preliminary contacts, an important goal is to obtain agreement from both partners to meet with the therapist for an initial joint meeting. The purpose is to provide a brief explanation of the treatment, while gaining initial couple commitment toward treatment engagement. Another goal is to also answer questions that the couple may have, assess for initial couple motivation, and obtain further commitment by scheduling for the next assessment.

Therapeutic Components of Stage 1

Assessment. Once the partners initially indicate that they are willing to explore this treatment, we minimally meet with them for an initial couple-based assessment and often include an additional two assessment sessions to provide more detailed assessment data. The purpose is to assess the partners regarding their appropriateness for this treatment and to obtain the information we use to drive case formulation. Much of this information can be gathered through clinical interview, although we also routinely use self-report measures as a way of augmenting clinical interview data.

During the couple-based assessment session, the goal is to establish rapport with the couple and to assess several major areas. We ask the partners their reason for seeking help now to establish motivation and circumstances affecting their decision to enter treatment. Alcohol and drug use by both partners is assessed, including recent types, quantities, and frequencies of substances used. Clinicians should also assess for extent of physiological dependence to determine need for medical detoxification. In addition, we ask about prior substance abuse treatment experiences, periods of sobriety, and what has been helpful in the past in achieving periods of sobriety. Finally, we assess for the effects of substance use on the couple and family, along with the individual's functioning.

Assessment also involves obtaining data on relationship commitment and stability. These data are important for establishing the likelihood that the couple will be able to complete and benefit from the treatment. It is fairly common for couples to report that this is seen as the final opportunity to make their relationship work. To be appropriate for this treatment, it is important that couples be initially committed enough to at least try treatment for several weeks.

Risk assessment is an important component of the evaluation. We focus upon two primary areas: risk for homicide/suicide and risk for partner physical violence. If either partner presents with substantial homicidal/

suicidal risk, then managing this risk clearly takes precedent. Regarding risk for partner physical violence, we believe that it is a good idea to also obtain questionnaire self-report data on these behaviors, and to meet with each partner separately to ask about violence occurrence (see Heyman, Taft, Howard, Macdonald, & Collins, Chapter 7, this volume, for additional information about couple violence risk assessment). Couples who present immediate risk for very severe partner violence that could cause serious injury or life threat are inappropriate for this treatment. However, our experience is that a very small percentage of cases are ruled out of this treatment due to very severe violence risk.

Gaining Commitment and Starting Treatment. When the partners return for the first session following the assessment, the therapist should start by exploring their reaction to the assessment. Therapists should specifically ask about the couple's commitment to starting treatment. If couples report being committed to starting, therapists should affirm this decision, then provide a preview of the initial session.

The next step is to provide the treatment rationale. We review the four specific domains that are common themes among couples with substance use disorders: alcohol and drug use, love and daily caring, fun together, and problems. We describe how active alcohol and drug use affects these domains and what happens with these domains during recovery. We then provide a brief preview of the interventions used to address each of these domains.

After reviewing the treatment rationale and answering questions about this, we review treatment expectations (e.g., showing up on time, being engaged in treatment). It is important to know that on the issue of missed sessions, BCT-SUD takes a different stance than that in other couples-based treatments. The approach in some other couples-based treatments is not to meet if only one partner can make it. However, given that missed sessions are a common precipitant to substance use relapse, the treatment philosophy is that it is better to meet with one partner than to meet with neither, with the goal of checking in about substance use issues and problem-solving factors that interfere with both partners attending.

Following one partner's absence and return to therapy, we review the concept of limited confidentiality, which is explained in the first session. In addition to the standard limits to confidentiality (e.g., to protect self or others from harm), we explain that in general we have a "no secrets policy," which means that we typically share information provided by one partner with the other partner. However, we explain that it is up to the therapist's discretion whether to choose to share information provided by one partner. This is to allow the therapist professional latitude in choosing to share specific information, while setting up the general understanding that the therapist is not going to be placed in the position of holding secrets.

The final piece to introducing the treatment is to explain and ask the couple to commit to the four promises. These promises are as follows: (1) no threats of divorce or separation, (2) no violence or threats of violence, (3) focusing on the present and future—not the past, (4) actively participating in all session and completing all homework assignments. These promises are viewed as basic requirements to allow the therapy to be successful by addressing fundamental negative relationship behaviors that undermine the partners' ability to work together. Regarding the promise of no threats of divorce or separation, couples frequently threaten divorce or separation out of anger and without much forethought, despite the fact that such threats have a very negative impact on the relationship. Of course, if one or both partners continue to have frequent thoughts of separation, this should be dealt with during a couple session. In addition, threats and occurrence of violence undermine the partners' ability to feel safe in sharing or working together to improve the relationship. We ask couples to focus on the present and future, not the past, because often couples with substance abuse disorders get caught in cycles of revisiting old wounds and grievances inflicted by the substance abuse rather than being able to move forward in the relationship. It is important to note that we ask couples to avoid negative, destructive arguments about the past at home, but we encourage discussion of past problems during couple sessions in which the therapist can help the partners communicate more effectively. Finally, it is imperative for both partners to be actively engaged in the treatment inside and outside of sessions.

Stage 2: Supporting Abstinence from Alcohol and Drugs

After initially engaging the couple, treatment quickly shifts toward helping the couple to initiate behaviors that promote abstinence from alcohol and drugs. As previously described, this principal treatment goal is a necessary precondition to addressing the secondary goal of improving the couple relationship. The primary intervention for promoting sobriety is the couple *recovery contract* (see Handout 10.1, at the end of this chapter), which is constructed during the first two "core" intervention sessions. (This and the other handouts included in this chapter are from a larger set of 31 reproducible forms provided by O'Farrell & Fals-Stewart, 2006.) The recovery contract then provides the partners with specific sobriety-related behaviors in which to engage throughout the remainder of treatment. In addition to the recovery contract, the protocol utilizes a number of interventions that promote sobriety: reviewing urges to use alcohol or drugs, decreasing exposure to alcohol or drugs, addressing stressful life problems that can serve as triggers for relapse, and decreasing the supporting partner's behaviors that reward substance use.

Treatment Challenges and Strategies

It is not uncommon for couples to struggle initially with carrying out some of the behaviors used to promote sobriety. Therapists should anticipate that these problems may arise and use these incidents as opportunities to reiterate the goals of the recovery contract and other behaviors aimed at promoting sobriety. Therapists should also help the couple to problem-solve issues that are getting in the way of carrying out these behaviors. One common barrier to completing the recovery contract occurs when the supporting partner views certain aspects of the contract in a negative way. For example, the supporting partner may believe that he or she is taking on too much of the burden of ensuring the substance-abusing partner's sobriety. In such cases, therapists should remind supporting partners that they are only responsible for their own behaviors, as indicated on the recovery contract, and that substance-abusing partners are responsible for their part. Despite agreeing to the promise of focusing on the present and the future, some supporting partners engage in bringing up past problems associated with their partners' substance-abusing behaviors. We have found that it is often effective to paraphrase supporting partners' statements, so that they feel understood. Therapists can then reframe these comments to make sure that partners with alcohol or drug problems understand the full impact of their prior negative behaviors.

Other problems can arise as a result of unintentional therapist behaviors. For example, therapists sometimes unintentionally contribute to couple noncompliance with the recovery contract by failing to provide detailed and repeated description regarding the purpose and expectations of treatment components. Therapists may also get sidetracked and fail to fully check all homework assignments. It is important to summarize briefly the rationale and specific details about homework when checking in each session. This helps to ensure that couples are reminded of the rationale, which can offset tendencies toward viewing it as not important. Therapists should also check all aspects of homework at the beginning of each session, so that couples receive the message that it is a high priority and feel consistently supported for their efforts.

Dealing with a relapse to alcohol or drugs is also a challenge that unfortunately is common, particularly in early sobriety. If a relapse does occur, couples should be encouraged to attend a session as soon as possible, since early intervention is important in trying to offset a longer relapse cycle. Sometimes couples may be hesitant to attend a session following a relapse out of embarrassment or because they are engaging in all-or-none thinking by viewing the therapy as being pointless, since sobriety was not sustained. Therapists should address this by empathizing with couples' disappointment and then explaining that relapses are not unusual within the context of recovery from alcohol or drug problems. Therapists should describe how it is important to get back on track following a relapse, and added practice can effectively help couples to achieve longer-term sobriety.

Therapeutic Components of Stage 2

Recovery Contract. The couple recovery contract (Handout 10.1) is the major method used to help couples engage in positive behaviors to promote sobriety. One important component is the daily trust discussion. A purpose of the daily trust discussion is to help the couple to reestablish trust regarding the substance-abusing partner's alcohol or drug use, which often has been highly compromised due to recurrent lies and attempts to cover up substance-using behaviors. Another purpose is to help the couple to reinforce efforts toward achieving sobriety, since past conversations are likely to have focused upon problems created by substance use. The daily trust discussion involves the substance-abusing partner asserting the following: "I have been alcohol and drug free for the last 24 hours and plan to remain alcohol and drug free for the next 24 hours. Thank you for listening and being supportive of my efforts to remain alcohol and drug free." The supporting partner then responds, "Thank you for staying alcohol and drug free for the past 24 hours. I appreciate your efforts in trying to stay clean and sober." If the person is taking a recovery-related medication (e.g., naltrexone), we encourage the substance-abusing partner to ingest the medication each day as part of the trust discussion. The trust discussion is rehearsed in session throughout treatment as a way of making sure that the couple stays on track in keeping with the important points when completing the trust discussion. In addition, the partners engage in the trust discussion each day and record their progress in completing the discussion, along with other important sobriety-promoting behaviors that we describe, on the *recovery contract calendar* (see Handout 10.2, at the end of this chapter). The recovery contract calendar helps the partners to remember to engage in their recovery-oriented commitments and to see their progress in completing these activities.

In addition to the daily trust discussion, there are several other components to the recovery contract. We explicitly indicate in the recovery contract the therapy promise to focus on the present and future—not the past, and ask the supporting partner not to bring up past or possible future substance use outside of session. This is meant to help partners to avoid arguments about substance use that escalate and keep them caught in conflictual patterns that are counterproductive to moving forward in recovery.

As part of the recovery contract, the partner with the substance use disorder is asked to consider making a commitment to self-help attendance (e.g., Alcoholics Anonymous [AA]), since engagement in self-help is shown to be positively related to treatment outcomes. Partners are also encouraged to consider support groups (e.g., Al-Anon) to help them to cope with issues they may face. Each partner indicates in the recovery contract the number of self-help meetings he or she is committing to attend and records attendance on the recovery contract calendar. If the partner with the substance use issue has a drug use problem, we encourage that urine drug screens also be incorporated into the recovery contract. If a couple agrees to this being part of the recovery contract, urine drug screens should be administered and reviewed during each session. Urine drug screen results provide objective data that can be used to strengthen the drug-abusing partner's progress in staying clean, while providing reassurance to the supporting partner. The final component to the recovery contract is to allow couples to add additional personalized ways of supporting sobriety (e.g., reading AA's *The Big Book* daily or engaging in exercise 3 days per week).

Other Support for Abstinence. Along with the recovery contract, this treatment provides other interventions to promote sobriety. One important strategy is to review urges or thoughts to drink or use drugs at each session. This is done at the beginning of each session, before discussion of other issues, because achieving sobriety is the primary goal of the treatment. This helps the couple to identify possible triggers to use and to develop strategies for coping with these. Another intervention is to utilize emergency sessions when a patient has relapsed or is at high risk of relapsing. These sessions occur outside of the regularly scheduled therapy sessions and are used to develop strategies to interrupt or prevent a relapse. This approach also helps couples to find ways to reduce the substance-abusing partner's exposure to alcohol or drugs, or to develop strategies for coping with unavoidable exposure. Finally, couples learn to identify and cease supporting partner behaviors that enable continued substance abuse (e.g., covering up when alcohol or drug use has occurred).

Stage 3: Improving the Relationship

Many BCT-SUD strategies for improving the relationship overlap with interventions found in other cognitive-behavioral approaches to treating couples, namely, interventions used to increase the frequency of positive couple activities and improve couple-based communication strategies. Due to this overlap, we provide a briefer description of Stage 3 treatment, and interested readers can look to other chapters in this book for descriptions of similar techniques applied to other presenting issues. Unlike other couple treatments, the purpose of these interventions in BCT-SUD is not only to improve the relationship but also to engage the couple in relationship behaviors that are thought to increase chances for sobriety. This added benefit to supporting sobriety may occur both directly (e.g., couple engages in shared rewarding activities that are inconsistent with substance use and that encourage sobriety) and indirectly (e.g., increased time engaging in shared rewarding activities improves relationship satisfaction, thereby reducing the likelihood of a return to substance use in response to low relationship satisfaction).

Treatment Challenges and Strategies

Couples occasionally view the initial focus on engaging in positive couple activities or utilizing positive or neutral topics in learning communication skills as meaning that the negative aspects of their relationship are being ignored or not addressed. In an effort to address such concerns, therapists should explain that the treatment initially focuses on increasing positive couple activities, since engagement in these activities is often absent or minimal when substance abuse is occurring. Therefore, the initial focus on engaging in positive relationship activities is to help the couple to practice behaviors they will find fun and rewarding, thereby increasing the chances at sobriety. Couples who are more satisfied are better able to work together on dealing with relationship problems and are more likely to achieve sobriety. Hence, the focus on increasing positive couple behaviors is setting the foundation for the partners to be able to better work effectively through their problems, while achieving sobriety.

Regarding the issue of using positive or neutral topics when introducing communication skills, therapists may use the analogy that learning communication skills is like learning to hit a baseball, crochet, or play an instrument. Learning these skills in the beginning can be difficult. Therefore, it is wise to practice with an easier setting, such as hitting a slow pitch in a batting cage rather than having a Major League pitcher throw 90 miles per hour at you. Couples should be told that once effectively learned, these skills can then be applied toward discussing more difficult topics, and couples should be encouraged to address these problems once they have obtained adequate practice and mastery using positive or neutral topics.

It is also important for the therapist to not ignore significant issues, if the couple reports a strong immediate need and desire to address these. In fact, the protocol has the therapist check in with the couple in setting the session agenda to see whether the partners would like to have time for discussing any significant relationship issues or other concerns. Unless the couple is bringing up a true emergency (e.g., relapse or violent incident), discussion of these issues should occur after checking in about substance use or urges to use, as well as last week's homework assignments, so as not to send the message that addressing the substance use or completing the homework assignments are of secondary importance.

Therapeutic Components of Stage 3

Increasing Positive Couple Behaviors. Several interventions for increasing positive couple behaviors that are found in other approaches have been adapted to BCT-SUD. One simple yet highly effective intervention for increasing positive relationship behaviors is the daily assignment to "catch your partner doing something nice." The goal is to help couples begin more regularly to notice positive couple behaviors within the relationship. This is followed with the introduction of the daily "catch your partner doing something nice and tell him or her (catch and tell)" exercise. This primary goal of "catch and tell" is to help couples begin regularly to encourage desirable relationship behaviors. Stage 3 also introduces the concept of planning and engaging in a weekly shared rewarding activity. Shared rewarding activities help to promote increased relationship satisfaction, while engaging the couple in enjoyable interests that do not involve alcohol or drug use. The couple is also introduced in to the concept of doing a "caring day" for one another. Using this approach, the partners surprises one another with a day in which they exhibit various caring gestures. The goal is to help them to engage in positive behaviors that are often lost in a relationship due to substance-abusing behaviors.

Improving Couple Communication. As with other cognitive-behavioral couples approaches, BCT-SUD provides couples with communication skills training. We believe that this is particularly relevant to substance-abusing couples, since they are shown to exhibit deficits in effective communication behaviors when compared to non-substance-abusing couples. Also, improvements in communication can help couples to address more effectively relationship issues or concerns, thereby reducing the chances of relapsing in response to interpersonal conflict. Fairly common communication skills training techniques are used, including coaching couples on nonverbal communication behaviors, direct communication of feelings, use of paraphrasing, and methods for problem solving. More basic communication skills (e.g., nonverbal communication behaviors) are introduced in earlier sessions and more advanced skills (e.g., problem solving), in later sessions.

Improving Couple Conflict Management. The couple time-out intervention, which is described in several other chapters of this book, is also incorporated in this protocol. This technique is one that we believe is especially germane to substance-abusing couples, given that various estimates of one year partner violence prevalence exceed 50% among individuals seeking substance abuse treatment (Murphy & Ting, 2010). Time-out provides the couple with a way of managing conflict when topics are becoming too heated by allowing partners an opportunity to step away from the situation, cool down, and then come back to address the issue in a more calm and collected manner.

Stage 4: Continuing Recovery

The final three sessions (Sessions 10 through 12) are primarily spent focusing upon planning for the couple's continuing recovery and discharge from weekly sessions. Many couples who have actively engaged in treatment find that they have achieved some success with sobriety and improving their relationship by the latter sessions. However, couples may begin to backslide if they stop or decrease activities that have supported these improvements. Therefore, planning for maintenance of treatment gains and prevention of relapse are thought to be critical.

Treatment Challenges and Strategies

Some couples may express reservations about ending weekly sessions. These concerns may arise out of fear that ending treatment will lead to an alcohol or drug relapse or the couple returning to negative couple interaction patterns. Therapists can address such concerns by affirming the positive treatment gains that the couple has made and pointing out that they are taking away from the therapy new skills that will help to reduce their likelihood of relapse or returning to negative couple interaction patterns. In addition, therapists should point out that a *continuing recovery plan* (see *My Continuing Recovery Plan*, Handout 10.3, at the end of this chapter) to help to keep them on track and an action plan to get back on track in the event of a relapse will be developed. Finally, we recommend couple checkup sessions or additional relapse prevention sessions following the end of the standard protocol, so couples do not need to feel that they are entirely on their own following treatment.

Therapeutic Components of Stage 4

Continuing Recovery Plan. The therapist helps the partners to compose their continuing recovery plan to maintain abstinence and positive relationship functioning. This plan essentially replaces the activities in which the partners were engaged during weekly treatment. This plan involves asking the couple to consider continuing with one or more interventions in each of the following areas: interventions from the recovery contract, positive activities, communication skills continuing recovery tools, other activities, and supporting the partner's role. In clinical practice, we encourage couples to consider following up with the therapist for a few checkup appointments every couple of months for the first 2 years following treatment. Based on data from a Veterans Administration (VA) sample suggesting that an additional 15 sessions of relapse prevention sessions improves outcomes for couples with more severe substance abuse problems (O'Farrell, Choquette, & Cutter, 1998), we recommend this more frequent contact for couples with more severe substance use problem severity.

Action Plan. The action plan is the plan that each partner will take in the event that a relapse to alcohol or drugs occurs. To introduce this, we typically use the simile that the action plan is like constructing a plan for evacuation in case of a fire. Just because the couple would have an evacuation plan for a fire does not mean that a fire is inevitable. Likewise, putting together an action plan in case of a relapse does not mean that the relapse is unavoidable. However, it is better to be safe and have a plan.

Factors Influencing Treatment

It is not uncommon for individuals with substance use disorders to have partners who also have substance use disorders. We have found anecdotally that the protocol can be effectively implemented among substance-abusing partners when both members are motivated to stop using alcohol or drugs. When implemented with substance-abusing couples, the recovery contract can be modified to use a dual recovery contract that includes a joint trust discussion and other recovery activities for each partner. Otherwise the standard protocol can be used with these cases. We believe that it would be difficult to implement this protocol effectively among these couples, unless both partners are willing to work on eliminating their problematic substance use. Therefore, among substance-abusing couples in which one partner is unwilling to commit to abstinence, we recommend trying other approaches, such as motivational enhancement prior to BCT-SUD, in order to increase the likelihood that a commitment to abstinence is reached.

Another factor that can influence treatment is when partners are living apart from one another due to not getting along. Sometimes non-substance-abusing partners will initiate a "trial period" of separation, with the understanding that the substance-abusing partner must demonstrate sobriety as a precondition of the return to living together. If it is the desire of the substance-abusing partner to reconcile and demonstrated sobriety is a prerequisite for reconciliation for the non-substance-abusing partner, this can sometimes be used as a motivation to get the substance-abusing partner to engage in sobriety-supporting behaviors (e.g., attending a self-help organization). Therapists may then want to meet with these partners to support progress toward meeting these preconditions to reconciliation but should hold off on starting this protocol until the partners reconcile and both members report commitment to work together toward positive change.

TAILORING TREATMENT TO ACTIVE DUTY OR VETERAN COUPLES

Structuring an Abbreviated Protocol

Situational factors may constrain the amount of time available to treat veterans or service members. In such cases, it may not be realistic to complete the full 12 weeks of the standard protocol. In such cases, there are several approaches that clinicians may consider. The first approach would be to deliver the standard 12 sessions, but do so in a condensed time frame, such as sessions twice per week for 6 weeks. The advantage to this approach is that couples have the opportunity to be exposed to the full protocol. A disadvantage is that this approach leaves little time for couples to practice newly acquired skills outside of session.

Rather than delivering all 12 sessions in a condensed time frame, an alternative approach is to structure an abbreviated protocol that cuts down the number of sessions. Our approach in such a scenario has been to maintain the components that focus on increasing chances for sobriety, while reducing the amount of time spent on increasing positive couple activities and improving communication. We have used this strategy because it maintains direct interventions aimed at improving the primary goal—abstinence from alcohol or drugs.

If time constraints prevent the non-substance-abusing partner from being able to complete the full protocol, there are other approaches that clinician can consider. An example of such as scenario occurs when the non-substance-abusing partner is a service member who is to be deployed in a short time frame but wants to be involved in treatment up until the deployment. One option would be to deliver the standard protocol in a condensed time frame, which would allow the supporting partner to participate fully. Then the clinician could consider augmenting with individual or group substance use treatment following the completion of BCT-SUD. Another option would be to condense the protocol by reducing the number of sessions, then augmenting with other formats of substance abuse treatment that can be attended by the substance-abusing partner alone. These are good options to consider when the substance-abusing partner is able to remain involved in treatment, because they provide the opportunity for the substance-abusing partner to receive continued care, while the supporting partner is able to have at least some levels of involvement in the treatment.

Addressing the Co-Occurrence of Posttraumatic Stress Disorder

As described in the beginning of this chapter, PTSD is a disorder that frequently co-occurs with substance use disorders for veterans and service members. Fortunately, there are data to suggest that the co-occurrence of PTSD does not necessarily impact negatively the effectiveness of this treatment in increasing sobriety and improving the relationship. In a study in a VA substance abuse treatment program, Rotunda, O'Farrell, Murphy, and Babey (2008) compared 19 veterans with a diagnosed substance abuse disorder and PTSD to a demographically case-matched group of 19 veterans with a substance abuse disorder but without PTSD. Both groups received BCT-SUD and were followed for 1 year following treatment. Results showed that both groups exhibited significant improvements in substance- and relationship-related outcomes. Furthermore, there were no differences between the group with PTSD and the group without PTSD on treatment outcomes. This may have been due to the small sample size, but it may also suggest that veterans with PTSD can achieve benefits from this treatment equal to those achieved by veterans without PTSD.

Despite these preliminary positive outcomes, the standard format of BCT-SUD does not focus upon helping veteran or military couples to reduce PTSD. In an effort to improve upon the this treatment model in treating veterans and service members who have both substance use disorders and PTSD, we are currently in the process of conducting a VA-funded pilot study that integrates BCT-SUD with components of cognitive-behavioral conjoint therapy (CBCT) for PTSD (see Monson, Fredman, & Riggs, Chapter 8, this volume). One aspect of the rationale behind developing this combined treatment is that integrated treatment for substance use and PTSD may help to address the common self-medicating cycle of using alcohol or drugs as a method for coping with PTSD symptoms. Furthermore, this integrated model shares the philosophy of BCT-SUD and CBCT for PTSD that relationship functioning has a bidirectional association with substance abuse and PTSD. Therefore, interventions aimed at improving the couple's relationship will have the added benefit of reducing substance abuse and PTSD symptoms.

Case Illustration

Stage 1

After entering medical detoxification at the local VA medical center, Jason was approached by a therapist named Anne, who asked him if it would be okay to contact his wife Cassie. Jason was initially unsure but felt relieved when Anne said she would tell his wife that his decision to seek treatment at this time showed motivation for change, and that he was progressing well in the treatment program. Anne called Cassie over the phone with Jason present, and Cassie agreed with the idea of meeting with Jason and Anne for a discharge planning session. Anne met with them the next day, and they agreed to meet with Anne following Jason's discharge from detoxification to further explore the possibility of BCT-SUD.

At the initial session following Jason's discharge from the detoxification unit, most of the session was spent on assessing the couple's reasons for seeking help, each partner's substance use history, and their current commitment to the relationship. At times during the session, Cassie became tearful in describing the damage that Jason's alcohol and marijuana use had caused to their family. They admitted to several incidents of pushing and slapping that had occurred when Jason was drinking and they began to argue over this. A further risk assessment revealed that the couple was not at risk for very severe violence, and that violence occurrence was tied to Jason's substance use behaviors. By the end of the session, Anne had determined that Jason and Cassie were appropriate to try BCT-SUD. Anne provided them with a brief overview of the treatment. Cassie reported that she felt like this could be their last chance to save their relationship, and Jason also said that he was hoping this could help.

The next week the couple attended the initial therapy session. Anne started by reaffirming the couple's commitment to starting treatment and described the "no secrets" policy. Anne then provided an overview of the treatment model and explained the four treatment promises. The partners reported that not bringing up the past would be difficult for them, but they would be willing to commit to do their best to adhere to this. After Anne explained and then modeled the trust discussion, Jason and Anne practiced this in session. Next they reviewed the couple recovery contract (see Handout 10.1). Jason would not agree to attend AA at that point, saying that he thought going to the groups and couples sessions would be enough. Jason was in agreement with Anne further exploring this issue with them as treatment progressed to see if this might fit better later on. Next they went over the "catch your partner doing something nice" exercise. Cassie was initially reluctant to engage in this exercise, saying that she was still too angry at Jason to notice anything positive that he did. Anne helped Cassie to see that noticing positives did not erase her frustrations over Jason's past drinking, but that if they worked together to improve their relationship, this could increase Jason's chances at sobriety. After hearing this, Cassie was more agreeable, and the partners took turns sharing with one another one positive behavior of the opposite partner over the course of the past week.

Stage 2

When Jason and Cassie returned for Session 2, their therapist Anne started by reviewing the typical sequence of sessions. Jason's urine screen results from the prior week were then reviewed, and Anne congratulated Jason on having a negative urine result. Cassie looked like she was relieved to hear about this result, and she verified this feeling when Anne asked her directly how she felt about this. Next they reviewed urges and thoughts to use alcohol or drugs, and Jason reported that he had thoughts about drinking after feeling frustrated by not being able to finish work on his car. Cassie couldn't believe that Jason would consider drinking, until Anne pointed out that thoughts of using in early recovery are normal, and that Jason had coped well by taking a walk. Anne praised each partner for efforts at keeping the treatment promises, although Cassie admitted to bringing up a past drinking episode on one occasion. Anne restated the rationale for not bringing up the past, and both partners committed to working on this again during the next week. In reviewing the couple's recovery contract calendar, Anne first praised the couple on completing the trust discussion on 5 of the past 7 days (see Handout 10.2). She then asked what got in the way on the 2 days the partners were unable to complete the trust discussion, and found out that this occurred after they had an argument. Anne explained the importance of completing the trust discussion daily, even if they were feeling anger toward one another, and the couple committed to try to do this daily during the next week. The remainder of the session went relatively well, with the "catch and tell" exercise being described, modeled, and practiced in session, and concluded with homework assignment and review.

Stage 3

After having several consecutive weeks of the therapy go relatively well, Cassie called Anne to report that Jason relapsed and had been drinking and smoking pot for the past several days. After experiencing an urge, Jason had decided to stop by an old drinking buddy's house, where he was offered beer and pot. This led to his using for several days in a row. At Anne's urging, the couple attended a crisis session that day and discussed a plan for preventing additional alcohol use. One good thing that arose from this experience was that Jason was now in agreement to try the AA group for veterans that met at the local VA hospital.

The couple returned for the next regular session. Anne checked in about thoughts or urges to use alcohol or drugs, reviewed the couple homework assignments, and further discussed ways that Jason could cope with the situation that led to the relapse if it reoccurred. In reviewing their progress, Anne congratulated Jason and Cassie for completing all of the commitments on their recovery contract. In addition, Jason found that he connected with some of the members from the AA group and was willing to continue with AA as part of the recovery contract.

Throughout the remainder of Stage 3, Anne introduced and built upon communication skills. At first, the in-session practice of the communication skills felt a bit awkward. However, Anne helped the partners quickly get used to this strategy by normalizing their initial feelings and providing corrective feedback by consistently affirming their positive communication strategies, while providing feedback for communication behaviors that needed improvement.

Stage 4

By Stage 4, the new skills that Jason and Cassie were learning as part of treatment began to feel more natural to them. Anne informed them that this was directly related to their hard work in repeatedly practicing these skills. Although Jason did still occasionally have urges to use alcohol or drugs, these were becoming less frequent, and he and Cassie attributed this to some of the sobriety skills they had learned, along with improvements in their relationship.

Anne spent the last several sessions helping Jason and Cassie to develop their continuing recovery plan, an action plan for dealing with a possible relapse, and summarizing their treatment progress. As part of his *continuing recovery plan*, Jason agreed to continue with AA meetings (see Handout 10.3). After discussing options for follow-up, the couple agreed to a 1-month follow-up appointment. Anne ended the session by congratulating them for their hard work and progress in treatment, and reminded them to call her prior to their 1-month follow-up appointment if Jason experienced a relapse, or if they experienced other significant issues.

SUMMARY

Substance disorders are a significant problem among substantial numbers of men and women who serve in the military and their families. Among individuals with substance use disorders, there typically exists a bidirectional relationship between the substance use disorder and the relationship functioning with their partners. BCT-SUD directly addresses this bidirectional relationship by targeting couple behaviors that improve the chances at sobriety and by using interventions that promote increased positive couple relationship behaviors and improved communication. This protocol is shown to be superior to individual-only approaches to treating substance use disorders, and this evidence includes studies with veterans. BCT-SUD has strong applicability to veterans and service members given that it is a flexible treatment that can be easily integrated with other treatments for substance use disorders.

RESOURCES

Kulka, R., Schlenger, W., Fairbank, J., Hough, R., Jordan, B., Marmar, C., et al. (1990). *Trauma and the Vietnam war generation: Report of findings from the National Vietnam Veterans Readjustment Study*. Philadelphia: Brunner/ Mazel.

Marshal, M. P. (2003). For better or worse?: The effects of alcohol use on marital functioning. *Clinical Psychology Review, 23*, 959–997.

Milliken, C. S., Auchterloine, J. L., & Hoge, C. W. (2007). Longitudinal assessment of mental health problems among active and reserve component soldiers returning from the Iraq War. *Journal of the American Medical Association, 298*, 2141–2148.

Murphy, C. M., & Ting, L. A. (2010). The effects of treatment for substance use problems on intimate partner violence: A review of empirical data. *Aggression and Violent Behavior, 15*, 325–333.

O'Farrell, T. J., Choquette, K. A., & Cutter, H. S. G. (1998). Couples relapse prevention sessions after behavioral marital therapy for male alcoholics: Outcomes during the three years after starting treatment. *Journal of Studies on Alcohol, 59*, 357–370.

O'Farrell, T. J., Choquette, K. A., Cutter, H. S. G., Brown, E., Bayog, R., McCourt, W., et al. (1996). Cost–benefit and cost-effectiveness analysis of behavioral martial therapy with and without relapse prevention sessions for alcoholics and their spouses. *Behavioral Therapy, 27*, 7–24.

O'Farrell, T. J., Cutter, H. S. G., Choquette, K. A., Floyd, F. J., & Bayog, R. D. (1992). Behavioral marital therapy for male alcoholics: Marital and drinking adjustment during the two years after treatment. *Behavior Therapy, 23*, 529–549.

O'Farrell, T. J., Cutter, H. S. G., & Floyd, F. J. (1985). Evaluating behavioral marital therapy for male alcoholics: Effects of marital adjustment from before to after treatment. *Behavior Therapy, 16*, 147–167.

O'Farrell, T. J., & Fals-Stewart, W. (2006). *Behavioral couples therapy for alcoholism and drug abuse*. New York: Guilford Press.

O'Farrell, T. J., Van Hutton, V., & Murphy, C. M. (1999). Domestic violence before and after alcoholism treatment: A two-year longitudinal study. *Journal of Studies on Alcohol, 60*, 317–321.

Rotunda, R. J., O'Farrell, J. J., Murphy, M., & Babey, S. H. (2008). Behavioral couples therapy for comorbid substance use disorders and combat-related posttraumatic stress disorder among male veterans: An initial evaluation. *Addictive Behaviors, 33*, 180–187.

HANDOUT 10.1

Recovery Contract

Instructions: Use this form to formalize each partner's responsibilities as part of the BCT recovery contract.

In order to help (patient) _____ with his or her recovery and to bring peace of mind to (partner) _____, we commit to the following.

Patient's responsibilities	Partner's responsibilities
❒ Daily Trust Discussion (with medication _____ if taking it)	
• States his or her intention to stay substance free that day (and takes medication if applicable).	• Records that the intention was shared (and medication taken if applicable) on calendar.
• Thanks partner for supporting his or her recovery.	• Thanks patient for his or her recovery efforts.
❒ Focus on Present and Future, Not Past	
• If necessary, requests that partner not mention past or possible future substance abuse outside of counseling sessions.	• Agrees not to mention past substance abuse or fears of future substance abuse outside of counseling sessions.
❒ Weekly Self-Help Meetings	
• Commitment to 12-Step meetings: _____ _____	• Commitment to 12-Step meetings: _____ _____
❒ Urine Drug Screens	
• Urine drug screens: _____ _____	

(continued)

☐ Other Recovery Support	
• _____	• _____

Early Warning System

If, at any time the trust discussion (with medication if taking it) does not take place for two days in a row, we will contact (therapist/phone #: _____) immediately.

Length of Contract

This agreement covers the time from today until the end of weekly therapy sessions, when it can be renewed. It cannot be changed unless all of those signing below discuss the changes together.

_____   _____
        Patient   Partner

_____   _____/_____/_____
       Therapist   Date

Recovery Contract Calendar

Instructions: Couples should complete this form to track their engagement in the daily trust discussion and other recovery contract activities.

☐ ✓ = Trust Discussion Done   ☐ A = AA or NA meeting   ☐ D = Drug Urine
+ or –

☐ ✓ = Trust Discussion with   ☐ = Al-Anon or Nar-Anon   ☐ O = Other
Medication (_____)   (_____)

Mo & Yr: _____							Mo & Yr: _____						
S	M	T	W	T	F	S	S	M	T	W	T	F	S
☐	☐	☐	☐	☐	☐	☐	☐	☐	☐	☐	☐	☐	☐
☐	☐	☐	☐	☐	☐	☐	☐	☐	☐	☐	☐	☐	☐
☐	☐	☐	☐	☐	☐	☐	☐	☐	☐	☐	☐	☐	☐
☐	☐	☐	☐	☐	☐	☐	☐	☐	☐	☐	☐	☐	☐
☐	☐	☐	☐	☐	☐	☐	☐	☐	☐	☐	☐	☐	☐
☐	☐	☐	☐	☐	☐	☐	☐	☐	☐	☐	☐	☐	☐

My Continuing Recovery Plan

Instructions: Partners should complete this form to indicate details of how they will continue to implement their skills learned as part of the therapy.

As part of my continuing recovery, I have checked the tools, activities and skills I will practice and use to maintain sobriety and continue to improve my relationship after weekly couples therapy ends.

1. Recovery Contract

_____ Trust discussion (daily)

_____ Take medication (_____) during trust discussion

_____ Regular support meetings

_____

_____

2. Positive Activities

_____ Catch and tell

_____ Shared rewarding activities (___ ×/week)

_____ Caring day (___ ×/week)

3. Communication Skills

_____ Communication sessions (___ ×/week)

_____ Listening and understanding

_____ "I" messages

_____ Relationship agreements (specify: _____)

_____ Problem solving

_____ Time-out—as needed

4. Continuing Recovery Tools

____ Action plan to prevent or minimize relapse

____ Couple check-up visits (1-month follow-up)

____ Couple relapse prevention sessions

5. Other

_____

_____

_____

6. Partner's Role (completed by partner)

_____

_____

_____

CHAPTER 11

Combat-Related
Traumatic Brain Injury

Shirley M. Glynn

Steve was in the U.S. Army Reserves in Iraq for a second deployment; he worked in Transportation. He and Cindy had been married 3 years and had a young son, Michael. As Steve was traveling with his buddies in a convoy about 5 weeks before he was to rotate home, his vehicle hit an improvised explosive device (IED) while he was driving. Usually Steve sat on the passenger side during the first half of the run. However, on this day he "wanted something to do" and told his crew he wanted to drive first. Two of Steve's buddies on the passenger side were killed and Steve was blown out of the humvee and smashed his head on the ground. Everything seemed like it was happening in slow motion and it took a few seconds, maybe a minute or two (he lost track of time), to understand what had occurred. Steve felt dazed. His head hurt but he checked himself—nothing seemed broken and he did not see blood. He ran over to his buddies but their bodies were a mess; there were medics in the convoy, and they said there was nothing to do but call for reinforcements, retrieve the bodies, and head back. When the medics asked Steve how he was, he told them fine—nothing broken. Steve was pretty shaken up—his head hurt, his ears were ringing, and he was nauseous. He could not remember much about the ride back to the base. He got checked out by medical staff on base but did not volunteer much about what he was experiencing. He was working very hard just to be calm but felt awful—he would have been killed if he had been in his usual place on the passenger side during the drive.

Steve did go home a month later. Cindy knew about his buddies who were killed and worried that he might have some posttraumatic stress disorder (PTSD) symptoms when he came home—he was jumpy, remote, irritable, had difficulty sleeping, and did not seem interested much in her or Michael. He was drinking more than he had and seemed distant. Even more striking, Steve seemed more disorganized, less motivated, and forgetful. He would say he would do something—pay the bills, repair the car—but it did not happen. He complained of headaches a lot and felt dizzy. He did not seem to be interested in school or work. Cindy thought Steve should do something—go talk to the chaplain on base or maybe the doctor at the Veterans Affairs Medical Center (VA)—but Steve was not willing. He did enroll at the local VA so he would be eligible for benefits and care, but he did not pursue any treatment. Steve knew (but did not tell Cindy) that he had screened positive for likely PTSD at his discharge; he was not inclined to get treatment and felt he would recover with time. Cindy and Steve argued more and more; she grew increasingly resentful and found it hard to be kind to him. She decided to call staff at the local Vet Center and see if they could help.

The struggles of service members and veterans with traumatic brain injury (TBI) can be stressful and disruptive to family members, and emerging data suggest that being exposed to highly stressed family members can impede recovery. In such a closed system, family intervention can be critical to improved functioning in the service member or veteran. This chapter begins with a brief description of the circumstances, incidence, and symptom patterns in TBI as typically found in combat veterans, with an emphasis on the recent conflicts. Family issues reported in relatives who care about someone who has experienced a TBI are then discussed, followed by a description of the mutual interplay of family and veteran factors that influence outcomes. The current state of research on family interventions for TBI is then discussed, followed by a description of an emerging best-practice, couple-based, phasic intervention. This time-limited couple-based intervention incorporates three components that appear essential to addressing the needs of a service member or veteran with TBI and his or her partner: (1) education about TBI, co-occurring disorders, and self-care; (2) developing problem-solving skills to address deficits and symptoms resulting from the TBI; and (3) targeted strategies to strengthen the couple's emotional intimacy. Moderating factors likely to influence treatment outcome are then outlined, with suggestions for how these interventions can be tailored to the needs of an active duty and veteran population. A description of Cindy and Steve's treatment, highlighting critical points made in the chapter, is interwoven into the text.

INCIDENCE AND IMPACT OF TBI IN OPERATION IRAQI FREEDOM/OPERATION ENDURING FREEDOM SERVICE MEMBERS AND VETERANS

In the current Operation Iraqi Freedom (OIF) and Operation Enduring Freedom (OEF) conflicts, the most common types of physical injuries result from blasts, land mines, and IEDs—homemade bombs, often placed in cars on the side of the road, that are detonated as service members drive by. Because most service members wear armored flak jackets, their trunks are protected. However, their limbs, necks, and heads are exposed, which means these are most commonly injured.

Blasts and IEDs often knock service members off their feet and blow them a distance. The pressure of the blast itself can cause injury, and service members may also take hard hits to their heads. While some service members may incur multiple injuries simultaneously, others may have no obvious wounds, but their heads may still have rocked hard back and forth in their helmets, causing their brains to sway in cerebral fluid and repeatedly hit the skull from within. These are called "concussive injuries," and they can be deceptive. The person with the injury may lose consciousness for only a brief period or not at all, and there may be no blood seen. However, the individual may still have sustained a TBI, especially to the frontal lobe, that part of the brain responsible for "executive processing"—that is, using strategies for planning for the future, reasoning, weighing options, and restraining impulses. A list of TBI symptoms is presented in Handout 11.1, *Facts about Combat-Related Traumatic Brain Injury*, at the end of this chapter.

TBIs are classified into mild–moderate–severe categories based on disorientation and uncommunicativeness at the time of the trauma, duration of posttraumatic amnesia, and length of loss of consciousness. Although severe TBIs are usually apparent at the time of the injury, the presence of mild to moderate TBI may not be recognized for days or weeks after the injury (often well after deployment), which can further complicate diagnosis and treatment. This chapter emphasizes mild to moderate TBIs, because these are most prevalent in the current conflicts. Those individuals with more severe TBIs likely have experienced polytrauma and have been seen in intensive medical facilities that direct specialized attention at family issues from the initiation of treatment.

One of the most widely cited studies of OIF/OEF veterans' health, conducted by the RAND Corporation (Tanielian & Jaycox, 2008), found a "probable" TBI prevalence of about 20%. Although these estimates may be high, because they are typically based on brief screens conducted retrospectively rather than by actual medical evaluations at the time of the injury, many OIF/OEF service members have acquired a TBI. Most persons sustaining a mild TBI make a complete recovery within 3–6 months, and thus there is little impact on long-term functioning; however, 10–30% of persons with a mild TBI continue to have residual difficulty, with gradual improvement over time (Management of Concussion/mTBI Working Group, 2009). Moderate and severe TBIs usually also improve gradually over time but often result in permanent impairments. Since the service member or veteran may not initially recognize or may be reluctant to acknowledge a problem, family members may be the ones most vocal about the reduced functioning resulting from the injury.

Combat-related TBI typically occurs within the context of a traumatic event; thus, symptoms of PTSD and TBI often co-occur. Some studies indicate that PTSD partially mediates concussive injury and subsequent symptoms. Given the overlap in symptoms in the two disorders (e.g., irritability, sleep problems, concentration difficulties), accurate diagnosis can be difficult, and comorbidity is common. Not surprisingly, many individuals with a TBI also become depressed or anxious and may use alcohol or drugs in an abusive manner to deal with their distress.

Family treatment for a combat-related TBI occurs within a system that is dealing with (or has dealt with) readjustment issues. The family that confronted stressors while the service member was deployed is now facing a new set of stressors when he or she returns home. Much has been written about the impact of multiple deployments, extended tours of duty, brief periods at home between deployments, real-time communication in the battlefield, and changed family roles during deployment on the readjustment processes (e.g., Institute of Medicine, 2010). It is critical that providers who see these couples consider these stressful background factors, while still targeting issues emanating from the TBI that affect the relationship.

To this point, there is little research on family issues and TBI of service member and veteran samples. Thus, the literature regarding adjustment in relatives of young adults who have incurred brain injuries in the civilian sector, augmented with the clinical experience acquired in Department of Defense (DoD) and VA Medical Centers, serves as the foundation for the couple intervention for combat-related TBI presented here. In extrapolating the work from civilian to service member and veteran samples, it is critical to remember that there are unique characteristics of the two populations. Research with civilians tends to comprise persons with moderate to severe TBI and their relatives, whereas service member and veteran samples are more likely primarily to comprise individuals with mild to moderate TBI. Furthermore, civilian studies vary dramatically in length of time from the injury; some studies evaluate the survivor and relatives days after the trauma, whereas others collect data years later. Finally, while the focus of this chapter is on couples issues, the majority of the civilian investigations enroll a cross-section of caregivers.

CONCEPTUAL AND EMPIRICAL UNDERPINNINGS

A review of the literature on partners of civilians who have experienced a TBI (Blais & Boisvert, 2005) reveals the following: (1) Heightened levels of distress include clinical conditions such as depression or anxiety, in partners of persons with a TBI, though typically less than half the sample report these problems; (2) relatives' distress is more accurately predicted by long-term impairment, especially behavioral and emotional problems resulting from the TBI, than by severity of initial injury; (3) partners' successful adaptation after a TBI is enhanced by problem-focused coping, positive reappraisal of stressful situations, and seeking social support (the latter especially among women); and (4) the couple's use of active coping skills is associated with better relationship satisfaction. There are data from civilian samples indicating higher divorce rates in couples in which a partner has experienced a TBI, but data regarding divorce from service members and veterans with TBI have not yet been reported.

Data collected from all types of TBI caregivers, not just partners, suggest that just as caring for a person with a TBI may impact negatively on the caregiver, the caregiver's behavior and attitudes may impact either positively or negatively on recovery from the TBI. Sander et al. (2002) found that family dysfunction assessed soon after admission to a postacute rehabilitation facility predicted less improvement, poorer functioning, and less vocational achievement 1 month after discharge in a sample of civilians with severe TBI. Drawing from the literature on the role of relatives' expressed emotion (i.e., criticism and overinvolvement) in predicting relapse in schizophrenia and bipolar illness, Weddell (2010) found that high expressed emotion in families was related to poorer outcomes in civilian patients with TBI. These data highlight the importance of helping families cope well with TBI, not just to reduce their own stress and burden, but to facilitate the recovery of their loved ones.

Evidence of Treatment Efficacy

A detailed review of the literature on family interventions in TBI is beyond the scope of this chapter. In brief, the methodology is highly variable, and there have been few randomized controlled trials. Most studies include a variety of relatives, with only one report thus far that has focused exclusively on partners in marriage or similar relationships; that study was a small successful feasibility trial of a Web-based intervention for female caregivers. Some studies have used individual family approaches and others have used multifamily groups. Although the interventions studied have differing components, the common elements include emphasis on problem solving and education about the disorder. Overall, the outcomes from most of the interventions have been modest, with studies reporting more benefits to caregivers than to TBI survivors; in part, this predominance of caregiver findings results from the fact that many studies have not collected data from the TBI survivor.

Taken together, the studies provide some insight into what an effective couple-based intervention for TBI might include, but only one has targeted the special problems of couples, and none has focused on combat-related TBI. As with any couple-based intervention to be delivered in the context of one member of the couple having an individual disorder, the clinician must first clarify the desired outcome of the couple work. Is the primary goal improvement in the individual disorder? Increase in couple satisfaction? Reduction in partner burden or distress? These are all worthy but different outcomes. The selection of a target treatment goal is a particularly salient issue in the field of TBI, as many of the published family interventions had their genesis in the physical rehabilitation and disability field. Common treatment goals, such as "reduction of caregiver distress" or "meeting unmet caregiving instrumental needs," predominate in that literature, with much less written about reducing psychopathology or addressing relationship dissatisfaction. Confronted with this lack of systematic information, clinicians working with couples in which one partner has a combat-related TBI will likely benefit most from integrating therapeutic approaches from empirically validated strategies to address the common symptoms of TBI. These common symptoms include cognitive and communication skills deficits, inappropriate affect, and behavioral excesses and deficits. Clinicians should also include techniques to reduce partner distress and strengthen the relationship. As suggested by Kreutzer, Marwitz, Godwin, and Arango-Lasprilla (2010), both cognitive-behavioral and family systems interventions can be useful in addressing the broad array of problems found in survivors of a combat-related TBI and their partners.

GUIDELINES FOR ASSESSMENT AND INTERVENTION

The couple-based intervention program outlined here incorporates three components that appear essential to addressing the needs of service members and veterans with TBI and their partners: (1) education about TBI, co-occurring disorders, and self-care; (2) addressing instrumental concerns through problem-solving skills training (e.g., developing compensatory strategies for TBI-related memory problems); and (3) focal strategies to increase the couple's emotional intimacy. Sessions are conducted conjointly. Some TBI family interventions have focused solely on circumscribed goals (e.g., improving problem solving) or have only included caregivers. A broader program that includes both partners and targets the TBI survivor's functioning, while simultaneously strengthening the relationship, is likely to be most effective.

Although the intervention begins with education, the order and relative emphasis of the other two components are guided by the couple's presenting problems and current strengths, as revealed in initial preintervention assessment sessions. Couples who are coping with many instrumental problems may prefer to do problem solving first, whereas those with a great deal of couple distress might benefit from work on strengthening the relationship first. Ideally, 50- minute sessions should be held weekly, because if too much time elapses between sessions, participants may forget the material. There is also more opportunity for perceived crises to emerge, which tend to derail the agenda and limit the opportunity for skills building. Nevertheless, families have competing demands and may not be able to schedule sessions every week. The couple's treatment should be embedded in a comprehensive program that includes case management, pharmacology, rehabilitation, and individual psychotherapy as warranted by the issues being experienced by the service member or veteran and his or her family. This is a time-limited but flexible length program. After the assessment, a minimum of 13 sessions is needed to cover the material, but some couples may benefit from more time because of the presence of complex problems or more severe deficits from the TBI.

Assessment Phase

Most typically, the couple therapist will not be making an initial diagnosis of TBI; this usually is done by a physician or neuropsychologist prior to the couple therapist becoming involved in the case. With the DoD and VA-mandated TBI screening of all returning OIF/OEF veterans in 2008, there is now a common point of entry for services and benefits. If couple therapists suspect undiagnosed TBI, they might administer brief screening tools, including questions to verify (1) exposure to a trauma that might have caused a TBI; (2) some indication of brain involvement at the time of the incident (e.g., loss of consciousness, confusion, amnesia, concussion); and (3) verification of present difficulties (e.g., memory problems, balance problems, or irritability). A positive screen would merit referral to a medical professional for further evaluation.

Over the course of the initial sessions, assessment of the following seven domains is critical to the development and implementation of an appropriate treatment plan: (1) the nature of the injury and current functioning, (2) comorbidities, (3) the past and current state of the dyadic relationship, (4) the role of other key supporters in the couple's life, (5) distress and coping in the partners, (6) joint understanding of the TBI, and (7) couple strengths. We encourage therapists to meet with the partners together for an initial session to begin developing an alliance, set the stage for further work, and start obtaining information on the areas outlined earlier. The tone can be conversational, and the therapist should encourage give and take between the partners. The therapist should use general queries that are typical of first sessions with all couples, such as "What made you decide to call for help now?" or "Who made the decision to call?" Time should also be allotted to begin collecting information in the seven domains outlined earlier. The session concludes with scheduling of a second assessment session in which the therapist meets with each partner individually. The goals of the therapy and how potential complicating issues raised in the individual sessions are also discussed. The clinician might say,

> "We have been talking about the possibility of couple therapy as one option for you, and that work is designed to move the two of you forward together. If the individual assessment uncovers information unknown to your partner that would compromise our work (e.g., an affair, unacknowledged spending or gambling debts), and I see issues that might be better dealt with individually first, I might recommend that option, and we would need to reconsider whether couple therapy is the best option at this time."

It is important that the therapist present a hopeful but realistic stance during the initial meeting. Because the treatment plan will evolve out of the assessment, committing to a course of couple work is delayed until the assessment is completed. It is essential to leave some leeway to recommend other options besides couple therapy if the assessment uncovers mitigating factors such as severe domestic violence or a lack of commitment to the relationship.

In the second assessment meeting, further information is collected in the seven domains noted earlier. One partner is interviewed while the other completes brief objective measures of mental health and relationship difficulties, and vice versa; the clinician clarifies that, based on his or her clinical judgment, information obtained in the individual interviews and assessments will be shared as necessary if they all decide together to proceed with the couple work. The assessment of comorbidities such as substance use; anxiety disorders, including PTSD; and depressive disorders is important as these problems may impact the progress of the couple work and may require additional individual attention (see Monson, Fredman, & Rigs, Chapter 8; Whisman & Sayers, Chapter 9; and Schumm & O'Farrell, Chapter 10, for suggested assessment strategies in this volume). In terms of dyadic functioning, assessing satisfaction, areas of conflict, and level of aggression is critical. Couples in which a high level of physical aggression is identified may be more appropriate for referral to programs targeting reduction of domestic violence, prior to work to address the issues raised by the TBI. The clinician must also be alert to safety planning issues if physical aggression is an issue in the relationship (see Heyman, Taft, Howard, Macdonald, & Collins, Chapter 7, this volume). Clinicians should also inquire about how instrumental tasks are being completed in the family and identify challenges in the completion of these tasks. Finally, as noted earlier, partners of persons with a TBI often experience high levels of distress themselves. It can be useful to have the partner complete measures of depression, anxiety, and substance use, as well to identify whether these problems will require special attention. It is also important for the clinician to elicit any feelings of resentment, discouragement, or guilt the partner may be having; to normalize these feelings; and to encourage self-care. Finally, open-ended interview queries can be useful in identifying accurate knowledge about TBI.

The clinician should review and integrate all of the data obtained in the first two sessions prior to a feedback session (typically, the third meeting). The goal is to identify areas of couple strengths and of problems or deficits, and to arrive at a consensus treatment plan for the next stage of intervention. In the feedback sessions, if the TBI-related couple work seems appropriate, brief descriptions of the three components of the intervention are presented, and the clinician and couple discuss their relevance to the couple's current situation and struggles. The order in which the interventions would most likely benefit the couple is determined. Ground rules regarding attendance, sharing of information, discussion of material outside of sessions, minimal number of sessions to be scheduled, importance of out-of-session practice, and the implications of couple rather than individual treatment are reviewed as well.

Case Illustration: Assessment Phase

Steve and Cindy arrived at the Vet Center on time for their initial assessment appointment. Cindy was very talkative during the interviews; Steve used mostly one- or two-word answers. Both indicated they had had a good life before Steve went to Iraq but now they were arguing a lot. Cindy felt burdened by school, work, and parenting their infant son Michael. The job Steve had as a delivery driver prior to being deployed to Iraq was not available when he came home—the company had been sold—and he was not putting much effort into finding a new job. He mostly hung around the house, watching TV during the day. This exasperated Cindy. Steve was having trouble sleeping and felt edgy. He was irritable with Cindy and the baby, and Cindy admitted, "I give as good as I get." They had had one shoving incident during an argument; otherwise physical aggression was not a problem. Finances were tight. Steve did not like going out much; he was very tense as he drove, but he did not want Cindy to drive. They almost never went out as a couple. Steve was drinking two to three beers a day to relax, although he denied symptoms of dependence.

During the feedback session, the therapist noted the couple's strengths: They still had good things to say about each other; they were committed to each other and their son; they both had good career prospects; and Steve was no longer in the Reserves, so they could settle down. The therapist noted the following deficits: Steve seemed aimless, unmotivated, and not able to get back on a path; Cindy was overburdened and had no time to relax; Steve seemed to have a number of symptoms of TBI and PTSD but was not getting treatment; and as a couple they were having many conflicts and did not seem able to defuse angry situations. The couple agreed with the formulation and to attend the couple treatment. Cindy was very concerned about their finances and Steve's not working; Steve admitted the problem but did not think he could be a driver anymore—his concentration was "shot" and he was too nervous. When the clinician and the couple discussed the possible order of treatment components, they decided to start with education, then to work on Steve's getting a job or something to do with his time, and to conclude with relationship strengthening.

Intervention Session Format

It is useful for the clinician to follow a standard agenda for each session: inquire about urgent issues that need to be addressed, briefly review material from the last session, follow-up on out-of-session assignments, present new material, and plan the next out-of-session assignment. In contrast to some other couple interventions, the program here is directive and structured. The ultimate objective is to promote skills and instill attitudes and beliefs that will support recovery from the TBI and shore up the intimate relationship.

Many families dealing with a TBI and readjustment issues are chaotic. It is important that the therapist recognize, but not get caught up in, the whirlwind of the relationship. The therapist is encouraged to follow the agenda and not get derailed by nonurgent issues. Strategies therapists can use to adhere to the format include (1) having a written agenda on a flipchart or whiteboard, so all participants can see the session plan each time; (2) keeping a formal running record of nonurgent topics that are collected by the therapist but deferred until later in the treatment (e.g., may be addressed again during problem solving); (3) reminding participants of the time-limited nature of the intervention, their prior agreement to the structure, and the wisdom of developing skills prior to tackling other issues. Of course, issues such as risk of harm to self or others, substance use increase or relapse, or treatment nonadherence are urgent and require immediate attention, even if that means delaying work planned for that session. Because TBI survivors are uniquely sensitive to ambient stress, the therapist should monitor and contain tension in the session to facilitate optimal learning. If conversations get overly heated, the therapist should rapidly intervene by interrupting, making a reframe, or calling a time-out as needed.

Phase I: Education and Self-Care

Treatment Challenges and Strategies

Unless there are compelling reasons to do otherwise, it is useful to begin the intervention with two sessions of education about TBI, augmented by a third session devoted to a discussion of the postdeployment experience if the couple was in their relationship during the deployment, and a fourth session on self-care. An additional session on education about PTSD should also be offered, if warranted. Although much of the formal TBI educational material can be covered in one session, scheduling time between sessions allows participants to bring up issues or questions they may not be able to access during the first session. In addition, this provides a slower pace for the session, which can be essential if the person with cognitive difficulties as a result of TBI is to absorb the information. Typically, to compensate for attentional and memory difficulties, verbal information is supplemented with take-home handouts that participants are encouraged to read between sessions. Some service members or veterans with TBI develop residual reading difficulties; in such cases, the noninjured partner is encouraged to take the lead in reviewing the written materials during out-of-session assignments.

Although it important to impart factual information during the education phase of the program, "learning facts" is primarily a means to greater therapeutic goals—partners' developing increased empathy for each other, developing attainable functional goals, and understanding the importance of following the recommended treatment plan. Normalization of their experience is also critical. The service member or veteran is identified as the "expert" on TBI from the phenomenological perspective, and he or she is encouraged to speak about living with it. Many families that may have read about TBI have not actually had a conversation in which the person with the injury discusses what it is like to be unable to follow a newspaper or movie anymore, or always to feel tired and have a headache, or to have no motivation. Conversely, the partner can talk about his or her worries and fears. The clinician is vigilant for opportunities to bolster any empathic

statements made by participants and to emphasize any strengths or rehabilitation successes identified.

Therapeutic Components

The format involves imparting information on TBI etiology, prognosis,
treatment, and factors that improve or impede outcome (see Handout 11.1).
Similar information should be presented on co-occurring disorders after
the discussion of TBI. In light of the high co-occurrence of PTSD and TBI,
clinicians should routinely plan to provide education on PTSD unless the
screening indicates it is not a factor (see Monson et al., Chapter 8, this volume). Information is communicated in an informal style, using the strategies and format promoted in the health risk communication literature (see
the VA/DoD's Management of Concussion/mTBI Working Group [2009]
for a discussion of health risk communication in TBI). Key principles of
effective health risk communication include demonstrating empathy, eliciting participants' perspectives, using shared decision making, and providing
honest and accurate information.

Clinicians benefit from using open-ended, Socratic questioning and
summaries of participants' statements as the primary intervention technique during these sessions; the goal is to elicit as much accurate information from the participants as possible, rather than to lecture. If this is a
new area of intervention, clinicians will need to learn about TBIs prior to
the session. In view of the wide variability in TBI symptom presentations,
talking to the survivor's neurologist or other members of the rehabilitation team can also be extremely helpful in deciding which information to
present and emphasize in the education. The second session concludes with
a discussion of the service member/veteran's current prescribed treatment
plan for TBI and other disorders. Components of the program, as well as
adherence issues, are identified and strategies to resolve problems are discussed.

Following the education sessions, a session is allotted to discussion
of the postdeployment experience, if the couple was together prior to the
deployment. The therapist asks the partners in turn to talk about (1) what
they had hoped the postdeployment period would be like, (2) what it has
actually been like for them, (3) what has been good, (4) what has been hard,
(5) how their partners have helped them, and (6) how they each would like
it to be going forward. The therapist lists the six topics on the board or
flipchart to guide the discussion. The therapist moderates the conversation, allowing partners to take turns sharing, and ensuring that each has
adequate time to speak. The goal is to facilitate the partners' reconnecting with each other based on shared expectations and desires for family
life. The therapist underscores any positive feelings or empathic statements

each partner expresses. As always, the therapist should be alert to signs of friction and intervene if the conversation involves personal attacks or argumentative comments.

A final educational session is devoted to developing self-care skills, which can be critical for both the person with the TBI and others assisting him or her. The tasks of this session are to have the partners identify the current stressors in their lives, list the current ways they deal with the stress, and commit to using two new positive coping behaviors to reduce stress levels over the course of the therapy. The session focuses on Handout 11.2, *Stress and Self-Care*, at the end of this chapter, which participants are asked to complete as an out-of-session assignment prior to the session. The therapist begins the self-care session by asking the couple why self-care is important. After the importance of self-care is highlighted, responses to Handout 11.2 are reviewed. Participants discuss their current stressors and ways of dealing with them, and the strategies they have agreed to practice during the couple treatment. If the participants are unfamiliar with the concept, the therapist can allot 10 minutes of the session to practicing deep breathing for relaxation. During this session, it is critical that the partner be allotted sufficient time to discuss the challenges of supporting the injured service member or veteran, and ways to obtain support for him- or herself. Referrals to appropriate support groups can also be helpful.

Case Illustration: Intervention Phase I

Although Steve was initially reluctant to acknowledge he was experiencing aftereffects from the IED attack, he did endorse a number of TBI symptoms after he read the related handout. Cindy had understood that his headaches and fatigue were likely related to his TBI but had not realized his amotivation and disorganization were also likely related. As she absorbed this, she began to be less strident with Steve. The therapist also noted that Steve seemed to be experiencing symptoms of PTSD—intrusive memories, numbing, avoidance, and irritability. Steve finally admitted to Cindy that he had screened positive for PTSD during the VA intake evaluation and that the evaluator had recommended that Steve pursue treatment, but he had thought things would improve over time and treatment scared him. The therapist inquired about what Steve knew about the treatment options for PTSD and TBI. Steve was not sure, and his therapist asked him to follow-up with the VA OIF/OEF Coordinator before the next session, so he could let Cindy know his options. The two agreed that they had expected the post-deployment period to be much different than it was—they thought they would be happy to be together again as a family as they prepared to buy a house and put down roots. Steve mentioned that he could not imagine being that settled anymore. He found it hard to think about the future, and he never felt well; nothing felt "important." Cindy got a little upset during the conversation—she was clearly ready to settle down—but the therapist was able to reframe Steve's reluctance to move ahead as a desire to do his best by Cindy and Michael, and not make a mistake in caring for them. Cindy grew calmer when she thought of it this way. When the couple discussed self-care, they both agreed that Cindy was carrying the bulk of the load and needed a break, and that if Steve could start taking care of Michael a couple of hours a week, Cindy could go out and see a friend or shop—just to have a few hours to herself. The thought of leaving the baby with Steve made Cindy a little anxious, but she offered to help Steve get more comfortable with the baby so that he could do it.

Phase II: Developing Problem-Solving Skills to Address Residual Deficits and Symptoms Resulting from the TBI

Treatment Challenges and Strategies

Through information collected in the assessment phase and observation in the educational sessions, the clinician now has a picture of which symptoms and deficits are causing the most strain for the service member or veteran and their partner. Although conducting a full rehabilitation program for the service member or veteran is outside the bounds of this treatment, the couple clinician can play a pivotal role in helping find solutions to common problems, as well as helping the couple implement solutions suggested by other healthcare professionals. Typically four to five sessions are devoted to this phase, and the problems addressed are those identified by the service member or veteran and partner as highest priority. Usually, one session is spent on each problem, with progress monitored at the beginning of subsequent sessions; typical problems might include addressing fatigue, developing strategies to remember important events or appointments, dealing with anger or irritability, or coping with urges to drink or use drugs. Sometimes problems are complicated and require work in multiple sessions. The problem-solving strategy proposed here is particularly useful for addressing practical or symptom-related issues—everything from remembering what to get at the store to deciding whether to continue in treatment. However, we find that this strategy works best with instrumental issues; couples' affiliative concerns are most effectively targeted by the third component of the program, which involves enhancing emotional intimacy.

A standard problem-solving training format, originally developed by D'Zurilla and Goldfried (1971), is implemented to address residual symptoms and difficulties, as well as to increase coping efforts. In the literature on family interventions for mental health disorders, there is wide variability in how much emphasis is placed on *teaching* participants to use a strategy to solve problems versus actually *solving* problems in the sessions. The goal in this program is to *teach* the skill, so participants can use it after they leave the program. This emphasis on teaching the skill sometimes delays arriving at the actual solution, but the benefits of providing a strategy that participants can use when they leave the program merit the effort and the brief delay to resolve an issue (typically just a few minutes or continuing on to the next session).

A final word about addressing common problems in TBI is in order. Persons with TBI can experience a wide variety of symptoms—amotivation, somatic complaints, anger problems, and impulsivity. These problems can be difficult to resolve and often require sustained work over time. Although problem solving can be an effective strategy in addressing these issues, it can also be helpful for the clinician to inform couples about strategies others have used to resolve these problems. Thus, clinicians working with service members or veterans with TBI and their partners benefit from learning multiple strategies to resolve typical TBI problems. The clinician can offer these ideas as solutions during the brainstorming phase of the problem solving, or can even direct the couple to these materials, if the content is relevant to them.

Therapeutic Components

As with all skills training, this technique is introduced by eliciting a rationale for improving the skill—that is, by asking participants how they usually solve problems and whether there might be any benefit to strengthening their problem-solving efforts. The steps of the six-step problem-solving technique are then reviewed, using a written handout (see Handout 11.3, *Problem-Solving/Goal-Setting Record*, at the end of this chapter). The training style is conversational, not didactic. The clinician asks the couple about each component of the skill (e.g., "What do you think it means to define the problem?"; "Why do you think it might be best to think of a few solutions prior to picking one?"). The objective in all these interactions is to enhance motivation to do the work by helping participants develop personalized understandings of the advantages of the process. The clinician can also give the participants a completed problem-solving sheet as an additional teaching tool. It is important to foster a problem-solving orientation throughout the therapy; that is, differences or challenges are viewed by the couple as problems to be solved rather than issues about which to argue.

The clinician then asks the couple to identify an initial problem for problem-solving. There are typically many possibilities—the couple and clinician will have the problems identified in the initial assessments, as well as topics or issues that were deferred in the education phase of the program. Consistent with a skills training approach, the goal is for the couple to have a mastery experience in working on the first problem, so optimally the problem selected is one that lends itself to a relatively easy solution. The couple is encouraged to start with a simple problem. The therapist can say, "This is the one where we are going to use training wheels before you take off on the bike on your own." In shaping an initial exemplar for training, optimal problems are those (1) that are more likely to increase the positive tone in the couple; (2) for which the therapist can think of a likely successful, implementable solution easily; and (3) for which there does not seem to be a great deal of conflict. Problems such as spending more time together (if the partners get along well when they are together), figuring out a way to take medication regularly, making doctors' appointments, and developing strategies to remember things better are often good as first training opportunities.

In training the skills, the clinician does not lead the discussion; he or she assumes more of a "coach" role in helping the couple go through the process and recording the information on the form. Typically, one member of the pair is asked to chair the problem-solving discussion each time. This role can rotate, but to facilitate the initial successful experience, it is optimal to select the participant who can most easily read and complete the form for the first problem. The clinician then prompts the Chair to lead a discussion on each step of the skills. For example, the clinician might say, "Okay, Chair, what is step 3? I see 'List the advantages and disadvantages of each solution.' So now you can lead a discussion on these and make sure to list them on the form." The clinician's comments are directed to the Chair, so that partner can learn how the process works and the couple can develop a sense of empowerment about it. It is important for the clinician to be alert to problems that may arise in implementing the procedure; typical sticking points include evaluating solutions before they are all generated and not fully developing, implementing, and monitoring the solution. Written records of the problem-solving efforts are kept, so that if there is an obstacle in implementing solutions between sessions, the form can be reviewed at the beginning of the next session and difficulties identified (e.g., the wrong problem was defined, or the plan for implementation was not sufficiently developed). The couple is encouraged to consider problem solving as an iterative process in which new attempts to resolve issues are made if the first attempt is unsuccessful.

Because the goal of this phase is mastering problem solving to resolve issues with the TBI, couples should complete at least three problem-solving efforts before ending this component of the treatment. Typically, successful resolution of a problem involves some work at home, so out-of-session assignments are an integral component of the problem-solving work. It is critical that the therapist and couple come to an explicit agreement about out-of-session work each week. As a routine part of the development of homework assignments, potential obstacles to completion should be identified and addressed *prior to leaving the session*. Couples are encouraged to continue using the strategy for other problems as they arise, and the clinician can do more problem solving in subsequent sessions if it appears warranted.

Case Illustration: Intervention Phase II

Steve and Cindy had opted to work on problem solving prior to working on emotional intimacy in their relationship. During the early part of the work, Steve was also exploring TBI and PTSD treatment options at the VA. Cindy wanted to work on getting more income into their marriage; thus, Steve had to figure out what to do about a job. The therapist encouraged them to "start small"; Steve was the Chair of the first problem-solving session, and they decided to pick an inexpensive activity they could do together as a family. They worked on the problem and decided to have a picnic in the park not far from the house, and to walk there so Steve could relax. Steve was surprised at how much he enjoyed being with Michael when they were out of the apartment. The couple then started working on the issue of Steve's job. They defined the problem as "finding a job for Steve that uses his driving skills but does not involve driving," since driving still made him apprehensive. Cindy chaired this problem solving session and they came up with some good solutions. Steve decided to look for an auto mechanic job. In addition to driving, he had helped to keep the vehicles in good shape in Iraq and thought that working with tools (rather than driving) would help his concentration. The couple made a plan for Steve to start getting a resumé together and putting in applications. Looking for work became part of Steve's out-of-session assignments.

Phase III: Focal Strategies to Increase Emotional Intimacy

Treatment Challenges and Strategies

For a couple, the TBI occurs against the backdrop of their relationship. Many couples will have known each other long before the service member or veteran experienced the TBI; thus, both members need to adjust to "the new normal"; other couples meet after the incident and do not have a shared preinjury life. Whether a couple has been together 10 months or 10 years, the experience of a TBI is likely to bring stressors into the relationship. The noninjured partner may need to compensate more for the partner with the TBI; role expectations and demands may shift. Whereas education and problem solving can reduce some of this stress and thereby improve the bond between the partners, it is essential that the couple-based intervention also focus on strengthening the relationship by increasing emotional intimacy. Although some of this work can be interwoven into all therapy components, allocating at least four sessions to specifically altering and improving the way the partners understand and interact with each other is recommended.

Strategies to Be Interwoven in the Therapy from the Beginning to Strengthen the Relationship

Throughout treatment, the therapist should identify and acknowledge any positive interactions or experiences noted by the couple. For example, if the partners mention having a nice evening or weekend, the therapist should express curiosity about that event and spend a few minutes eliciting specific details to help the partners identify their strengths and promote hope and optimism; for example, "That's good to hear. What made it so good? What do you do (partner X) to contribute to that? How about you (partner Y)?"

Increasing empathy between partners is also a critical aspect of strengthening the relationship. The therapist should be alert to opportunities to underscore "soft feelings" or vulnerabilities that each member spontaneously expresses; these include feelings such as "being hurt," "feeling sad," "being disappointed," "being discouraged," "being worried" (rather than being "angry," "pissed off," or "mad"). One easy way to highlight these feelings is for the therapist to stop the discussion briefly when these feelings are articulated, paraphrase the statement, and then inquire briefly about it, especially from the listener. Was this new information? Did it make the partners feel closer?

Finally, during education and problem-solving efforts, the therapist can differentially attend to issues that are likely to strengthen the couple's relationship. For example, from the assessment it will become clear whether misunderstandings about the legitimacy of symptoms are contributing to relationship conflict. The partner who may not understand that amotivation is a typical symptom of TBI may attribute lack of effort to "laziness." Clarifying this inaccurate characterological appraisal is an important part of the education work. Similarly, in selecting issues for problem solving, the clinician can encourage tackling issues that appear to have the most impact on the relationship. These might include problems that both partners identify as a stressor on the relationship (e.g., anger problems or lack of time together).

Sessions Primarily Devoted to Increasing Emotional Intimacy

Many couples dealing with a combat-related TBI are highly distressed. They are often young and have been living with the uncertainties and stressors of military life and war (e.g., relocation, limited financial resources, separations, possibility of injury or death); they often have young children and are now dealing with difficulties caused by TBI and (often) PTSD. In working with couples experiencing high levels of relationship distress, the reader may also wish to consult basic texts in this area (e.g., Jacobson & Christensen, 1993). However, even in a conjoint treatment targeting symptoms of TBI, we believe attention to strengthening the relationship is in order.

Therapeutic Components

There are two primary goals in this phase of the work: (1) to increase immediate positive reinforcement in the relationship through the use of a behavioral exchange exercise, and (2) to increase the probability of long-term satisfaction within the relationship by improving empathic communication. After the results of the problem-solving strategies are reviewed, the behavioral exchange exercise, as modified by Jacobson and Christensen (1993), is begun. A rationale of partners working independently over the next few weeks to increase their satisfaction in the relationship is first discussed, eliciting as much of a rationale from the couple as possible. Each participant is then asked, before the next session, to make a list of actions that convey love and caring to the other person. Each is instructed that the partner *should not* be consulted in creating the list and should have no input at this point. The list of items generated should range in intensity from small (e.g., making coffee in the morning) to large (e.g., letting the partner select where the couple lives). The partners bring their respective lists to the next session (or spend some time completing the list at the beginning of the next session, if they did not do it), then spend the bulk of the session discussing the lists. The therapist inquires about the specifics of each item (e.g., "Why do you think this means love and caring?") and helps to shape any vague items into clear behaviors that can be observed. Again, the partner who will be the recipient of these behaviors is not queried at this point; he or she only listens. However, the therapist can work to expand the list if the potential recipient of the behaviors has made a request not mentioned on the list. The other partner's list is reviewed in the same way. Then, each partner is asked to use the list to increase the other's satisfaction until the next session. Again, the participants are instructed not to discuss the activities with each other and are told that their effort is not contingent on the other's behavior (i.e., not "tit for tat"). Rather, each is working independently to improve the life of the other. As with all out-of-session assignments, it is useful to spend some time troubleshooting before the couple leaves the session (e.g., "What could go wrong? How could we prevent that?").

During the next session, the results of the exercise are discussed. The therapist inquires what it was like for each "giver" and each "receiver." Successes are highlighted, and problems are acknowledged as well. The receiver is now also queried about the items on the giver's list and can indicate whether each item is "a keeper," "minor but still pleasing," or "off the mark." The list is refined, and the receiver is also given the opportunity to suggest other items for the partner's list. The out-of-session assignment to practice the work at home again is given. This exercise is then routinely assigned throughout the remaining therapy sessions. At each subsequent session, the clinician briefly queries about how that behavioral exchange effort is proceeding and reminds the couple at the end of the session to keep working on the exercise.

The second goal in this phase of the therapy is to promote empathic communication through communication skills training. As with all skills training, the process begins by eliciting a rationale for the skills training from the participants—in this case, by asking the partners why it might be beneficial to "sharpen up" their communication. This language avoids implying that their communication is currently deficient and may therefore reduce resistance. In addition to whatever reasons the partners identify for improving their communication, the need to compensate for attentional and memory problems accruing from the TBI is also noted. The clinician then asks the couple to define the characteristics of good communication, looking for approximations of the key features outlined in Handout 11.4, *Good Communication Elements*, at the end of this chapter.

The clinician provides the partners with the handout on good communication and, to increase commitment to using the skills, asks them why each feature is important. The clinician then demonstrates the first skill and obtains feedback about the partners' observations of this skill. The therapist then sets up the first practice for the couple. This role play involves practicing active listening. The clinician outlines the characteristics of active listening (i.e., good eye contact, nodding one's head, saying "uh uh", asking clarifying questions, summarizing what was heard). Each partner is given the opportunity to express a positive feeling about an experience or characteristic of the other partner, and that partner practices his or her active listening skills. The speaking partner is then prompted to give feedback to the listening partner about his or her use of the skills; the goal is to provide positive feedback first. One simple way to elicit this positive feedback is to ask the partner, "What did you like about that?" If the speaking partner has a difficult time identifying positive feedback for the listener, the clinician should focus on the specifics the listener evidenced (e.g., "What did you like about his or her eye contact? Was he looking at you?"). If the listener demonstrates good use of skills, the roles reverse, the listener becomes the speaker, and the process is repeated. If the listener has difficulty performing the skill adequately, he or she is given a prompt about how to improve during a second trial (e.g., "This time when you do it, I want you to be sure to paraphrase—summarize—what she said. Any questions about that? Okay, let's begin") and the role play is completed a second time, with the same round of positive, constructive feedback. A third role play may be necessary.

Active listening, expressing a positive feeling, making a positive request, and expressing a negative feeling are all practiced. This typically requires at least two sessions, and participants are asked to practice between sessions and can be given a sheet on which to record the results. Many couples struggling with TBI may benefit from more practice or work on advanced skills such as "requesting a time-out" and "compromise and negotiation." If so, the reader is referred to the section on communication skills training in Mueser and Glynn (1999) for details on developing more complex problem-solving and communication skills.

The goal of this phase of the treatment has been identified as the development of empathic communication. Active listening can be a cornerstone of empathic communication, but couples are also encouraged, as their skills develop, to move from simple paraphrasing of comments to adding a statement about the speaker's likely feelings. This is demonstrated below.

Case Illustration: Intervention Phase III

As Cindy and Steve entered the final phase of the couple work, some things were going very well; Cindy was glad Steve was applying for jobs and seemed to be enjoying his time with Michael. Cindy was trying to get out of the house for a couple of hours alone each week, although she was only able to manage to do this about half of the time. Steve had finally started seeing a psychiatrist at the VA and was now prescribed medication for sleep; he had been offered individual psychotherapy but was not sure he wanted to pursue it. Steve and Cindy had a difficult time with the beginning of the behavioral exchange exercise. Steve had a hard time thinking of things that pleased Cindy, and she was hurt by that. She thought that if Steve really cared for her, he would know what she liked. However, the therapist helped Steve put items on his list that Cindy had mentioned during the therapy, reminding Cindy that because TBI often results in memory difficulties it would be good not to hold these against Steve. Once they started doing the behavioral exchange exercises, they felt more connected with each other.

Then they started the communication skills training; here is an example from that session.

THERAPIST: So, Cindy, now it is your turn to express a concern or negative feeling to Steve, and Steve, you are going to use your active listening. Remind me again, Steve, what the tools of active listening are?

STEVE: Keep my mouth shut!!! Face her—look her in the eye—repeat what she says—ask a question if I do not understand.

THERAPIST: Great Steve—just right. Okay, Cindy, and what were the key parts of expressing a negative feeling?

CINDY: I should look at him—be clear and specific about what I am upset about—use an "I" statement—and tell him how he could prevent this in the future.

THERAPIST: Great, Cindy, you got all the points. You can begin.

CINDY: (*looking at Steve*) Steve, I am really angry you are drinking again. You know the doctor told you to cut down.

STEVE: A couple of beers will not hurt. You nag me too much.

THERAPIST: Steve, active listening, right? Look at the sheet.

STEVE: Right, okay. You are angry because I was drinking last week. And I guess you are worried, too, since the doctor told me to stop because it is not good with my meds.

THERAPIST: Is that right, Cindy? Worried, too?

CINDY: Yes, really worried. If he starts drinking a lot—I mean I like a drink, too—but then we fight. I am tired of the fighting.

THERAPIST: So he caught you were angry and worried—great, Steve. Cindy, you don't want to fight anymore—you want to be close to Steve. And Cindy, how about the other points of active listening? Did Steve get those? What did you like?

CINDY: Well, not the first time. But he did the second time. He looked at me and did not interrupt and repeated what I said.

THERAPIST: And how did you feel about the fact he understood you were worried even though you did not say it?

CINDY: Like he understood me—he knows I am concerned.

THERAPIST: Thanks, Cindy. He knows you. Steve—just right the second time. And it was great you also identified that Cindy was worried—even though she said angry. Let's do it again and this time, Steve, I want you to use the active listening tools right after Cindy stops, and make sure you get in she looks worried, too, even if she does not say it.

The clinician continued with the exercise even when there were opportunities to get derailed, focused on the positive, prompted Steve and Cindy to give specific feedback to each other, structured multiple role plays, and highlighted statements that reflected empathy.

Steve and Cindy concentrated on improving their communication skills in the next three sessions, then felt ready to end the therapy as planned. Steve had not found a job, but he had a couple of interviews and was hopeful. He also felt more connected to Michael and Cindy, though it was still hard for him to find the words to express how he felt, and he hated being so forgetful. Cindy was pleased that they completed the entire program, had decided to lighten her courseload a bit to give herself a chance to "breathe," and understood more about Steve's challenges. She was happy that he was going to the VA and sleeping a little better, although she still worried about his drinking. Both thought they were arguing less often and that they knew how to stop things when it got heated.

FACTORS INFLUENCING TREATMENT

At least three issues that merit attention in the TBI-related couple work may influence whether it is a viable treatment alternative. The first of these is the severity of the TBI. This chapter has emphasized mild to moderate TBI, but some service members or veterans acquire more debilitating TBI, which more seriously compromises their ability to function. Although education, problem solving, and communication skills training can assist them and their families, the limitations imposed by the TBI often mean that the underlying structure of the family must change. The noninjured partner often must assume greater responsibility for the sustenance of the family and meeting its instrumental and nurturance needs, especially if there are children involved. Ensuring the survival of the family, rather than strengthening the couple's bond, becomes the primary goal. In such cases, the noninjured partner may benefit more from individual supportive sessions in which he or she can vent frustration, resentments (if any), and loss, without stressing the injured partner. These are also useful venues for obtaining information on resources to help with basic needs such as disability applications or respite care.

A second moderating factor is the strength of the relationship prior to the TBI. If the partners knew each other before the injury, they will have established a set of implicit and explicit rules about how things "work" in their relationship (e.g., partners are kind or critical, trustworthy or not, competent or not). If the TBI occurs within the context of a strong relationship, there are resources to draw upon to bolster the participants during the recovery phase. If the TBI occurs in the context of a relationship already marked by strife, the couple may have fewer resources to bring to this stressful period. Couple therapy for TBI assumes that the noninjured partner is willing to provide the injured partner support and sustenance during the recovery phase. Although the noninjured partner must have some needs met in the therapy, the format and treatment goals of the therapy recognize that the participants are not "on a level playing field," and that one needs greater assistance and attention than the other. Individuals whose baseline levels of relationship satisfaction or interpersonal functioning are so low that they do not want or cannot make the kinds of accommodations required to support the partner in recovery often have difficulty in the therapy. For example, the wife of a veteran with TBI may be depressed and have little energy to work on the relationship if she was also unhappy in the marriage before the injury. These issues are often apparent during the initial assessment sessions, wherein the noninjured partner may express little warmth, perspective-taking ability, or empathy for the TBI survivor, even with probing. In such a situation, the clinician can offer the couple a few TBI educational sessions and then reconsider the treatment plan. These early sessions may meet some of the couple's needs and will provide more data for the clinician to determine whether the more extended couple treatment will be a viable alternative, or if the couple might benefit more from a traditional couple intervention or individual therapy.

A third, complicating issue involves feelings of grief and loss about "how things used to be." These feelings vary dramatically across families. Although severity of the residual impairment plays a role, *perception* of the change is at least, if not more, important. The therapist must acknowledge and honor the perceived loss, but also can use cognitive reframing to highlight any benefits of the change. For example, not being able to pursue a career aggressively may mean a TBI survivor has more time to nurture his or her children.

TAILORING TREATMENTS TO ACTIVE DUTY OR VETERAN COUPLES

Adapting the Protocol to Abbreviated Interventions

This treatment is designed to be administered in about 4 months of weekly sessions, usually to include three assessment sessions (with feedback) and 13 intervention sessions. If a couple's relationship is conflictual, it typically takes the full allotment of sessions, and additional boosters may be helpful. Some couples may have a difficult time attending weekly sessions because of transportation or scheduling constraints. In such cases, two adaptations of the model are helpful. With some couples, meeting every other week in person for longer sessions can be useful. Extending these sessions to 90 minutes permits coverage of the material in an expeditious fashion. In these circumstances, a brief, scheduled phone session with the couple between sessions to check on progress or problems with out-of-session assignments and scheduled breaks during the face-to-face sessions to address concentration issues can facilitate learning. As a second option, the therapist can continue weekly sessions but alternate between meetings in the clinic and sessions conducted over the phone, as long as the partners have two lines or a speaker phone, so they can be on the phone simultaneously. A number of family groups in the VA who are now using the phone or even the Internet for family sessions are reporting success with these strategies. The key is planning in advance for the couple to have access to all of the paperwork and out-of-session assignments and handouts, until they see the clinician again, and inquiring about what the experience on the phone is like for them.

Tailoring Treatment to Separated or Deployed Couples

Couples who are separated but wish to continue to work on their relationship are candidates for this intervention, as long as they agree to do out-of-session assignments together as appropriate. In working with these couples, the clinician should augment the initial interview with directive questions so that she or he can understand how the partners evaluate a potential for reconciliation (or even mutual support). If either partner does not seem willing or capable of committing to working with the other in a 4-month program, then this is likely not the appropriate intervention. Deployment of service members with a significant TBI does not occur frequently. If deployment occurs, deferring couple treatment until partners can attend together rather than trying to accommodate separation and distance issues is recommended.

SUMMARY

Both the VA and the DoD are working to create treatments to remediate the symptoms of TBI. Often, the work involves developing effective compensatory strategies to overcome cognitive and emotional deficits, and couple interventions can be an ideal vehicle for this work. As it becomes more and more apparent that family attitudes and behaviors play a critical role in influencing recovery in TBI survivors, programs to help couples develop the skills and beliefs to move forward in their lives are becoming increasingly viable and necessary.

RESOURCES

Blais, M., & Boisvert, J. (2005). Psychological and marital adjustment in couples following a traumatic brain injury (TBI): A critical review. *Brian Injury, 19*, 1223–1235.

D'Zurilla, T. J., & Goldfried, M. R. (1971). Problem-solving and behavior modification. *Journal of Abnormal Psychology, 78*, 107–126.

Institute of Medicine. (2010). *Returning home from Iraq and Afghanistan: Preliminary assessment of readjustment needs of veterans, service members, and their families.* Washington, DC: National Academies Press.

Jacobson, N. S., & Christensen, A. (1993). *Acceptance and change in couple therapy: A therapist's guide to transforming relationships.* New York: Norton.

Kreutzer, J. S., Marwitz, J. H., Godwin, E. E., & Arango-Lasprilla, J. C. (2010). Practical approaches to effective family intervention after brain injury. *Journal of Head Trauma Rehabilitation, 25*, 113–120.

Management of Concussion/mTBI Working Group. (2009). *VA/DoD clinical practice guidelines for management of concussion/mild traumatic brain injury (mTBI).* Retrieved November 1, 2011, from *www.healthquality.va.gov/mtbi/concussion_mtbi_full_1_0.pdf.*

Mueser, K. T., & Glynn, S. M. (1999). *Behavioral family therapy for psychiatric disorders.* Oakland, CA: New Harbinger.

Sander, A. M., Caroselli, J. S., High, W. M., Jr., Becker, C., Neese, L., & Scheibel, R. (2002). Relationship of family functioning to progress in a post-acute rehabilitation programme following traumatic brain injury. *Brian Injury, 16*, 649–657.

Tanielian, T., & Jaycox, L. H. (2008). *Invisible wounds of war: Psychological and cognitive injuries, their consequences, and services to assist recovery.* Arlington, VA: RAND Corporation.

Weddell, R. A. (2010). Relatives' criticism influences adjustment and outcome after traumatic brain injury. *Archives of Physical Medicine and Rehabilitation, 91*, 897–904.

Facts about Combat-Related Traumatic Brain Injury

Instructions: Use this handout to provide information about the common effects of traumatic brain injury (TBI), the severity levels of TBI, and commons symptoms of TBI.

TBI is the most common physical injury in the OIF/OEF conflicts.

There are estimates that 10–20% of OIF/OEF service members have incurred a TBI.

Most OIF/OEF TBI results from closed head injuries—such as being hit with something or hitting the head after an explosion, or just being close to a big explosion and being exposed to the percussive pressure waves.

There are many kinds of TBI symptoms.

Common Effects of a TBI			
Physical:	**Cognitive:**	**Communication:**	**Behavioral and Emotional:**
Headache, sleep changes, fatigue/ loss of stamina, dizziness, balance problems (tendency to fall), sensory changes	Confusion, slowed speed of processing, attention problems, difficulties with memory, planning and organization problems, difficulty with decision making and problem solving, recalling events that did not actually happen	Difficulty speaking clearly, problems starting a conversation, word-finding problems, problems following a conversation, reading comprehension problems	Frustration, increased anger/ aggressiveness, impulsivity or difficulties in self-control, poor judgment, reduced or lack of initiative, repetitive behaviors, less effective social skills, changes in sexual behaviors, lack of self-awareness

(continued)

Multiple exposures to head trauma likely make symptoms worse.

TBIs can be classified as mild, moderate, or severe. TBIs are classified in severity based on what happened at the time of injury.

Severity Grades of TBI		
Mild (Grade 1)	**Moderate (Grade 2)**	**Severe (Grade 3 & 4)**
Altered or loss of consciousness (LOC) < 30 minutes With normal CT & MRI	LOC < 6 hours with abnormal computed tomography (CT) or magnetic resonance imaging (MRI)	LOC > 6 hours with abnormal CT or MRI
Glasow Coma Scale (GCS) score 13–15	GCS 9–12	GCS < 9
Posttrauma amnesia (PTA) < 24 hours	PTA < 7 days	PTA > 7 days

Most of the TBIs suffered by service members in Iraq and Afghanistan are in the mild–moderate range.

Typical symptoms of a mild TBI (also called a *concussive injury*) are listed in the table below. It is important to note that *mild* refers to the circumstances at the time of the injury, not to the impact of the symptoms on the service member or veteran and his or her family.

Postconcussion/Mild TBI-Related Symptoms		
Physical Symptoms: Headache, dizziness, balance disorders, nausea, fatigue, sleep disturbance, blurred vision, sensitivity to light, hearing difficulties/ loss, sensitivity to noise, seizure, transient neurological abnormalities, numbness or tingling	**Cognitive Symptoms:** Difficulties in attention, concentration, memory, speed of processing, judgment, executive control	**Behavior/Emotional Symptoms:** Depression, anxiety, agitation, irritability, impulsivity, aggression

(continued)

At least 70% of persons with a mild TBI recover within about 3 to 6 months. It is not yet known why a subset does not recover as quickly. Some have argued that ongoing symptoms may be more related to other physical health and psychological problems such as posttraumatic stress disorder (PTSD).

Clinicians cannot predict who will make a full recovery from a TBI and who will not.

It is important to have hope. People can recover from TBIs. Often, survivors experience slow but gradual improvements over months and even years.

Treatment for a TBI involves rehabilitation—targeted efforts at specific problems such as memory, irritability, and so forth. There are no medications to cure TBI, but some help to improve symptoms such as poor concentration.

Many people with a TBI also develop other problems—PTSD, depression, anxiety, and substance use are most common. These can often be treated with medication or psychotherapy.

Loving someone with a TBI can be hard. Survivors usually do better if their families can develop accepting and supportive, positive attitudes, become good problem solvers, and take care of themselves as well. Trying to avoid existing problems is usually not a good strategy.

Stress and Self-Care

Instructions: Use this handout to help partners consider stressors that they are facing and healthy ways for them to cope with their stress.

We all live with stress and it can be hard to deal with. Partners coping with a TBI do better if they find positive ways to cope with stress. What are some of the stressors you are currently facing? _____

_____

How do you cope with them? _____

_____

_____

Which of these strategies are you willing to try to reduce stress as you go through the couple treatment? Circle at least two you will try this week. If they help, we would like to continue using them. If not, we would like you to try new ones.

Guided imagery

Do physical exercise

Take a nap

Talk with friends or family

Read a book, newspaper, or magazine

Make a list, prioritize, and do one thing on the list each day

Don't be a perfectionist; good enough is often good enough

Try deep breathing

Eat nutritiously

Other _____

Concentrate on what is controllable, not on what's not controllable

Do a favorite hobby

Go for a drive

Say "no" when you are overwhelmed

Let the little things go

Go for a walk or a run

Look for the positives

Pray

Take a short break

Do some problem solving

Get enough sleep

Do (or plan) something fun

Problem-Solving/Goal-Setting Record

Instructions: Use this handout to facilitate the couple's problem-solving or goal-setting discussions. Remind the partners to wait to evaluate their solutions until they consider advantages and disadvantages of each solution.

1. Discuss the problem or goal. Get everyone's opinion. Try to reach agreement on exactly what the problem/goal is. Write down specifically what the problem /goal is. _____

2. Brainstorm at least three possible solutions (five is better). Do not evaluate them at this time—wait until Step 3._____

3. Briefly evaluate each solution. List major advantages and disadvantages.

Advantages   **Disadvantages**

_____

_____

_____

_____

4. Choose the best solution(s). Consider how easy it would be to implement each solution and how likely it is to be effective. _____

5. Plan the implementation. When will it be implemented?_____

What resources are needed and how will they be obtained?_____

Who will do what to implement the solution? _____

List what might go wrong in the implementation and how to overcome it.

_____

Practice any difficult parts of the plan. _____

Who will check that all the steps of the plan have been implemented?

_____

6. Review implementation at next meeting (Date: _____). Revise as needed.

Good Communication Elements

Instructions: Use this list of good communication elements to teach partners how to better communicate with one another. Encourage them to review these elements as they practice communicating outside of session.

- Maintain good eye contact.
- Use "I" statements ("I feel _____when you _____").
- Be specific about the event or behavior upon which you are commenting.
- Make sure you are close enough to hear each other.

Examples:
Active Listening
- Look the speaker in the eyes.
- Nod your head.
- Say "Uh huh."
- Paraphrase what you have heard.

Expressing Positive Feelings
- "I feel happy that you cleaned the bathroom."
- "I felt relieved that you called the family meeting when you said you would."

Making a Positive Request
- "I would appreciate it if you would pick up your clothes off the floor. It would make me feel happier if we shared the responsibilities."
- "I would feel proud if you really tried to complete the school semester without any more absences."
- Expressing Negative Feelings (usually combined with a positive request)
- "I am hurt that you criticized me in front of the kids. In the future, I would feel less upset if you would wait until we were alone."
- "I am frustrated that you forgot to pay the rent again. I would feel calmer if you would make sure you pay it a day or two before it's due."

CHAPTER 12

Grief and Loss

David M. Scheider, Lance Sneath,
and Thomas C. Waynick

Staff Sergeant Anderson and his wife, Anna, had struggled emotionally for a year since their daughter Maria was killed in an automobile accident during their last assignment in Germany. They
had recently endured the anniversary of her death and decided to
pursue therapy together to manage their loss more effectively. Sergeant Anderson admitted that, in the midst of their shared pain,
he and his wife had withdrawn from each other. Their isolation
had been interrupted by intermittent episodes in which one or
the other tried unsuccessfully to engage the other. These attempts
usually erupted into a volcano of anger that always seemed to end
in threats of divorce. They had grown more despondent and now
wondered if they could ever find happiness together. However,
they had two other children and could not imagine confronting
them with even more loss than they had already endured. Both
parents successfully provided comfort to their children; now they
needed help to support each other.

The Andersons are illustrative of a normal couple experiencing an atypical
family life event. In this age of superior healthcare, couples are often ill
equipped to accept that their children could precede them in death. Partners can often effectively comfort each other in the event of a more predictable loss, where one member suffers a loss and the other provides care.
However, when both are in despair and unavailable to the other, resentments can build, and a sense of mutual abandonment often replaces intimate bonds.

Any couple who loses a child faces the grief of their catastrophic loss, and military life can complicate that already complex grief dynamic. Such was the case for the Andersons. Their loss occurred far from their present duty station, overseas where they had been stationed less than a year. Because of the death, the military gave them the option of returning stateside. Unfortunately, due to Sergeant Anderson's job skills, the assignment had to be on the other side of the United States from where their extended families resided. No one at their current duty station had been in the community where the accident occurred; indeed, few knew of their loss. Some days Anna sat and cried, remembering the place off the autobahn where the accident happened. She felt that part of her had been left there 7,000 miles away. Although it was common in her culture to return to the scene of a death and even place roadside remembrances, because the couple was tied to the military, this was not possible.

Service members, veterans, and their families often manage multiple losses simultaneously. They grieve for losses from frequent moves, normal life changes, combat deaths of friends, and reduction of mutual support that come after each combat tour. They grieve losses of physical functioning accompanying serious combat-related injuries. In many respects, the military is a culture with expected grieving. Such multiple losses render military families more susceptible to protracted and complicated grief.

Because both members of a couple often grieve multiple losses, military couples may find that neither partner is available to provide support to the other. Although numerous resources offer guidance for counseling individual military members or surviving spouses experiencing grief, and some for counseling couples outside the military or veteran setting (e.g., Wills, 2003), few resources are available for guiding grief therapy with military and veteran couples specifically. In this chapter we describe an approach that is informed by recent meta-analyses of grief therapy that treats couples with complicated grief with interventions that strengthen the marital bond and encourage partners in their search for meaning. We conceptualize these issues in an interpersonal framework and illustrate the intervention with a case study. We also discuss resources that are available to the clinician in supporting the grieving military or veteran couple.

THE INCIDENCE AND IMPACT
OF COMPLICATED AND NORMATIVE GRIEF

Specifying the incidence and impact of complicated grief and normal variants of grief and loss in either civilian or military/veteran samples presents unique challenges. First, as discussed further below, the operational criteria for distinguishing normal from complicated grief are ambiguous at best and vary considerably across cultural and subcultural contexts—including those defined by ethnic, religious, and familial backgrounds. Second, the precipitating events that result in grief responses are conceptualized and categorized in diverse and inconsistent ways. From a narrow perspective, these may be restricted to deaths of members of the immediate or extended family. More broadly, precipitants may include deaths of close friends or others in a shared community (including a military unit). However, significant losses and complicated grief responses frequently follow events other than death—including nonlethal physical injuries (loss of limb or either motor or sensory function), loss of community (including geographic moves or separation from work or military service), loss of status or role, and other transitions that involve loss of either an emotional attachment or substantive aspects of one's own identity.

The terms "grief," "mourning," and "bereavement" are frequently used interchangeably but have important distinctions (Stroebe, Hansson, Schut, & Stroebe, 2008). "Bereavement" is commonly used to denote the objective situation of having lost someone significant through death. "Grief" is a term applied primarily to the emotional reaction to the loss of a loved one through death or some equally impactful loss. "Mourning" is often distinguished from grief, and refers to the public or social expressions or acts of expressive grief that are shaped by the beliefs and practices of a given society or group.

The text revision of the fourth edition of the *Diagnostic and Statistical Manual of Mental Disorders* (DSM-IV-TR) suggests that expressions of bereavement often mirror those of a major depressive disorder, but notes that grief responses may be considered to deviate from a normative response if any of the following is present: (1) symptoms are still present 2 months after the loss; (2) guilt about things other than actions taken or not taken by the survivor at the time of death; (3) thoughts of death other than the survivor feeling that he or she would be better off dead or should have died with the deceased person; (4) morbid preoccupation with worthlessness; (5) marked psychomotor retardation; (6) prolonged and marked functional impairment; or (7) hallucinatory experiences other than thinking that he or she hears the voice, or transiently sees the image, of the deceased person.

Others (e.g., Prigerson, Vanderwerker, & Maciejewski, 2008) have argued for a separate diagnosis of prolonged grief disorder. Prigerson et al. estimate that in U.S. civilian samples, on average, four persons are significantly affected by another person's death, and that 11% do not progress through normal grief. Whereas normal grieving typically involves significant reduction in symptoms such as disbelief, yearning, or despair after 6 months and significant progress toward acceptance within 24 months, by contrast persons exhibiting prolonged grief disorder have enduring and intense "longing and yearning for the person who died . . . feel bitter over the loss and wish desperately that their life could revert back to the time

when they were together . . . have little hope that he or she will find fulfill-
ment in the future . . . feel that life lacks meaning and purpose without
the deceased, and find it extremely difficult to move on with their lives
by forming other interpersonal relationships and engaging in potentially
rewarding activities" (p. 170).

Against this conceptual backdrop, the following statistics can be cited.
As of 2011, since the initiation of Operation Iraqi Freedom (OIF) in 2003—
and including Operation Enduring Freedom (OEF) beginning in 2001—
there have been over 4,800 combat-related deaths among U.S. service members. The number of recorded significant injuries is considerably higher,
with more than 46,000 from these combined operations. Reflected in these
statistics is neither the number of affected family members—spouses, parents, children—nor the number of service members or veterans impacted by
comrades killed or injured in action. Also not reflected in these statistics are
equally profound complicated grief reactions to nonphysical injuries—the
broad array of emotional traumas and their sequelae—experienced by service members and veterans, and resulting in significant, enduring impairment in their individual and relationship lives.

Like most cultures, the military is often insensitive to the longevity
of the grieving process. Once the service member returns from emergency
leave to bury the dead, supervisors expect a high level of functioning. In the
past, grieving personnel were often unsupported by supervisors, who felt
that it was time to get on with normal life and work. Currently, the military has a heightened awareness of grief, trauma, and depression. Supervisors are now encouraged to provide counseling support for those who are
not functioning well because of combat or relational problems. With an
inflated suicide rate, the message is becoming increasingly clear that referring service members to counseling is to everyone's advantage.

However, like all systems, there is a need for continual education and
accountability. The most obvious inhibitor to grieving in the military is
the lack of emotional support from extended family and friends. Because
military families move frequently, many are geographically separated from
families of origin and their communities. Likewise, many military and veteran families break connections with the religious structures of their child-
hoods. Lacking emotional support and a worldview in which to make sense
of their losses, many are at elevated risk for complicated or prolonged grief
compared to their civilian counterparts.

CONCEPTUAL AND EMPIRICAL UNDERPINNINGS

The model we advocate here for addressing both normative and complicated grief represents a best-practice approach, informed by literature
regarding crisis intervention, psychoeducational components typical of

grief counseling from a secondary prevention perspective, as well as more intensive therapeutic interventions aimed at enduring or complicated grief. The therapeutic model we advocate reflects an integration of diverse theoretical perspectives targeting emotional components of the couple's relationship, pragmatic aspects of adjusting to objective changes resulting from traumatic events, as well as subjective challenges of finding personal meaning following a painful loss. Our approach is also informed by empirical research on the efficacy of treatments for normal versus complicated grief.

The empirical literature raises important questions about routinely implementing intensive intervention protocols in situations of normative grief. One meta-analysis of 14 studies of complicated grief following death of a loved one found a significant positive effect from treatment, with the average effect size increasing at follow-up (Wittouck, Van Autreve, De Jaegere, Portzky, & Van Heeringen, 2011); however, prevention programs targeting specific risk groups (e.g., suicide survivors and widows) did not yield significant benefits compared to no intervention. In a larger meta-analysis of 61 controlled treatment outcome studies of interventions targeting grief and loss, Currier, Neimeyer, and Berman (2008) found only modest overall effects at posttreatment, with diminishing benefits and a lack of statistical significance at follow-up assessments. However, the efficacy of these interventions varied as a function of the targeted population. Specifically, Currier et al. distinguished among three classes of treatments: (1) universal interventions targeting anyone experiencing bereavement; (2) selective interventions targeting particular groups of bereaved individuals facing a heightened risk of experiencing acute distress—such as parents losing a child to a violent death; and (3) indicated interventions restricted to those individuals exhibiting problems adapting to loss—including symptoms of an established psychiatric disorder or other clinically significant difficulties. This meta-analysis offered little empirical support for the efficacy of universal or selective interventions but did find support for interventions targeting individuals in the indicated group exhibiting adaptation difficulties.

Commenting further on these findings, Neimeyer and Currier (2009) concluded that "grief therapy can be helpful to a range of people contending with a range of losses, ameliorating many forms of distress in the near and long-term aftermath of bereavement, regardless of how they enter therapy, if they are assessed as contending with substantial clinical distress to begin with" (p. 355). However, they also emphasized that many individuals experiencing significant loss respond with remarkable resilience without any professional assistance; that is, normal grief progresses and resolves naturally when met with emotional support from family, friends, and others in the social environment.

In light of these findings, the model we advocate comprises a multitiered approach in which the level of intervention is tailored to the specific needs of the individual or couple presenting with grief; the duration of the grief response, as well as enduring adverse impacts in diverse domains of individual or relationship functioning; and comorbidity with other significant emotional or behavioral dysfunction. From this perspective, all individuals experiencing grief or loss may benefit from time-limited "grief counseling" interventions aimed at providing information and support primarily for the purposes of preventing more enduring or complicated grief reactions (Worden, 2008). For a military subculture that is typically distant from families and communities of origin, such brief psychoeducational interventions can help fill the emotional and information gap, and help couples navigate the strange new world of grief. Such an approach does not pathologize grief, but rather conceptualizes it as a normal response to loss, with predictable experiences and challenges.

For some individuals, reactions to traumatic loss extend beyond normal grieving and involve more significant disruption of emotional or behavioral functioning. Left unchecked, this initial crisis response can either escalate in the short term to major difficulties in managing day-to-day responsibilities or gradually progress over the long term to more generalized or enduring dysfunction. Hence, when initial grief counseling adopting a psychoeducational approach fails to resolve more serious aspects of individual or relationship dysfunction, we adopt a crisis intervention approach along the lines advocated by Aguilera (1998). As described more fully in the subsequent section detailing intervention guidelines, this crisis intervention approach promotes restabilization by targeting three core domains of "balancing" factors: (1) the individual's or couple's interpretations of the crisis, (2) currently available emotional support, and (3) specific coping mechanisms.

Finally, the overall intervention approach advocated here recognizes that despite initial grief counseling and crisis intervention, some individuals dissolve into a protracted and complicated grief response characterized by enduring disruption of emotional or behavioral functioning across diverse domains of their individual or relationship lives. The meta-analytic findings described by Currier et al. (2008) suggest that for such individuals contending with substantial clinical distress, more extensive grief therapy protocols can yield significant benefits. We draw heavily on a grief intervention model for use with military and veteran families proposed by Hall (2008). This model articulates specific foci and tasks across stages of transition from grief to recovery, including (1) working through the ending of a previous relationship or other significant loss; (2) addressing the new reality and adapting to both emotional and pragmatic demands resulting from the loss; and (3) finding new meaning, then envisioning and investing in the future.

GUIDELINES FOR ASSESSMENT AND INTERVENTION

Initial Assessment

It is our experience that most military families request assistance when they are in the throes of crisis. We respond immediately to their need by setting up an initial session as soon as possible. Often other disciplines that have identified them as a family in crisis are sources of referral. We believe that waiting for more than a few days is unreasonable for people with severe emotional pain. When we are not able to schedule an immediate session, we make referrals to other agencies that are able to help quickly.

The first session involves joining with the couples in their present crisis. Typically this is a time to hear of their loss, to provide care, and to offer an initial formulation of their struggles and an intervention model for helping them to move forward. For many couples, the next session or two are planned for brief psychoeducational interventions. Because most couples grieve naturally with adequate support, more intensive therapy is not necessary. Indeed, some research suggests that therapy for grieving couples is often not helpful and in some cases may inhibit partners from the natural grief process (Currier et al., 2008).

The assessment phase of therapy includes one session with the couple followed by an individual session with each partner. Attention is given to both the individual symptoms of grief and the interaction style in which the partners engage each other while under stress or in conflict. When conducting individual assessments we routinely ask about safety, other persons involved in providing emotional support to the individual, and the nature of that relationship. We also want to know about other potential comorbid conditions including posttraumatic stress disorder (PTSD), suicidality, alcohol or other substance abuse, and other behaviors or disorders that could interfere with or complicate therapy. Objective screening measures frequently used in military and veteran settings, such as the PTSD Checklist—Military (PCL-M), Patient Health Questionnaire (PHQ), and Alcohol Use Disorders Identification Test (AUDIT) can be helpful in this regard. (See also Monson, Fredman, & Riggs, Chapters 8, Whisman & Sayers, Chapter 9, and Schumm & O'Farrell, Chapter 10, this volume, for additional assessment recommendations.) It is not unusual for individuals with complicated grief to exhibit symptoms of other disorders, and additional individual or couple-based interventions are incorporated to address these concerns as warranted.

Intervention

Overview

We organize our grief intervention protocol for military and veteran couples and families into four stages. Consistent with the previous empirical findings, we note that the first stage of this intervention may be all that is necessary for the majority of couples.

- *Stage 1:* Psychoeducation about normative grief processes, stages of transition (endings, intermediate or neutral phase, and new beginnings), and balancing factors (interpretations of the situation, emotional support, and specific coping mechanisms). Such secondary prevention grief counseling is offered to all couples who have experienced significant loss, and is designed both to manage the immediate crisis and to provide a model for negotiating the transitions that the loss requires.

For couples who show significant disruption in individual or relationship functioning, or for those in which one or both partners struggle with significant grief lasting for more than 6 months, the following additional stages of intervention should be implemented:

- *Stage 2:* Stabilization and shared understanding of the traumatic loss and its impact on the marriage or family system; understanding assigned meanings and reframing the problem in relationship terms. Partners are helped to understand that their inability to support each other emotionally stems at least in part from their inability to find energy for anything more than focusing on their grief.
- *Stage 3:* Restructuring partners' interactions to promote mutual support and strengthen their emotional bond. This stage focuses on helping the couple to connect emotionally by promoting more intimate emotional disclosures and empathic responses, and by assisting partners to approach one another in a softened manner and to engage in difficult but meaningful discussions rather than to retreat.
- *Stage 4:* Facilitating new solutions and methods of coping, and promoting integration of these emergent interactions into sustained relationship patterns facilitating intimacy and adaptability. Strengthening patterns of engagement during times of stress; recognizing and resisting previous patterns of escalation or withdrawal.

Throughout the entire intervention, partners are encouraged to co-construct the meaning of the loss. The therapist resists imposing answers or meanings and instead uses questions to help partners recognize their own and each other's emotional experiences and to develop a new shared meaning of their own.

Sessions are designed to be 50 minutes in length. Although occasional assignments may be given for individual partners or the couple to complete outside of session (e.g., structuring activities promoting more emotional connection or enlisting additional resources for strategic support), the emphasis is on facilitating emotional connection and new meaning within sessions. The partners then decide what to do with these changes between sessions and report on their progress, at the beginning of the next session. We consider grief therapy for couples to be systemic; that is, we define the *relationship* to be both the medium and focus for change, while concurrently working to relieve grief-related symptoms. The concepts introduced to partners during this intervention are intended to externalize the problems they are experiencing, from the individual partners themselves to their interactional patterns.

Stage 1: Psychoeducational Interventions

In our experience, the typical couple referred for grief support has recently experienced the loss of a family member through death, incarceration, or court-ordered removal from the home. In other cases, individual partners may have experienced loss of a limb, psychological function, or emotional control as a result of combat injuries. Most of these couples require crisis counseling and psychoeducation to help them manage their emotions and their decisions during the short-term adjustment to their loss. They also seek assistance to help them navigate the emotional turmoil this unwelcome change has brought into their lives.

The stance of the therapist at this stage is decisive and compassionate. After hearing the narrative of loss and grief, the counselor assesses how each person perceives the loss, the emotional and instrumental support structure available to each, and how each person copes with his or her emotions. Providing the partners with a formulation that normalizes their grief and highlights the challenges of transition helps to externalize the problem and challenges them to work as a team to navigate the changes they face. We often use a brief handout about grief and loss as a way of introducing this discussion (see Handout 12.1, *Understanding Grief and Loss*, at the end of this chapter). The goal is to educate the couple regarding the grief process and to encourage partners to use the social support and coping mechanisms they already have. If there are deficiencies in either support or coping mechanisms, the counselor schedules more sessions to explore possible solutions and to teach skills. Examples of promoting emotional and instrumental support include constructing a chart or visual schematic of the social system that highlights people in the extended family or community who have special skills or experience in grief. Coping mechanisms that are helpful during grief include journaling, exercise, meditation, bibliotherapy, and prayer.

Typically couples in grief are unaware of the lengthy process involved and the emotional turmoil normally associated with adjusting to their loss.

Many couples who arrive in counseling blame each other for not being emotionally available. In other words, rather than identifying their grief as the problem, they label the partner as the problem. The counselor educates partners about the normative grieving process and helps them to articulate ways of coping with this natural process while it works its way through their relationship. An essential part of coping involves partners being present for each other, while also understanding that the other partner is also in crisis and therefore may not be sufficiently available. It is important to draw upon others in the community who can provide support; it is equally vital to have self-regulating coping skills to alleviate pressure on the couple's relationship. Individuals who expect their partner to be their only support and coping mechanism for managing grief are at risk individually and relationally. Goal setting in this stage involves identifying multiple resources of emotional and instrumental support, and exploring various mechanisms for coping with stress, grief, and logistic consequences of specific losses.

A helpful component of this psychoeducational stage is helping the couple to think of recovery as passing through phases or transitions—each with its own unique challenges and tasks (Hall, 2008). The initial phase of recovery requires experiencing and tolerating the painful emotions related to the loss, finding emotional and instrumental support, and dealing with practical consequences of the loss. Because many persons may be inclined to end the counseling once the worst of the initial pain subsides, interventions during this psychoeducational stage encourage them to anticipate additional challenges and opportunities later in the recovery process. For example, during an intermediate or neutral phase, the primary challenges involve establishing new patterns required by the loss (e.g., expanded relationships, gradual reexposure to situations or events previously associated with the loss, or compensatory mechanisms for dealing with lost physical functions). Part of stepping up to the new reality involves developing new plans or goals. Consideration of new goals leads naturally to the final phase of recovery characterized by deriving new meanings in one's life and reinvesting in one's marriage, family, or broader community.

Stage 2: Stabilization

For couples who show significant disruption in functioning or continue to struggle with prolonged grief, Stage 2 involves more intensive interventions extending beyond psychoeducation to promote stabilization. In this second stage, the therapist assists the partners to stabilize and mutually understand the impact of their experience. Two conceptual bases inform this stage of intervention. The first draws upon tenets of crisis intervention theory (e.g., Aguilera, 1998) and emphasizes restoration of emotional and behavioral balance. The second derives from understanding that emotional support undergirds much of the natural grieving process, and hence draws upon tenets of emotionally focused couple therapy (Johnson, 2004) as a basis for strengthening this core component of the couple's relationship.

From a crisis intervention perspective, the counselor helps partners identify any unmet needs that could facilitate recovery of a balance in their emotions and life. The three domains of balancing factors that can prevent someone from falling more deeply into crisis are the person's interpretation of the crisis, currently available emotional support, and coping mechanisms (Aguilera, 1998). With regard to the first domain, does each partner have a reasonably accurate perception of what is going on in the situation? Some couples label the symptoms of grief as the problem and make them into a moral dilemma—for example, "If he would simply stop the emotional outbursts, excessive drinking, and running away, then everything would return to normal." The counselor listens respectfully to partners' interpretations of the problem and guides them to new understandings as needed. If partners resist facing the problem directly, the counselor can explore unspoken fears that keep them from identifying the situation accurately. Assisting both partners to express difficult emotions helps them to move toward accepting a formulation of their problem as struggles with grieving. This simple reframing of the problem, from seeing their struggles as a moral or relationship failure to seeing them as expressions of grief, helps them to regain hope.

Second, do both partners have outside support available to them during this period of grieving? People with strong support systems function better in times of crisis. Essential to this stage of intervention is building up both emotional and instrumental support resources for the grieving partners. This may include formal support systems available through the military or other organizations, or accessing informal support resources in the extended family or community. When the loss involves the death of a service member, social support may begin with a ceremony for members of the unit at the installation's chapel. In addition to a unit ceremony, the chaplain and significant members of the unit may attend the family's funeral and provide comfort to the bereaved. In the event of a family member death, a chaplain may also offer a religious service or other memorial ceremony, so that all who are affected by the loss or wish to provide support may attend.

The third balancing factor involves various specific mechanisms or strategies for coping with grief. Coping mechanisms include those skills that help the person approach the problem in an active and solution-focused manner, as well as occasionally stepping away from the problem to get a break. Examples of mechanisms for getting a break from the problem can be easily identified by asking, "Before this loss hijacked your life, what activities did you enjoy?" Restoring grieving persons to as many positive features of their previous life as possible, with its multiple routines and activities, successfully reconnects them to those things that represent safety and security.

A new Army program provides services to survivors of fallen soldiers. Survivor Outreach Services (SOS) is a long-term case management program designed to embrace and assure survivors that they will be a part of the Army family as long as they desire. In so doing, SOS provides support coordinators and financial counselors to help survivors gain the resiliency they need on their grief journey. Some of the many resources available are assistance in locating counseling services and support groups, life skills training, investment and estate planning education, and employment or education support services. The SOS teams reach out to survivors and provide services closest to where the survivor resides. Links to the Army SOS program webpage and a services locater can be found on the My Army One Source website (*www.myarmyonesource.com*). Although SOS is an Army-funded program, survivors from other military services who seek assistance are not turned away. There are also many nongovernment agencies that assist survivors, and links to quite a few of them may be found on the SOS webpage.

However, both service members and veterans experience numerous losses other than death and, regretfully, formal structures for dealing with these other losses are often lacking. Moreover, from a couple-based perspective, in the long-term the most important source of emotional support is likely to be one's spouse or intimate partner. Hence, an important component of promoting stabilization for the individual or couple involves strengthening the intimate and secure bonds in that relationship. A useful theoretical perspective for achieving this goal is provided by emotionally focused couple therapy (Johnson, 2004). Adopting this approach, the therapist promotes a therapeutic alliance by making the therapeutic relationship one of safety, trustworthiness, and emotional stability and responsiveness for both partners. The therapist maintains empathic attunement to each partner, accepting and validating each person's journey. As the therapist models validation of each partner's subjective experiences, partners begin to see each other as fellow pilgrims in different aspects of the same experience.

The therapist also reframes many of the relationship problems that arise during complicated grief as resulting from negative interactional cycles within the couple's relationship. For example, the therapist helps the couple to understand how one partner may turn to the other for emotional stability at a time when the other partner feels overwhelmed, and how the resulting emotional interaction is perceived as rejection when, in reality, the other person is simply immobilized with grief. This common pattern is normalized as a typical response to grief and loss, and the therapist helps partners to understand their own and each other's emotions as resulting from attempts to gain safe, secure connection. When this reframing of the part-ners' interactions succeeds, negativity declines, because partners see with greater clarity how the loss experience they have been through has hijacked their relationship and brought significant pain and confusion to their lives. Understanding both their distress and struggles from this altered perspec-tive can promote a unified stance and hope in the potential for change.

Stage 3: Restructuring Partners' Interactions

In the third stage of grief therapy, with some of the more basic misunder-standings clarified and negativity reduced, couples are now at a point where they are ready to discuss deeper existential questions that they have not discussed because of the instability in their relationship. The therapist uses both reflection and questions to heighten and deepen emotions to facilitate greater self-awareness, as well as promote mutual awareness of the under-lying emotions driving partners' interactional process. The desire for inti-mate and secure emotional connection is heightened when it is expressed within session so as to help partners remember what they once had before their loss. The therapist also empathically identifies the fear of rejection and loneliness when it is experienced, and facilitates enactments between the partners to share deeper fears of loneliness, abandonment, or even death. The therapist looks for soft and genuine emotions during these enactments to heighten and replay for the purpose of amplifying their impact for part-ners in promoting intimate connection. Restoring or creating a close and secure relationship, in which sadness, hurt, and deep fears can be expressed and understood, provides a context in which the natural healing process of grieving can unfold. Previously critical partners typically demonstrate significant softening toward each other, and withdrawing partners char-acteristically increase their engagement when the couple experiences this secure and deeper connection.

The therapist uses the couple's increased emotional connection to facilitate dialogue about deeper issues of identity, meaning, and existen-tial struggles that grief-related experiences frequently raise for individu-als. These may include discussions about the role of suffering or pain, the nature of injustice or evil in the world, questions of personal redemption, or finding greater purpose and appreciation for life in the face of tragic loss. Because change evolves slowly with successive risks and achievements, the therapist needs to caution partners about being too ambitious in their ini-tial discussions; gradually working up to more difficult issues is wise. The therapist knows that the couple is ready to move on to Stage 4 when they report significant changes at home, such as mutually satisfying intimacy, extended discussions involving the exchange of deep feelings, and shared visioning of their future together.

Stage 4: Integration

In the final stage of grief therapy, the counselor helps the partners to observe and reflect upon their journey together, both prior to therapy during the couple's experience of loss and throughout therapy as the partners processed what has changed and how they are now different both as individuals and as a couple. This stage is a time for celebrating their victory of transition from loss and stress to growth and renewal. Many couples choose to commemorate this time with some form of meaningful event that signifies the restoration of their relationship and decision to move forward. For example, the couple described at the beginning of this chapter, who had lost their daughter during a deployment overseas, arranged with city officials in the community where they had grown up to create a small alcove in the city park with a bench and rose bushes in memory of their daughter—knowing they would have opportunities over the years to revisit that special place.

FACTORS INFLUENCING TREATMENT

A variety of factors can influence the course of therapy for complicated grief in a military or veteran couple. We categorize these influences here according to individual, unit, and spiritual factors. With regard to individual factors, the most common issue complicating treatment is the presence of one or more comorbid conditions. It is not unusual for one or both partners—but particularly often the service member or veteran—to show features of or meet diagnostic criteria for major depression, PTSD, or substance abuse. Oftentimes, the PTSD stems from the same event(s) related to the traumatic loss precipitating the partner's complicated grief. The emotional dysregulation that is characteristic of PTSD—including both emotional numbing and heightened reactivity—and flashbacks and other cognitive intrusions need to be assessed for their impact on both the individual and interactions with his or her partner (see guidelines in Monson et al., Chapter 8, this volume). Similarly, major depression may co-occur with complicated grief and invariably renders grief therapy more difficult and protracted. Traumatic loss is more difficult to absorb in individuals who are vulnerable to depressive disorders, and the impoverished emotional and physical energy characteristic of depression often undermines the couple's efforts to promote intimate connection. Similarly, alcohol or other substance abuse often follows traumatic loss as an effort at self-medication, but it may also precede the loss and serve as a preexisting vulnerability to complicated grief. In either case, the counselor may draw upon detailed guidelines for assessment and intervention offered elsewhere in this volume (e.g., Whisman & Sayers, Chapter 9, on depression, or Schumm & O'Farrell, Chapter 10, on substance use) and integrate these techniques into the grief therapy, or may refer either partner to collateral individual treatment as warranted.

Both service members and veterans must often negotiate with their supervisor for flexibility in scheduling sessions and time away from work during extended treatment. In both the military setting and civilian workplace there is often an expectation that grief should be completed within weeks rather than months. Because complicated grief is manifest after 6 months, many persons in the partners' lives do not interpret their behavior as symptoms connected to their loss. In such cases, the therapist may seek permission from one or both partners to speak with the respective supervisor or employer regarding the nature of their struggles in order to offer education and elicit better understanding and more compassionate support. Within the military, for the most part, senior officers and enlisted members heed warnings against blocking mental health interventions. However, the risk persists that younger or less informed officers or others who supervise those most in need may not be adequately sensitive to the process and course of complicated grief recovery. As in all systems, there may be individuals in supervisory or administrative roles who require continued education and accountability.

In our clinical experience, not all couples search for the meaning of their loss. However, for the majority who wonder why they have such a loss to endure, their search pushes the boundaries of traditional medicine and psychology. Answering existential questions of life and death involves some use of philosophy and theology. We find that the content of these answers is best found by the partners within their own worldview or faith community. However, the process of these discussions is not only appropriate but also sometimes essential within the therapeutic environment and not available in other venues. It is important for the counselor to distinguish between advocating a particular theological or spiritual perspective and facilitating partners' exploration of these issues in a reflective and supportive manner. It makes no more sense (and is no more defensible) to ignore issues of spirituality for clients struggling with issues of grief and loss than it would be to ignore issues of sexuality for clients dealing with difficulties of sexual desire or arousal.

As the partners and the therapist engage in discussions of purpose and meaning, the conversation may include anger toward their higher power, disillusionment with this higher power's lack of protection for them, and a sense of abandonment by their faith community. Listening to and slowly encouraging the partners to explore their beliefs or engage their community of faith with their anger and disappointment may allow some growth to occur over time. Specifically, in Judaism and Christianity, the tradition of angry prayers has clear precedence, with numerous scriptural accounts of characters expressing anger toward a God who gives those who are griev-ing permission to vent. Consider, for example, the depth of suffering and accusations against God in the book of Job or the numerous psalms of lamentation—including the first verse of Psalm 22—expressing feelings of abandonment that Jesus also uttered while on the cross. Honest and open discussions about spiritual dilemmas provide a safe context in which these deep, personal issues can be explored and potentially resolved. Disillusion-ment often dissolves into a more accepting worldview in which the patterns of life and death do not destroy couples' ability to feel safe and enjoy the opportunities their relationship and life provide them.

TAILORING TREATMENT TO ACTIVE DUTY
AND VETERAN COUPLES

In our practice with active duty service members and their families, we often adjust therapy to accommodate separations for training, temporary duty, or deployments. When there is phone connection for the deployed spouse, we have used a speaker phone for the absent member to engage in therapy. Depending on resources, videoconferencing to conduct sessions may be possible. When there are no direct communication resources avail-able, we shift to individual counseling with the nondeployed spouse and make a referral to a chaplain or mental health professional deployed or stationed in near proximity to the other partner. We encourage partners to use e-mail as a way of staying emotionally connected and sharing in each other's respective progress through the grief recovery.

Case Illustration:
"They Took the Man I Married, and Gave Me You!"

Mike and Judy grew up in a small, conservative town of about 5,000 in the midwestern United States—one of those little "Mayberry towns" where everybody knows everybody. Mike and Judy were both 21 years old, and had attended both public school and church together. They met at their church youth group, where they had found respite from their respective abusive families, and dreamed of rearing children together in a healthy and safe home. They spent time having picnics and fishing together by the river bank on weekends, fell in love, and married immediately upon finishing high school.

Mike talked Judy into letting him join the Army shortly after being married, and before they knew it he had completed basic training and was deployed to Iraq, where he would serve with an infantry unit for 12 months.

In their first 2 years of marriage, they were together less than 3 months. When Mike returned from Iraq, Judy noticed immediately that he was not the same. He had lost all interest in church and refused to talk about issues of faith and God, as they had so often in the past while strolling on long walks or fishing together at the river. Mike had lost more than some of his buddies during combat; he had lost his faith and sense of purpose.

A few months after his return, Mike helped one of his fellow soldiers who had deployed with him to get the house next door on the post when it became empty. The couple now seemed to spend time every day with their neighbors, and to Judy it seemed they didn't share even the most basic values. Every weekend seemed to be one big party with the next door neighbors, and Mike became verbally abusive when he was drunk. The neighbor's wife dressed and spoke in sexually provocative ways that offended Judy, but Mike seemed to defend such behavior rather than respecting or supporting Judy and her values. Judy felt alone and longed for the husband she had known before his deployment. When she threatened to pursue a separation unless Mike agreed to accompany her to talk with someone about what was happening between them, he reluctantly consented.

In their first session, the counselor focused on normalizing the feelings of hurt, loss, and confusion that each partner described, providing information about complicated grief and a model for recovery that offered them a sense of direction in the midst of their chaos and confusion. Consistent with the treatment model described earlier, their therapist conducted individual assessments targeting both partners' perception of their situation, their respective coping skills, and sources of emotional and instrumental support. The therapist also educated the couple about various stages of transition characterizing recovery from grief, and asked where the partners currently saw themselves in this process. The therapist helped them to understand that the initial romantic fantasy they shared about their relationship had ended with the husband's deployment. Judy wanted their military experience to be over and for Mike to be back home emotionally, as well as physically. It was clear that Mike was experiencing symptoms of PTSD, but he did not want to let go of the Army and his unit, noting that he felt more at ease with the military than with the civilians back home.

The couple agreed to an initial trial of six sessions but expressed openness to extending this to 10–12 sessions if warranted. Over the following month, counseling sessions focused on challenges of stabilization and promotion of a shared understanding of the impact of various losses on their marriage. In the fifth session, Mike disclosed that he had been struggling intensely with events that had occurred during his deployment but didn't yet feel safe discussing these with Judy. In response, their therapist agreed to integrate individual sessions with their couple sessions over the next month; both partners agreed that whatever was discussed in individual sessions could eventually be brought back into their conjoint couple sessions at their therapist's discretion. Although most of these individual sessions were conducted with Mike to explore traumatic experiences during deployment, some were offered to Judy to provide a safe context for exploring her own feelings of disillusionment and abandonment.

Mike was able to share in individual therapy the shame he felt regularly for blowing up a car that would not stop at a checkpoint, resulting in the death of the child in it. He felt so ashamed that he felt unable to discuss this event with his wife. While not yet discussing the specific content of this event, their therapist was able to use couple sessions to help the partners recognize dynamics of their negative interaction pattern. Specifically, they came to understand that many of Mike's hurtful comments to Judy when drunk, especially his own threats of divorce, were intended to push Judy away so that he did not have to deal with his deep pain; Judy had known something was wrong and kept trying to get Mike to open up to her. Reaching this understanding comprised a key change event, as expressed in the following exchange:

MIKE: We made some real progress this weekend. I got drunk, but I didn't say anything really hurtful. At least I didn't say the "D" word.

JUDY: (*looking at Mike half-smiling, but then looking at the therapist in a more serious manner*) We still can't seem to talk about anything deep. How long are we going to have to settle for defining a good weekend as just being Mike's not threatening to divorce me when he's drunk?

THERAPIST: Your relationship has changed a lot since you were first married, and you seem concerned that the direction of the marriage isn't going back to the marriage you remember it to be.

JUDY: The Army took my husband, and gave me him! (*Leans over and kisses Mike very quickly and pats him, saying "I still love you!"*)

THERAPIST: That's so significant what you just said. Let's freeze-frame that for a moment. "The army took my husband, and gave me him!" Then you leaned over and kissed and patted him. What a courageous risk you took to say that. What are you feeling as we reflect back on that statement together?

JUDY: (*now tearfully*) I feel scared about how Mike's going to take it. I'm also sick that I feel this way—that things are so bad right now after he's been back.

THERAPIST: (*to Mike*) What were you feeling, Mike, when you heard Judy say this?

MIKE: I'm okay with it. I'm feeling pretty dark right now inside. It scares me how dark I am inside since I got back from downrange. I don't like it, and I don't know if I'm ever going to be the same. But I'm here working on it, and doing the best I can.

THERAPIST: If there were one thing you could tell Judy right now that would help her cope with this shared sense of despair or darkness from what this deployment did to your relationship, what would that be?

MIKE: (*turning to Judy and taking both of her hands*) I know, Judy, that I've said some things that have hurt you deeply, and I hope you'll forgive me. I want you to know that I'm here, and I want our marriage to last and be everything we always wanted it to be. I don't have any plans to go anywhere, but I just need time and some help to get over what happened to me, and I can't make any promises about how long that will take.

JUDY: (*reaching toward Mike and the couple embracing*) That's what I needed to hear. I'll try to do my part and be more understanding of how much this has changed both of us.

THERAPIST: Just feel this embrace, and stay in the moment together. (*Allows the couple time.*) This war took a lot from both of you, but with this kind of sharing and openness you've shown here today, I believe these moments can strengthen each of you and your relationship.

In subsequent sessions, the therapy transitioned from stabilization to understanding impact and exploring meaning. Mike eventually confessed that because of his deployment and combat experience, his understanding of God had been reduced to a role "similar to that of the Joker—a God who can no longer be trusted." Mike acknowledged that his thoughts and feelings about God were challenged by his grieving process, but he also expressed his need for the freedom "not to believe" in the traditional Biblical God in which Judy so adamantly believed. Judy expressed her willingness to accept that the war had changed Mike's spiritual perspectives, and said that she could back off of the topic and remain tolerant of Mike's continued doubts and explorations of faith issues.

As the therapy progressed, Mike and Judy came to sessions with smiles on their faces and affirmed that they were no longer experiencing the kinds of crises they had earlier. They were more playful, and wondered aloud whether it might be time to end the counseling. It is important at such times for therapists to inform couples with complicated grief that they may experience continued "flashbacks"—not only to original

traumatic events but also to subsequent painful experiences in their relationship. Couples need to be able to anticipate such experiences and painful remembrances, and to practice even in session using their relationship
as a source of support for their underlying personal losses. Hence, the
therapist uses sessions to replay these events, to help couples discern the
triggers for emotional reactivity, to recognize the emergence of their previous negative emotional cycle, and its connection to underlying grief. In
Mike and Judy's case, this involved helping them to understand that Mike
sometimes turned to their neighbors and other soldiers because he was
feeling alone and ashamed of what happened in Iraq. In group settings
he allowed himself to be surrounded by other drunken people who could
identify with his pain and not talk about it. Here's how the therapist processed that event in session:

JUDY: What do we do about Mike going to these parties during the
weekends? We both agree that he shouldn't drink as much, and
that drinking makes it worse. I don't want to seem like a parent
and nag him, and I want to help him.

THERAPIST: So, Judy, it doesn't sound like you want to be a controlling
person, yet you recognize the potential harm for Mike and want
him to see you as part of the solution, not part of the problem, is
that right?

JUDY: I would really love for him to come and tell me how he feels,
what he wants from me. I mean, if he comes to me and says that he
feels like he just wants to be with his party crowd and needs some
space, or that he's feeling dark inside and just needs to do this,
that would be fine. I also would want him to know that if he said
that he was feeling dark and just wanted some pampering from
me, I would love to do that. I would put on some Victoria's Secret,
play some sexy music, and give him the time of his life.

MIKE: (*jokingly*) Hey, can we go home now? This therapy stuff is really
working!

The couple learned from exchanges similar to this one that they really
did care for each other and that their relationship was responsive enough
to take care of the new needs that emerged in response to the stresses and
trauma of deployment. Each had experienced critical losses—including
their romantic illusions of marriage, specific elements of the religious faith
they had previously shared, Mike's loss of comrades in combat, and his
damaged sense of personal integrity stemming from his own behaviors during deployment. But in the face of these losses, through a shared grieving

process, both partners came to a fuller and richer understanding of themselves and each other. Mike learned that he had a secure source of love and comfort from Judy at home. Judy's openness to physical intimacy even in the face of relationship struggles mirrored his own needs for reconnecting on an emotional level and sharing some of his deeper, dark secrets. Both partners found renewed emotional and physical intimacy to serve as a secure foundation for recovery and restoration.

In the final sessions with Mike and Judy, their therapist facilitated discussions about how they had changed, and how they had grown from both their traumatic losses and the therapeutic journey. The couple reflected on hidden resources they had unlocked in their relationship that empowered them to make it through their most difficult moments of grief. They celebrated their own newfound tools and saw themselves as stronger, more resilient, and as having a deepened appreciation for life.

In many respects, the couple therapy provided opportunities for important grief recovery that could not have been obtained in separate, individual work. Pursuing grief recovery through a couple-based perspective not only provided incremental opportunity for Judy to explore her own feelings of loss related to Mike's deployment but also actively promoted and then utilized the couple's own relationship as a vehicle for emotional support and healing. Their marriage became the safe container in which their grief could resolve.

SUMMARY

The complex and varied demands of the deployment cycle and traumatic losses that frequently occur for military families often result in enduring, complicated grief for service members and veterans alike, as well as their partners. For many couples, brief psychoeducational interventions regarding the grieving process promote a sense of shared understanding and connection offering a secure base of emotional support in which recovery unfolds naturally. For other couples, protracted or complicated grief requires more intensive interventions that recognize both individual and relationship factors interfering with recovery. A couple-based approach to grief therapy explores the impact of grief and loss on the couple's relationship and, more importantly, promotes restoration of an intimate and secure connection that becomes the mechanism for healing. The multitiered approach advocated here goes beyond providing information and initial stabilization to promote partners' new understanding of themselves and their relationship, then uses their altered experience of loss as an opportunity for discovering deeper and enduring meaning in their lives.

RESOURCES

Aguilera, D. C. (1998). *Crisis intervention: Theory and methodology.* St. Louis: Mosby.

Currier, J. M., Neimeyer, R. A., & Berman, J. S. (2008). The effectiveness of psychotherapeutic interventions for bereaved persons: A comprehensive quantitative review. *Psychological Bulletin, 134*, 648–661.

Hall, L. K. (2008). *Counseling military families: What mental health professionals need to know.* New York: Routledge.

Johnson, S. M. (2004). *The practice of emotionally focused couple therapy (2nd ed.).* New York: Brunner/Routledge.

Neimeyer, R. A., & Currier, J. M. (2009). Grief therapy: Evidence of efficacy and emerging directions. *Current Directions in Psychological Science, 18*, 352–356.

Prigerson, H. G., Vanderwerker, L. C., & Maciejewski, P. K. (2008). A case for inclusion of prolonged grief disorder in DSM-V. In M. S. Stroebe, R. O. Hansson, H. Schut, & W. Stroebe (Eds.), *Handbook of bereavement research and practice: Advances in theory and intervention* (pp. 165–186). Washington, DC: American Psychological Association.

Stroebe, M. S., Hansson, R. O., Schut, H., & Stroebe, W. (2008). Bereavement research: Contemporary perspectives. In M. S. Stroebe, R. O. Hansson, H. Schut, & W. Stroebe (Eds.), *Handbook of bereavement research and practice: Advances in theory and intervention* (pp. 3–25). Washington, DC: American Psychological Association.

Wills, R. M. (2003). Bereavement and complicated grief. In D. K. Snyder & M. A. Whisman (Eds.), *Treating difficult couples: Helping clients with coexisting mental and relationship disorders* (pp. 392–415). New York: Guilford Press.

Wittouck, C., Van Autreve, S., De Jaegere, E., Portzky, G., & Van Heeringen, K. (2011). The prevention and treatment of complicated grief: A meta-analysis. *Clinical Psychology Review, 31*, 69–78.

Worden, J. W. (2008). *Grief counseling and grief therapy: A handbook for the mental health practitioner* (4th ed.). New York: Springer.

Understanding Grief and Loss

Instructions: Use this handout to provide information about the normal grief process and to encourage discussion about challenges each partner is experiencing and how to pursue additional emotional and instrumental support.

What is grief?

Grief is a normal response to loss. Events commonly triggering grief include

- Death of a family member, friend, coworker, or fellow service member/veteran
- Illness or injury that results in loss or impairment of physical abilities
- Loss of community due to moves, or separation from work or military service
- Loss of status or role, including changes in intimate relationships or family life

What does grief look like?

Everyone grieves in his or her own way.

- Common feelings include sadness, loneliness, despair, guilt, anger, fear, numbness
- Common thoughts include hopelessness for the future, undue responsibility for the past
- Common behaviors include retreat or withdrawal, irritability or unpredictable reactions

Will the grief ever go away?

Feelings of sadness or hurt may never go away entirely. But for most persons, when offered adequate emotional and instrumental support from others around them, grief diminishes after a few months.

(continued)

The recovery process varies from person to person. But common phases include
- Denial: "I can't believe this has happened to me."
- Anger: "*Why* did this happen? Who's to blame?"
- Bargaining: "Just make this go away, and in return I will _____."
- Depression: "I can't go on. I just don't have the emotional or physical energy necessary."
- Acceptance: "I can find meaning in this, and regain direction and purpose in life."

Grieving individuals may experience all, none, or only some of these phrases.

Can any good come from grieving?

Although unwelcomed, grieving presents opportunities for growth:
- Forming new or deepened connections with other persons
- Creating new understandings and meanings about life

How can someone care for another person who is grieving?

- Just listen. Recognize and support feelings, and refrain from offering advice.
- Offer practical support, such as providing assistance with meals, laundry, child care, or simply time off from other responsibilities.

How can individuals care for themselves during times of grief?

- Don't isolate yourself. Seek out and accept emotional support from others:
  - Lean on family members, friends, and others who care about you.
  - If you follow a religious tradition, draw on the rituals that bring caring persons together.

- Seek out and accept instrumental help from others:
  - Consider asking for help at work, or for temporary reduction in hours or responsibilities.
  - Ask for occasional help at home—with meals, yard work, or child care.
  - This is a time to draw on friends and neighbors, or members of your church.
  - Become familiar with special resources available to service members and veterans.

- Take care of yourself emotionally and physically:
  - Allow yourself to experience and express your difficult feelings.
  - Make sure you're getting enough sleep and good nutrition.
  - Avoid alcohol or illicit drugs to numb the pain of grief.

- Anticipate grief triggers such as anniversaries or holidays
  - Plan to be with others or engaged in positive activities when those occasions arise.

- Be patient with yourself:
  - The grieving process takes time, and no one experiences it exactly the same way.
  - Be prepared for unexpected reminders and other setbacks when the grief resurfaces or surges unexpectedly.
  - Find an outlet for your feelings. Cry, walk, write about your experience, or talk with a friend.

Remember that your spouse, partner, or family member may also be grieving.

- Understand that your partner may not always be able to support you in your grief, and at times may need your support as well.
- Try to find ways of grieving together—for example, by spending time together quietly, or by participating in events that bring each of you comfort or joy.
- Allow each other to experience grief in your own unique ways and time lines.

How do I know if I need additional professional help?

Most persons can benefit from professional counseling at one time or another. Getting help now to deal with grief may prevent difficulties down the road. Consider getting some additional help from a professional if

- You're experiencing thoughts of suicide or dying
- Your grief is interfering with your close relationships
- Your grief is interfering with your ability to function at work or at home
- The frequency or intensity of painful grief reactions doesn't diminish or it actually increases
- You're feeling numb and disconnected from others for more than a few weeks

PART III

Integration
and Implications

CHAPTER 13

Integration and Implications for Clinical Practice and Research

Douglas K. Snyder and Candice M. Monson

Findings regarding the prevalence and elevated risk for emotional and behavioral difficulties among service members, veterans, and their families provide a compelling argument for expanding delivery of effective mental health services to military and veteran families. Since September 11, 2001, over 2 million individual service members have deployed to Iraq or Afghanistan, with nearly 800,000 deploying multiple times. More than 4,800 service members have been killed in action, and over 46,000 have been wounded (U.S. Department of Defense, 2011). On average, each service member has 1.5 dependents (primarily spouses or children) who also experience the challenges that deployment brings. Although many service members and their families demonstrate remarkable resilience in response to the service member's deployment to a combat theater, many others do not. In a large study of veterans serving in Iraq and Afghanistan, 37% received a mental health diagnosis, 22% were diagnosed with posttraumatic stress disorder (PTSD), and 17% with depression (Seal et al., 2009). In addition, multiple deployments result in relatively higher risk for anxiety, depression, alcohol use, and acute stress. Improved medical technology and decreased combat morbidity have resulted in the highest casualty survival rates in the history of U.S. conflicts but also a correspondingly high number of severely wounded veterans who need ongoing care and support from their families (Gawande, 2004; see also Glynn, Chapter 11, this volume).

The potential adverse effects of deployment extend beyond service members. Currently, about 71% of officers and 52% of enlisted personnel are married, and 43% of all service members have children (U.S. Department of Defense, 2007). Wives of deployed service members show increased risk of depression, anxiety, sleep disorders, and acute stress reaction and adjustment disorders compared to wives of personnel not deployed (Mansfield et al., 2010). More than 2 million children have experienced the deployment of at least one parent (see DeVoe, Paris, & Ross, Chapter 5, this volume), with increasing likelihood that the deploying parent may be the child's mother (given that women now comprise about 14% of the military force). Research indicates that the largest segment of this group—involving children 5 years of age or younger—has significantly higher rates of emotional and behavioral problems relative to their peers (Chartrand, Frank, White, & Shope, 2008; Esposito-Smythers et al., 2011). Some studies also suggest increased risks of child neglect and maltreatment during deployment (e.g., McCarroll, Ursano, Fan, & Newby, 2008).

Service members' and veterans' marriages and similar committed relationships also demonstrate increased risks from repeated or prolonged deployment. Findings from the U.S. Army's Mental Health Advisory Team (MHAT-V, 2008) indicate that the proportion of married service members planning divorce or separation increased in proportion with the length of time deployed, particularly among enlisted personnel. Trauma symptoms in soldiers, particularly sexual problems, dissociation, and sleep disturbance, predict poorer relationship functioning (Nelson Goff, Crow, Reisbig, & Hamilton, 2007). In a study of veterans referred to a Veterans Affairs (VA) behavioral health service, over 75% reported family readjustment problems (Sayers, Farrow, Ross, & Oslin, 2009). Another study found soldiers' reports of interpersonal conflicts with spouse, family, and others to increase fourfold between an assessment immediately following deployment and reassessment 3–6 months later (Milliken, Auchterlonie, & Hoge, 2007).

Complicating the need for mental health services across the deployment cycle are troublesome findings regarding both the availability and utilization of appropriate services. In a sample of 448 soldiers and Marines screening positive for a mental disorder 3 to 4 months following deployment to Iraq or Afghanistan, only 19% had sought help from a mental health professional in the prior year—although more than twice that percentage (41%) expressed interest in receiving such help, and the majority (81%) acknowledged having a mental health problem (Hoge et al., 2004). Because service members with psychological problems are more likely to leave the military in the year following deployment, the responsibility of providing mental healthcare to these veterans and their families may be expected to shift to both the VA healthcare system and the civilian sector (Sheppard, Malatras, & Israel, 2010).

What are the implications of these aggregate findings for meeting the mental health needs of service members, veterans, and their families?

Given the comorbidity of individual and relationship problems, and their prevalence in both military and veteran samples, how should couple-based interventions be integrated into traditional healthcare systems and services emphasizing individual treatments? How do we equip mental health providers in both the military/veteran and civilian communities to deliver best-practice or evidence-based couple interventions? What basic elements of emotional and behavioral challenges or impairments across the deployment cycle require more intensive study to guide effective interventions? What individual and relationship factors contribute to resilience, and what steps can be implemented to promote them across the deployment cycle? Based on work highlighted in the previous chapters, we propose here some guidelines to help direct further research in addressing these questions and facilitate clinical practice in meeting the mental health needs of service members and veterans.

• *Couple-based interventions need to be integrated systematically into service settings historically emphasizing individual treatments for service members and veterans.* The comorbidity of individual emotional or behavioral difficulties and relationship problems in military and veteran populations affirms well-documented findings in the general population—particularly for mood, anxiety, and alcohol or substance abuse problems (Snyder & Whisman, 2003; Whisman & Uebelacker, 2006). Veterans diagnosed with PTSD and their intimate partners report more numerous and severe relationship problems, more parenting troubles, and poorer family adjustment (Galovski & Lyons, 2004; Monson, Taft, & Fredman, 2009). In a study of U.S. Air Force security forces deployed to Iraq, predeployment levels of depression, PTSD, and alcohol use each predicted levels of marital or intimate relationship distress—and these associations increased in magnitude at 6- to 9-month follow-up after a 1-year deployment (Cigrang, Talcott, Snyder, Baker, & McGeary, 2009; Cigrang et al., 2011). Emerging anecdotal evidence points to the impact of a service member's or veteran's emotional functioning on the couple's ability to co-parent effectively, to cope with the challenges of traumatic brain injury, or to work through difficult grief and loss processes following deployment. In short, the comorbidity of individual mental health and relationship problems in military and veteran populations demands treatment approaches that effectively address critical difficulties in each of these domains.

Failure to address interpersonal difficulties not only leaves service members' or veterans' intimate relationships at risk but also jeopardizes their own individual functioning or response to treatment for individual mental health problems. Studies have shown that marital discord predicts longitudinal changes in psychiatric symptoms and the prevalence and incidence of mood, anxiety, and substance use disorders in population-based samples. Moreover, marital discord is associated with poorer treatment outcome for mood, anxiety, and substance use disorders, and with relapse and recurrence following treatment (Whisman, Snyder, & Beach, 2009).

The rationale for integrating couple-based interventions in treating individual emotional, behavioral, or physical health problems flows from the recursive influences that difficulties in either area are likely to exert on problems in the other. Just as living with or caring for a service member or veteran with a mental disorder may impact an intimate partner negatively, so too that partner's behavior and attitudes may impact either positively or negatively the other's management of, or recovery from, that disorder. The previous chapters in this volume note that intimate partners may be among the first to notice emotional or behavioral difficulties of the service member or veteran, or the first to bring these problems to the attention of helping professionals. Having both partners available enables the mental health professional to inquire about specific thoughts or feelings—and to observe specific interactions—that could contribute to, maintain, or exacerbate clinical concerns in the service member. Couple sessions potentially enable partners to adopt a new perspective, modify expectations or attributions that fuel resentment or despair, and develop shared strategies for modifying interactions that are distressing to both.

Couple-based interventions for treating individual mental or physical health problems generally adopt one of three strategies (Baucom, Shoham, Mueser, Daiuto, & Stickle, 1998). In disorder-specific interventions, the focus of treatment is on the individual partner's disorder, but couple relationship issues are introduced to the extent that they impact the disorder or are impacted by the disorder. Examples include partners' inadvertent enabling or reinforcement of maladaptive avoidance behaviors in various anxiety disorders, failure to adhere to deescalation strategies in treatment of intimate partner violence, or indirectly undermining efforts toward sobriety. In a second strategy involving partner-assisted interventions, the intimate partner acts as a surrogate therapist, coaching the individual to complete homework assignments and providing support. Examples include having the intimate partner facilitate a service member's approach toward trauma-related stimuli, construct menus of pleasurable activities to pursue separately or together, or brainstorm strategies to minimize adverse impacts of combat-related physical or cognitive impairments. The third strategy incorporates couple interventions as a means of reducing global relationship distress resulting from or contributing to the service member's or veteran's individual difficulties. In addition to the benefits of reducing couple distress in its own right—either as a contributing factor or as a consequence of one partner's disorder—reducing global relationship distress may be necessary before engaging in partner-assisted or disorder-specific interventions as a means of fostering partners' collaboration.

Hence, from both the conceptual perspective of reciprocal partner influences in couple relationships and empirical findings regarding comorbidity of individual and relationship problems, couple-based interventions should comprise a core strategy for addressing individual disorders. The empirical literature provides clear evidence for the efficacy of couple interventions for individual disorders in civilian samples (Snyder & Whisman, 2003). Previous chapters in this volume document emerging evidence of their effectiveness with both military and veteran samples. These findings complement an extensive literature over several decades indicating the effectiveness of a variety of couple therapy approaches for reducing general couple distress (Halford & Snyder, 2012; Snyder, Castellani, & Whisman, 2006). Where empirically supported protocols tailored specifically to service members or veterans do not yet exist, evidence-based approaches drawing from studies with civilian samples or best-practice approaches based on integration of specific treatment components having empirical support may guide treatment.

A prevailing approach *not* warranted on the basis of empirical findings is the singular reliance on individual treatments and the exclusion of couple-based interventions in one format or another.

• *Mental health providers in the military or veteran environment and the civilian sector need to be trained in the delivery of effective couple-based interventions.* This assertion derives as a corollary of the preceding guideline and has two components. The first involves disseminating evidence-based couple assessment and intervention strategies throughout the military and VA healthcare systems. Failure to recognize and respond to the interplay between individual and relationship functioning at each juncture of the mental health, social services, and medical healthcare delivery systems guarantees incomplete assessment protocols and suboptimal treatment for a broad spectrum of consumers. For example, as noted by Heyman, Taft, Howard, Macdonald, and Collins (see Chapter 7, this volume), intimate partner violence (IPV) has a high prevalence in both civilian and military populations and frequently goes underreported, even among couples presenting for therapy. Although advances have been gained in operationalizing reliable and valid indicators of IPV, systematic screening across mental and physical healthcare units has yet to be achieved—despite evidence linking IPV to length of deployment, as well as to individual disorders such as PTSD and alcohol or substance abuse.

Effectively evaluating and treating relationship distress goes beyond its comorbidity with individual mental health disorders. It relates to operational readiness, as well as retention of service members. In a survey of 140 U.S. Air Force Security Forces deployed to Iraq, over 33% reported that ongoing conflicts with their spouse or partner back home distracted them from focusing on their job or mission, and 18% reported that these relationship problems created stress leading to arguments with members of their unit or command in-theater (Cigrang et al., 2011). Maintaining an effective all-volunteer Armed Forces requires caring for those intimate relationships most important to the service member's well-being and his or her willingness to make the individual and family sacrifices accompanying deployment and the military lifestyle.

Progress in this regard is evident on several fronts. The 2008 congressional mandate (Public Law 110-387; U.S. 110th Congress, 2007) that VA medical centers provide marital and family therapy reflects a significant departure from previous policies limiting such services in the treatment of a veteran's diagnosed mental disorder. In response, the VA has engaged in disseminating empirically supported couple treatments such as integrative behavioral couple therapy (IBCT; Christensen et al., 2004). Similarly, training of mental health providers in cognitive-behavioral couple therapy for PTSD (see Monson, Fredman, & Riggs, Chapter 8, this volume) and alcohol or other substance abuse (see Schumm & O'Farrell, Chapter 10, this volume) has been extended to clinicians in both Department of Defense (DoD) and VA healthcare systems. Not all efforts have been confined to traditional mental health providers. For example, training in an empirically supported intervention to address both individual and relationship adverse impact from infidelity (see Snyder, Baucom, Gordon, & Doss, Chapter 6, this volume) has been provided to military chaplains, with preliminary evidence supporting the training protocol. Nevertheless, these efforts represent just a small impact relative to the magnitude of need and predominant culture of individual-focused treatments.

The second component of this guideline regards training of civilian providers in not only relevant couple-based interventions but also aspects of the military and veteran context relevant to treatment. As noted by the DoD's Task Force on Mental Health (2007), mental health care for service members and veterans should be provided by professionals familiar with military life. At issue is the "cultural competence" that is essential to effective delivery of services to members of any particular culture with its own norms, roles, and expectations distinct from the general population. The DoD's Task Force noted that "the military is a unique cultural context, and the psychological health problems experienced by service members and their families are inextricable from the unique experiences of military service" (p. 42). The Task Force also concluded that "the community-based network of providers is not consistently knowledgeable about military life stressors, and is not readily accessible in many locales, particularly in rural communities where many military installations are located" (pp. 42–43).

As noted by Whisman and Sayers (Chapter 9, this volume), clinicians should familiarize themselves with military culture sufficiently to assess the relevant aspects of military life and military deployments (see also Martin & Sherman, Chapter 2, this volume). Key aspects include the length and location of assignments, the specific jobs or responsibilities of the service member, exposure to combat, and experiences with the military and veteran healthcare systems. Marital and family-related aspects of military life include the arrangements made by the partners during extended training and deployments of the service member for managing their household, the nature and source of supports for the nondeployed partner during these times, and the perceptions of both partners regarding their functioning prior to and following deployments.

Even familiarity with common military terms or acronyms, military ranks, or basic organizational structure within branches is essential to establishing credibility with the military or veteran client. Appendices B–E at the end of this volume are intended to facilitate such familiarity at a rudimentary level. Also critical to effective intervention is knowledge of available resources across diverse domains and formats (see Slone, Friedman, & Thompson, Chapter 3, this volume). Appendix A in this volume provides an annotated listing of key resources, including websites, books, and programs, providing supplemental information for many of the issues highlighted throughout this book.

• *Both institutionally based providers as well as individual clinicians need to identify and reduce potential barriers to care.* Barriers to couple-based interventions occur at both institutional and individual-provider levels, and operate through both formal and informal mechanisms. For example, specific resources may target veterans, but not service members who are still on active duty, or vice versa. Some services available to military members may also be available to their families but, as Slone and colleagues note (Chapter 3, this volume), what defines a "family member" at times remains unclear. Married partners and dependent children may be included, but what about nonmarried intimate partners, married partners of the same sex, or sibling or parental caregivers? Although Public Law 110-387 mandates extension of couple and family therapy within the VA, healthcare systems and third-party payers in the civilian sector often implement reimbursement policies that discourage couple- and family-based treatments, despite evidence of their superior efficacy to individual interventions for some disorders (Snyder & Whisman, 2003).

Just as troublesome and perhaps more pervasive are informal barriers to care. Access to couple-based treatments depends on selection of personnel (e.g., licensed marital and family therapists or clinicians with specific training in couple interventions), on where personnel are assigned (e.g., in mental health clinics versus primary care or social service units providing greater access and outreach), and on specific assignment of provider responsibilities (i.e., prioritizing couple or family interventions over traditional individual treatments). Access to local clinics or community providers may be limited for service members or veterans in more rural settings, and ability to take time off from assigned responsibilities varies tremendously across unit command structures. Similar informal barriers impacting couple-based services in particular include hours of services (with evening hours more critical to dual-wage-earner couples) and provision of child care during appointments.

Promoting adoption of couple-based interventions in military and civilian healthcare systems and training providers in delivering these treatments does not ensure that service members or veterans will avail themselves of these services. (Unlike the narrative in the 1989 movie *Field of Dreams*, it is not necessarily the case that "If you build it, he will come.") The military culture is one that emphasizes toughness, self-reliance, and the ability to master stress without difficulty—all admirable traits but also norms that potentially connote weakness among those seeking mental health services (Bryan & Morrow, 2011). Many service members are concerned about stigma. In one survey of service members who had just returned from combat and met screening criteria for a mental disorder, about 60% were concerned that their fellow soldiers or commanding officers would lose trust in them or treat them differently if they sought treatment, and 65% stated that seeking treatment made them appear "weak" (Hoge et al., 2004). Concerns about possible stigmatization were nearly twice as high among individuals screening positive for a mental disorder compared to service members who did not; in the former group, only 23 to 40% sought mental health services during the study period. In a related study, nearly 60% of soldiers and 50% of Marines reported that leadership would treat them more negatively if they sought counseling (Wright et al., 2009).

One of the barriers to seeking mental health treatment is concern regarding confidentiality. For example, only military chaplains have explicit policies ensuring absolute confidentiality, an important consideration given that a variety of presenting problems (e.g., sexual affairs) constitute potential violations of the Uniform Code of Military Justice and could negatively impact the service member's career. A survey of service members deployed to Afghanistan found that whereas 87% reported sharing personal concerns with unit commanders, only about half trusted those commanders to respect confidentiality regarding those concerns. Issues regarding confidentiality can be reduced by articulating and adhering to clear, explicit guidelines about what will be held in confidence and what must be reported, and by training providers throughout the healthcare system, as well as supervisors along the entire chain of command, about standards regarding confidentiality. Other means of reducing stigmatization include providing different levels of intervention (e.g., brief written guidelines on communication skills; one-visit consultations with paraprofessionals; psychoeducational groups; or more intensive couple treatment) across diverse settings (e.g., day care centers, primary care settings, social service or mental health clinics) at times and in formats most readily accessible to potential military or veteran consumers.

Despite concerns about stigmatization, available evidence indicates that substantial numbers of service members will make use of mental health services when these are made available and other barriers are reduced. A large epidemiological study found that, within the first year after combat, 35% of military personnel serving in Iraq sought mental health services (Hoge, Auchterlonie, & Milliken, 2006). Among U.S. Air Force Security Forces returning from a 1-year deployment to Iraq, 37% had sought individual counseling for a psychological or relationship problem; contrary to findings by Hoge et al. (2004), utilization rates were highest among those airmen showing greatest impairment on a composite measure of psychological functioning (Cigrang et al., 2011).

- *Providing optimal intervention and prevention protocols to those individuals most likely to benefit requires timely and effective screening.* The goal should be to ensure that the best treatments are delivered to the right consumers, at a time when they are most likely to utilize and benefit from these services. As Slone and colleagues note (see Chapter 3, this volume), assessment of the service member or veteran requires understanding the context that surrounds individuals and their family members, including the military culture; discovering the particular stressors affecting individuals and their families; and understanding the unique barriers to care that individuals must overcome. Beyond this conceptual framework, it also requires brief screening measures with high diagnostic efficiency across domains of both individual and relationship functioning.

Timing of the assessment is critical. For example, in a large study of over 56,000 soldiers assessed immediately postdeployment and again 3–6 months later, self-reported symptom severity sufficient to warrant referral for formal evaluation by a mental health provider more than doubled, from 4.4% upon soldiers' immediate return to 9.3% when assessed again at 3- to 6-month follow-up (Milliken et al., 2007). Also critical is consistent screening for both individual psychological and relationship problems, regardless of the service setting. There are well-documented trends for marital and family therapists to neglect or underdetect individual mental health disorders, just as clinicians emphasizing individual treatments tend to neglect important interpersonal problems. Brief screening measures of both intrapersonal and interpersonal functioning can rectify this assessment bias when consistently used across diverse mental health and primary care settings (Snyder, Heyman, & Haynes, 2008).

Finally, intimate partners or other family members are often the first (or only) person to recognize difficulties of the service member or veteran; similarly, they may be the first to report these to healthcare agents and be most influential in bringing the service member to treatment. Hence, screening measures should be adapted for informant report, with separate thresholds or criteria established for diagnostic or treatment decisions.

The goal of such screenings is to facilitate access to services for those individuals who could potentially benefit. Hence, decision rules or thresholds for referral should emphasize sensitivity over specificity, even if this contributes to initial referral of individuals subsequently determined to have relatively low need for specific services. Additional criteria for evaluating screening strategies proposed by Rona, Hyams, and Wessely (2005) are that screening measures should be simple and precise, clinically and socially acceptable, appropriately implemented across relevant staff and facilities, and able to facilitate interventions demonstrated to have clear benefit.

• *Couple-based interventions are enhanced by identifying specific active components and developing guidelines for integration and adaptation across diverse disorders and populations.* The various couple-based interventions for diverse individual disorders described in earlier chapters share some striking similarities. For example, each emphasizes the importance of first targeting individual and relationship crises that disrupt basic functioning and impede use or acquisition of more adaptive coping strategies. Although specific interventions depend on the particular crisis—whether managing suicidality, containing intimate partner violence, medicating for psychotic symptoms, or briefly hospitalizing for drug or alcohol detoxification—the sequencing of interventions frequently requires crisis intervention and stabilization prior to skills-building and relationship enhancement.

Most of the interventions described in this volume adopt a predominantly cognitive-behavioral approach, reflecting a skills-building orientation consistent with the military culture, as well as the empirical foundations from which these intervention programs have evolved. Hence, specific intervention components, such as using constructive time-outs to regulate negative interactions, promoting problem-solving and decision-making communication skills, increasing positive interactions in rewarding activities in and outside the home, providing information and building skills in specific domains such as parenting and sexuality, and enhancing intimate connection by facilitating emotional expressiveness and empathic responding—all comprise modular elements of intervention that generalize across diverse individual disorders or relationship difficulties.

Each of the intervention protocols described in this volume also contains elements specific to the individual and relational characteristics of a particular disorder. Whether promoting sobriety, managing PTSD symptomatology, coping with sequelae of traumatic brain injury, or rebuilding trust following infidelity, understanding unique characteristics of the underlying phenomenon and having the expertise to provide specific interventions for addressing those characteristics are essential to providing competent care. Some of the specific intervention components targeting elements of one disorder may be sufficiently "portable" for incorporation into treatment protocols for other disorders. For example, intervention strategies developed for grief and loss (see Scheider, Sneath, & Waynick, Chapter 12, this volume)—including those from philosophical or theological perspectives—may be useful for couples struggling to cope with the impact of traumatic brain injury. Similarly, interventions aimed at rebuilding trust following infidelity (see Snyder et al., Chapter 6, this volume) may be useful for couples struggling with repeated deception and broken promises characteristic of relapses in treatment of alcohol or substance abuse.

Consistent with clinical complexity resulting from the comorbidity of individual and relationship problems generally, and from situational stressors linked to the military experience specifically, one could expect the requirements for integrative approaches to be the rule rather than the exception when working with military and veteran couples and families. When drawing upon diverse treatment modalities to address complex clinical problems, the clinician needs to determine which specific interventions to incorporate, in which order to implement them, and how to pace them. Issues relevant to these tasks have been described elsewhere (e.g., Halford & Snyder, 2012; Snyder, Schneider, & Castellani, 2003). Less clear from the literature is how to adapt couple-based treatments across diverse situational circumstances or subgroups within the military and veteran population. For example, because of rhythms in the deployment cycle, for many military couples there is greater risk of treatment being interrupted or shortened; consequently, adaptations of standard intervention protocols may require abbreviated formats that reflect changes in pacing or selection of specific treatment components, or use of evolving technologies to deliver couple-based interventions conjointly while one partner is deployed.

Separate from modifications demanded by the deployment cycle are treatment adaptations tailored to specific groups of service members or veterans. For example, about 27% of service members deployed to Iraq or Afghanistan have been members of the National Guard or the Reserves, who face the added challenge of departing from and returning to civilian communities and jobs (see Beasley, MacDermid Wadsworth, & Watts, Chapter 4, this volume). The families of such service members may be especially challenged because of relatively shorter preparation time or limited access to critical information, resources, and social supports otherwise available to installation-based families (MacDermid, 2006). Indeed, rates of PTSD in Reservists have been found to be 50% higher than rates in active duty soldiers within 3 to 6 months postdeployment (Milliken et al., 2007). Similarly, women now comprise a greater percentage of veterans compared to previous veteran cohorts, and their expanding service roles make it increasingly likely that these women have been exposed to combat-related trauma. Moreover, the marriages of women service members appear at even greater risk than those of men; a recent study showed that for both enlisted personnel and officers, women service members were more than twice as likely as men to divorce. Anecdotal evidence suggests that dual-military couples may be at higher risk than couples for whom only one partner is active military, and that service members who deploy individually rather than as intact units may also be at elevated risk for postdeployment difficulties. Unclear is whether variations in the individual or relationship difficulties themselves, or differences in resources available in the family or community, dictate adaptation of intervention strategies with service members in these specific groups.

• *Both researchers and clinicians need to distinguish between psychological disorders and normal adaptations across the deployment cycle, then identify mechanisms influencing each.* Responses to the challenges and stressors of deployment can be considered to fall within three general classes. Some service members, as well as their families, evidence little if any adverse impact and, in fact, may demonstrate both personal and relationship growth in developing new skills and deepened appreciation for their own and each other's capacities to thrive in the face of hardship. Others, as evidenced by statistics highlighted under the previous guidelines, develop significant emotional or behavioral disorders or suffer deterioration or failure of their intimate relationships. However, a large third group survives the challenges of deployment or exposure to combat without experiencing a mental disorder or failed relationship, but nevertheless experience a variety of normative individual or relational challenges, with a range of adverse impact or suboptimal functioning.

There is no single portrayal of the deployment cycle that fits all individuals or families. For heuristic purposes, it is useful to distinguish among various phases of deployment—whether as few as three (pre-, during, and postdeployment) or as many as the seven identified by the Army (train-up/preparation, mobilization, deployment, employment, redeployment, postdeployment, and reconstitution). Each phase, however operationally defined, presents its own individual and relational challenges to the service member and his or her family—such as preparing emotionally for separation, surviving life-threatening events in theater, coping as a spouse or youngster for extended periods in a single-parent home, managing financial and other logistic stressors associated with the deployment cycle, or becoming reacquainted as intimate partners or family members (Pavlicin, 2003). Veterans who have deployed to Afghanistan or Iraq frequently describe themselves as "different" or "changed"—regardless of whether such impact manifests itself in emotional or behavioral difficulties postdeployment (see Martin & Sherman, Chapter 2, this volume).

Better research that identifies normative challenges and coping strategies across the deployment cycle can inform prevention and intervention strategies that are evidence-based and offer a range of formats tailored to levels of need, delivered by diverse providers (e.g., training naturally occurring social support providers within enlisted units to deliver low-intensity evidence-based psychoeducation) at times when service members are most apt to receive and use the information.

What factors place service members or their families at higher risk for developing suboptimal functioning across different phases of deployment? Although many of these risk factors likely occur at the personal or relationship level, others likely reflect systemic influences within individual command units or the military environment more generally. Conversely, what factors promote resilience among service members and their families— again at individual, relational, or more systemic levels? Moreover, are risk and resilience factors the same or different? Available evidence suggests that, not unexpectedly, military families' quality of postdeployment functioning is strongly related to levels of individual and relational functioning prior to deployment (see Beasley et al., Chapter 4, this volume). Other factors that likely influence individual and relationship outcomes include the nature of deployment experiences (e.g., exposure to traumatic events); number, duration, and spacing of deployments; and availability and utilization of individual and family support resources across the deployment cycle.

Not only should the moderators of postdeployment functioning be identified, but also those mediating mechanisms contributing to individual and relationship outcomes. For example, which components or mechanisms of social support mediate the relation between exposure to combat and subsequent PTSD symptomatology, or the relation between combat-related loss and subsequent grief response? Does disclosure of traumatic experiences to a spouse or intimate partner reduce subjective distress in the service member, and are potential benefits of such disclosure influenced by the quality of that intimate relationship or specific listening/response strategies of the partner? Research on such questions could better inform efforts to educate intimate partners about postdeployment challenges and optimal reintegration strategies.

- *Programs intended to promote couple and family well-being during and following deployment should be evaluated for their effectiveness and to enhance their dissemination and utilization.* As of 2010, the DoD was spending more than $1 billion per year to improve the quality of life of service members and their families (see Slone et al., Chapter 3, this volume), including Family Readiness Groups (providing unit-specific information and emotional support across the deployment cycle), Army Community Services (providing practical assistance with issues such as relocation, spouse employment, financial strains, or transitions back to civilian life), and Family Assistance Centers (providing information and referrals to diverse community resources). Particularly noteworthy is the Army's "Resilience Training" program, formerly known as BATTLE-MIND (U.S. Army Medical Command, 2011), offering a constellation of resilience training modules for soldiers and command leaders related to deployment and the military setting, as well as for soldiers and their families to facilitate preparing for and managing challenges of the deployment cycle and reintegration.

A major challenge is to move toward a set of comprehensive, integrated, and evidence-based programs and services linked to outcomes that support service members and veterans throughout all phases of the military and subsequent civilian life. Although well-conceived, many of the resource programs intended to support service members and their families have yet to be subjected to objective evaluation of their effectiveness or means for improving dissemination or utilization. For example, although a majority of service members believe that some form of short-term (1–5 days) decompression in a third location is a good idea following deployment to a combat theater before returning home, to date no empirical evidence demonstrates that such programs confer any advantage over returning home directly, let alone identifying which components of these programs (e.g., psychoeducational components regarding challenges of reintegration vs. opportunities for mental and physical respite) could potentially mediate intended benefits (Adler, Zamorski, & Britt, 2011).

- *Additional information should be gathered on the impact of military service generally, and mental health difficulties of the service member specifically, on the well-being of family members.* Relatively few studies have documented the mental health status of military family members (Riviere & Merrill, 2011). A study with a large sample of military spouses, conducted at various phases of the deployment cycle, found that 20% exceeded criteria for major depression or generalized anxiety disorder and 10% exceeded criteria for PTSD (Eaton et al., 2008). Military spouses also report emotional challenges such as worry and loneliness, in addition to economic and logistical challenges (e.g., serving as a single parent).

Although findings from studies regarding rates of emotional or behavioral disorders among children or adolescents of deployed parents are mixed (Card et al., 2011), anecdotal evidence points to an abundance of unique challenges they encounter relative to their civilian counterparts throughout each phase of the deployment cycle. Preparing for emotional and physical separation, and living in a "geographically single-parent" home during deployment, bring their own challenges. Following deployment, younger children may not recognize their service member parent; adolescents may resist changes in rules or routines as the returning parent is reintegrated into the family (see DeVoe, Paris, & Ross, Chapter 5, this volume). Better information regarding the impact of military life and, more specifically, challenges of deployment and reintegration on military and veteran families, will be essential not only for developing effective prevention and intervention programs for these family members, but also for optimizing their participation in interventions targeting service members' own emotional or physical well-being.

SUMMARY

Since 2001, the U.S. Armed Forces have experienced the most frequent and protracted deployments in the history of the volunteer military. More than 2 million service members have deployed, and an estimate of other family members impacted by their deployment is several times that number. Even after the current conflicts wind down, history informs us that new conflicts and military obligations will emerge. Over one-third of veterans returning from deployment have a mental health diagnosis, and many more struggle with challenges of reintegration to family and civilian life. Individual emotional, behavioral, and physical health challenges of service members have a high comorbidity with relationship problems—and each can contribute to the development, exacerbation, or maintenance of the other. Hence, providers of mental health services to military and veteran families must be well-equipped to assess, conceptualize, and treat these difficulties, drawing upon couple-based interventions most likely to impact both individual and relationship domains.

As noted in the DoD's Task Force on Mental Health (2007),

A thorough review of available staffing data and findings from site visits to 38 military installations around the world clearly established that current mental health staff are unable to provide services to active members and their families in a timely manner, do not have sufficient resources to provide newer evidence-based interventions in the manner prescribed, and do not have the resources to provide prevention and training for service members or leaders that could build resilience and ameliorate the long-term adverse effects of extreme stress. (p. 43)

The men and women who have risked their lives for their country, and the family members who love and care for them, deserve better. Effective interventions drawing on both individual and relationship processes have been developed; others are emerging or will become available in the foreseeable future. It now rests on the shoulders of mental health providers within the military, veteran healthcare, and civilian communities to become proficient in these couple-based interventions and to bring them to the military and veteran families they have been entrusted to serve.

RESOURCES

Adler, A. B., Zamorski, M., & Britt, T. W. (2011). The psychology of transition: Adapting to home after deployment. In A. B. Adler, P. D. Bliese, & C. A. Castro (Eds.), *Deployment psychology: Evidence-based strategies to promote mental health in the military* (pp. 153–174). Washington, DC: American Psychological Association.

Baucom, D. H., Shoham, V., Mueser, K. T., Daiuto, A. D., & Stickle, T. R. (1998). Empirically supported couple and family interventions for marital distress and adult mental health problems. *Journal of Consulting and Clinical Psychology, 66,* 53–88.

Bryan, C. J., & Morrow, C. E. (2011). Circumventing mental health stigma by embracing the warrior culture: Lessons learned from the Defender's Edge program. *Professional Psychology: Research and Practice, 42,* 16–23.

Card, N. A., Bosch, L., Casper, D. M., Bracamonte Wiggs, C., Hawkins, S. A., Schlomer, G. L., et al. (2011). A meta-analytic review of internalizing, externalizing, and academic adjustment among children of deployed military service members. *Journal of Family Psychology, 25,* 508–520.

Chartrand, M. M., Frank, D. A., White, L. F., & Shope, T. R. (2008). Effect of parents' wartime deployment on the behavior of young children in military families. *Archives of Pediatric and Adolescent Medicine, 162,* 1009–1014.

Christensen, A., Atkins, D. C., Berns, S., Wheeler, J., Baucom, D. H., & Simpson, L. E. (2004). Traditional versus integrative behavioral couple therapy for significantly and chronically distressed married couples. *Journal of Consulting and Clinical Psychology, 72,* 76–191.

Cigrang, J. A., Talcott, G. W., Snyder, D. K., Baker, M., & McGeary, D. (2009, November). Individual psychological health and intimate relationship functioning in a cohort of active-duty service members prior to OIF deployment. In S. Sayers (Chair), *Understanding the marital context of the impact of combat deployment.* Symposium presented at the annual meeting of the Association for Behavioral and Cognitive Therapies, New York, NY.

Cigrang, J., Talcott, G. W., Tatum, J., Baker, M., Cassidy, D., Sonnek, S., et al. (2011, November). Psychological health and intimate relationship functioning across the deployment cycle in a cohort of active-duty service members. In D. K. Snyder (Chair), *Emerging evidence regarding post-traumatic stress disorder and relationship functioning in OEF/OIF combat veterans*. Symposium presented at the annual meeting of the Association for Behavioral and Cognitive Therapies, Toronto, ON.

Eaton, K. M., Hoge, C. W., Messer, S. C., Whitt, A. A., Cabrera, O. A., McGurk, D., et al. (2008). Prevalence of mental health problems, treatment need, and barriers to care among primary care-seeking spouses of military service members involved in Iraq and Afghanistan deployments. *Military Medicine, 173,* 1051–1056.

Esposito-Smythers, C., Wolff, J., Lemmon, K. M., Bodzy, M., Swenson, R. R., & Spirito, A. (2011). Military youth and the deployment cycle: Emotional health consequences and recommendations for intervention. *Journal of Family Psychology, 25,* 497–507.

Galovski, T., & Lyons, J. A. (2004). Psychological sequelae of combat violence: A review of the impact of PTSD on the veteran's family and possible interventions. *Aggression and Violent Behavior, 9,* 477–501.

Gawande, A. (2004). Casualties of war: Military care for the wounded in Iraq and Afghanistan. *New England Journal of Medicine, 351,* 2471–2475.

Halford, W. K., & Snyder, D. K. (in press). Universal processes and common factors in couple therapy and relationship education: Introduction to the Special Series. *Behavior Therapy, 43,* 1–12.

Hoge, C. W., Auchterlonie, J. L., & Milliken, C. S. (2006). Mental health problems, use of mental health services, and attrition from military service after returning from deployment to Iraq or Afghanistan. *Journal of the American Medical Association, 295,* 1023–1032.

Hoge, C. W., Castro, C. A., Messer, S. C., McGurk, D., Cotting, D. I., & Koffman, R. L. (2004). Combat duty in Iraq and Afghanistan, mental health problems, and barriers to care. *New England Journal of Medicine, 351,* 13–22.

MacDermid, S. M. (2006, June 22). *Multiple transitions of deployment and reunion for military families*. Unpublished presentation, Purdue University, West Lafayette, IN. Retrieved November 1, 2011, from *www.cfs.purdue.edu/mfri/deployreunion.ppt*.

Mansfield, A. J., Kaufman, J. S., Marshall, S. W., Gaynes, B. N., Morrissey, J. P., & Engel, C. C. (2010). Deployment and the use of mental health services among U.S. Army wives. *New England Journal of Medicine, 362,* 101–109.

McCarroll, J. E., Ursano, R. J., Fan, Z., & Newby, J. H. (2008). Trends in U.S. Army child maltreatment reports: 1990–2004. *Child Abuse Review, 17,* 108–118.

Mental Health Advisory Team (MHAT-V). (2008). *Operation Iraqi Freedom 06–08 final report. Office of the Surgeon Multinational Force–Iraq and Office of the Surgeon General United States Army Medical Command*. Retrieved November 1, 2011, from *www.armymedicine.army.mil/reports/mhat/mhat_v/mhat-v.cfm*.

Milliken, C. S., Auchterlonie, J. L., & Hoge, C. W. (2007). Longitudinal assessment of mental health problems among active and reserve component soldiers returning from the Iraq war. *Journal of the American Medical Association, 298,* 2141–2148.

Monson, C. M., Taft, C. T., & Fredman, S. J. (2009). Military-related PTSD and intimate relationships: From description to theory-driven research and intervention development. *Clinical Psychology Review, 29,* 707–714.

Nelson Goff, B. S., Crow, J. R., Reisbig, A. M. J., & Hamilton, S. (2007). The impact of individual trauma symptoms of deployed soldiers on relationship satisfaction. *Journal of Family Psychology, 21,* 344–353.

Pavlicin, K. M. (2003). *Surviving deployment: A guide for military families.* St. Paul, MN: Elva Resa.

Riviere, L. A., & Merrill, J. C. (2011). The impact of combat deployment on military families. In A. B. Adler, P. D. Bliese, & C. A. Castro (Eds.), *Deployment psychology: Evidence-based strategies to promote mental health in the military* (pp. 125–149). Washington, DC: American Psychological Association.

Rona, R. J., Hyams, K. C., & Wessely, S. (2005). Screening for psychological illness in military personnel. *Journal of the American Medical Association, 293,* 1257–1260.

Sayers, S. L., Farrow, V. A., Ross, J., & Oslin, D. W. (2009). Family problems among recently returned military veterans referred for a mental health evaluation. *Journal of Clinical Psychiatry, 70,* 163–170.

Seal, K. H., Metzler, T. J., Gima, K. S., Bertenthal, D., Maguen, S., & Marmar, C. R. (2009). Trends and risk factors for mental health diagnoses among Iraq and Afghanistan veterans using Department of Veterans Affairs health care, 2002–2008. *American Journal of Public Health, 99,* 1651–1658.

Sheppard, S. C., Malatras, J. W., & Israel, A. C. (2010). The impact of deployment on U.S. military families. *American Psychologist, 65,* 599–609.

Snyder, D. K., Castellani, A. M., & Whisman, M. A. (2006). Current status and future directions in couple therapy. *Annual Review of Psychology, 57,* 317–344.

Snyder, D. K., Heyman, R. E., & Haynes, S. N. (2008). Assessing couple distress. In J. Hunsley & E. Mash (Eds.), *A guide to assessments that work* (pp. 439–463). New York: Oxford University.

Snyder, D. K., Schneider, W. J., & Castellani, A. M. (2003). Tailoring couple therapy to individual differences: A conceptual approach. In D. K. Snyder & M. A. Whisman (Eds.), *Treating difficult couples: Helping clients with coexisting mental and relationship disorders* (pp. 27–51). New York: Guilford Press.

Snyder, D. K., & Whisman, M. A. (Eds.). (2003). *Treating difficult couples: Helping clients with coexisting mental and relationship disorders.* New York: Guilford Press.

U.S. Army Medical Command. (2011). *Resilience training.* Retrieved November 1, 2011, from *www.resilience.army.mil.*

U.S. 110th Congress. (2007). Veterans' mental health and other care improvements Act of 2008. In *Database of Federal Legislation.* Retrieved November 1, 2011, from *www.govtrack.us/congress/bill.xpd?bill=s110-2162.*

U.S. Department of Defense. (2007). *Demographics 2007: Profile of the military community.* Retrieved November 1, 2011 from *www.militaryhomefront.dod. mil/12038/project%20documents/militaryhomefront/reports/2007%20 demographics.pdf.*

U.S. Department of Defense. (2011). *Defenselink casualty report 2011.09.30.* Retrieved November 1, 2011 from *www.defense.gov/news/casualty.pdf.*

U.S. Department of Defense Task Force on Mental Health. (2007). *An achievable vision: Report of the Department of Defense Task Force on Mental Health.* Falls Church, VA: Defense Health Board.

Whisman, M. A., Snyder, D. K., & Beach, S. R. H. (2009). Screening for marital and relationship discord. *Journal of Family Psychology, 23,* 247–254.

Whisman, M. A., & Uebelacker, L. A. (2006). Impairment and distress associated with relationship discord in a national sample of married or cohabiting adults. *Journal of Family Psychology, 20,* 369–377.

Wright, K. M., Cabrera, O. A., Bliese, P. D., Adler, A. B., Hoge, C. W., & Castro, C. A. (2009). Stigma and barriers to care in soldiers postcombat. *Psychological Services, 6,* 108–116.

Appendices

Philippe Shnaider, Valerie Vorstenbosch, and Sonya G. Wanklyn

Resources for Military and Veteran Couples and Families

This appendix provides resources including websites, books, and programs that provide supplemental information for many of the issues highlighted throughout this book. The majority of these resources are geared toward military personnel, veterans, and their families. For clinician-based resources, please refer to the resources provided at the end of each chapter. Web-based resources evolve continuously; some listed below may disappear, while many other new resources emerge. The more general websites often provide links to more focused resources. Inclusion of resources listed below does not constitute endorsement of specific content.

THE BASICS

211 Information and Referral
Website: *www.211.org*

The 211 Information and Referral search engine provides confidential referrals for a number of different services, including help with food, employment, and health.

Defense Centers of Excellence for Psychological Health and Traumatic Brain Injuries
Website: *www.dcoe.health.mil*

The website aims to improve clinical care, education and training, and provide patient and family outreach for psychological health problems and traumatic brain injury.

Military Homefront
Website: *www.militaryhomefront.dod.mil*

Military Homefront offers support for military families through programs focused on child care, youth programs, family advocacy, relocation, and deployment.

Military OneSource
Website: *www.militaryonesource.com*
Toll free (referral service hotline): 1-800-342-9647

Military OneSource provides support and educational materials for military personnel and their families. Services provided include a telephone referral service, free short-term counseling, telephone consultation, webinars, podcasts, and discussion boards.

National Resource Directory
Website: *www.nationalresourcedirectory.gov*

This website aims to provide a variety of support and informational material to service members and their loved ones. Information regarding benefits, compensation, health, family support, and additional resources can be found on this website.

CRISIS RESOURCES

Alcohol and Substance Use

National Helpline for Substance Abuse
Toll free: 1-800-821-4357

This hotline helps individuals locate substance abuse treatment facilities in their surrounding area.

Domestic Violence

National Child Abuse Hotline
Toll free: 1-800-4-A-CHILD (1-800-422-4453)

This hotline provides assistance to children who are experiencing abuse. Crisis intervention, information, and additional resources are provided to callers. Calls are confidential and anonymous. The hotline should be contacted if you know of or suspect that a child is being abused.

National Domestic Violence Hotline
Website: *www.ndvh.org*
Toll free: 1-800-799-SAFE (1-800-799-7233)

This hotline provides confidential and anonymous support for individuals experiencing domestic violence (emotional, verbal, sexual, and physical).

Suicide

National Suicide Prevention Lifeline
Website: *www.suicidepreventionlifeline.org*
Toll free: 1-800-273-TALK (1-800-273-8255)

This hotline provides free and confidential support for individuals experiencing suicidal thoughts or emotional distress.

1-800-SUICIDE

Toll free: 1-800-SUICIDE (1-800-784-2433)

EDUCATIONAL INFORMATION

Alcohol and Substance Abuse

National Institute on Drug Abuse (NIDA)
Website: *www.nida.nih.gov/medstaff.html*

NIDA provides information about commonly abused drugs, as well as the prevention and treatment of drug abuse.

Substance Abuse and Mental Health Services Administration (SAMHSA)
Website: *www.findtreatment.samhsa.gov*
Toll free: 1-800-662-HELP (1-800-662-4357)

SAMHSA provides information regarding drug and alcohol abuse treatment facilities in your surrounding area.

Children and Adolescents

Military Child Education Coalition
Website: *www.militarychild.org*

This website contains information for parents about various difficulties associated with being a military child, including deployment, education, and parenting advice.

Sesame Workshop
Website: *www.sesameworkshop.org/initiatives/emotion/tlc*

Sesame Workshop provides child-friendly videos to help children learn more about issues related to deployment, homecoming, changes, and grief.

Zero to Three
Website: *www.zerotothree.org*

This organization strives to provide information to healthcare professionals and parents about how to best care for infants and toddlers. Their initiatives include Coming Together Around Military Families, a program dedicated to increasing awareness about the importance of effectively caring for young children of military families.

Depression

Allaboutdepression.com
Website: *www.allaboutdepression.com*

This website provides information about the causes, symptoms, and treatments for depression.

Depression-guide.com
Website: *www.depression-guide.com*

This website provides information about depression symptoms, psychological and pharmacological treatments, and associated psychological disorders.

Grief and Loss

Operation Healthy Reunions: Bereavement and Grief
Website: *www.mentalhealthamerica.net/reunions/infowargrief.cfm*

This website provides information about bereavement and grief for military families and communities. Topics include living with grief, helping others grieve, helping children grieve, and helping resources.

Mental and Physical Health

MyHealtheVet
Website: *www.myhealth.va.gov*

This website, provided by the U.S. Department of Veterans Affairs, provides veterans with a better way to manage their healthcare. This website gives veterans access to their VA scheduled appointments, as well as access to secure messaging with their healthcare team.

U.S. Department of Veterans Affairs: Mental Health
Website: *www.mentalhealth.va.gov*

This website provides mental health information for veterans, their families, and providers. Topics include depression, military sexual abuse, posttraumatic stress disorder, substance abuse, and suicide prevention.

Posttraumatic Stress Disorder

Center for the Study of Traumatic Stress (CSTS)
Website: *www.centerforthestudyoftraumaticstress.org*

CSTS conducts research on the psychological effects of trauma exposure and works to inform and advance trauma care. It provides information to the public, as well as consults with private and public agencies to disseminate and apply their research findings.

International Society for Traumatic Stress Studies (ISTSS)
Website: *www.istss.org/publiceducationpamphlets2/3234.htm*

The ISTSS website provides public education pamphlets that cover topics including trauma, PTSD, and associated problems, such as relationship dissatisfaction, substance use, and children and trauma.

National Center for PTSD
Website: *www.ptsd.va.gov*

This center provides online educational resources including articles and videos that explain PTSD, common reactions to trauma, treatments, self-help and coping, as well as the effects of trauma on family members and close friends.

Sexual Assault

Military.com
Website: *www.military.com/benefits/veterans-health-care/sexual-trauma*

This website provides information about available benefits and compensation to military personnel who have suffered a sexual trauma while on active duty.

Rape, Abuse and Incest National Network (RAINN)
Website: *www.rainn.org*

RAINN provides education about sexual assault and resources for victims.

Sexual Assault Prevention and Response Office (SAPRO)
Website: *www.sapr.mil*

SAPRO provides information to military personnel about dealing with sexual assaults that occur within the military. This website addresses topics that include reporting of sexual assaults, training on how to respond to these situations, treatment and support for victims, prevention, and confidentiality involved in reporting.

Suicide

Air Force Suicide Prevention Program (AFSPP)
Website: *afspp.afms.mil*

AFSPP provides information to military personnel in order to reduce the occurrence of suicide within the Air Force.

Transitioning to and from Deployment

Afterdeployment.org
Website: *www.afterdeployment.org*

This website provides numerous resources for service members, veterans, families, and providers. Topics include depression, PTSD, anger, substance use, family relationships, physical injury, traumatic brain injury, and sexual abuse. Clinical practice guidelines are also provided for professionals.

Deployment Health and Family Readiness Library
Website: *deploymenthealthlibrary.fhp.osd.mil*

This online library for service members, families, and healthcare providers includes fact sheets, guides, and other materials that discuss deployment readiness.

Iraq and Afghanistan Veterans of America
Website: *supportyourvet.org*

This website provides information to families and friends of military personnel deployed in Afghanistan and Iraq to help with reintegration upon their return home.

Traumatic Brain Injury and Other Physical Injury

Brainline.org
Website: *www.brainline.org*

This website aims to increase the understanding of traumatic brain injury (TBI) via articles and videos for individuals with TBIs, their families, and mental health professionals.

Courage to Care Courage to Talk
Website: *www.couragetotalk.org*

This website provides information for providers, families, and friends on how to deal effectively with war injuries. Topics include talking with children and obtaining resources for recovery.

Military in-Step: Dealing with Grief and Depression
Website: *www.amputee-coalition.org/military-instep/dealing-grief-depression.
html*

This website contains information about grief and depression for amputees. Topics include stages of grief, signs and symptoms of depression, and overcoming depression.

SOCIAL SUPPORT

Support for Veterans and Families

Strong Bonds
Website: *www.strongbonds.org*

Strong Bonds, a program offered to service members and their families, assists in preparing them for deployment, as well as with other stressors associated with a military lifestyle.

Veterans Support Organization (VSO)
Website: *www.theveteranssupport.org*

The VSO, a nonprofit organization, provides social support to needy veterans. It deals with issues such as veteran homelessness, financial need, and funding programs for veterans.

Vets 4 Vets
Website: *www.vets4vets.us*

Vets 4 Vets is a program that provides peer support to Iraq- and Afghanistan-era war veterans with mental health conditions. Its mission includes helping veterans overcome the challenges associated with reintegration. The program is provided free of cost.

Vet to Vet
Website: *vet2vetusa.org*

Vet to Vet is a peer counseling program in which veterans who have been consumers of VA mental health services provide support to others veterans.

Support for Children and Adolescents

Comfort Zone Camp (CZC)
Website: *www.comfortzonecamp.org*

CZC is a free, year-round, bereavement camp for children ages 7–17 who have lost a family member. This camp provides support groups and confidence-building programs to help children during this emotionally difficult period.

DAY-TO-DAY LIFE RESOURCES AND SERVICES

Alcohol and Substance Use

Al-Anon/Alateen
Website: *www.al-anon.alateen.org*

Al-Anon/Alateen is a support group for families and friends of problem drinkers. This site and hotline provides information on meetings throughout the United States and Canada.

Alcoholics Anonymous (AA)
Website: *www.aa.org*

AA is a support group to help individuals who have a desire to stop drinking. This site provides information on meetings throughout the United States and Canada.

Other Substance Use Problems

Cocaine Anonymous (CA)
Website: *www.ca.org*

Narcotics Anonymous (NA)
Website: *www.na.org*

Partnership at Drugfree.org
Website: *www.drugfree.org*

This nonprofit organization provides information to help parents prevent, intervene, and find treatment opportunities for their children who are abusing drugs or alcohol.

Children and Adolescents

Army Reserve Child and Youth Services (CYS)
Website: *www.arfp.org/cys*

CYS provides online tools and resources for day-to-day issues and military-related stressors for parents and children of Army Reserve soldiers. Resources are provided for both young children and teenagers.

Deploymentkids.com
Website: *www.deploymentkids.com*

This website contains activities to help children understand and cope with the deployment of a parent.

Military K–12 Partners
Website: *www.militaryk12partners.dodea.edu*

This website provides resources for parents of military children to ease the transition of relocation. Available resources promote quality education, seamless transitions, and deployment support.

National Military Family Association: Operation Purple Program
Website: *www.operationpurple.org*

The Operation Purple program is comprised of camps to give military children and families tools to deal with the stressors associated with a military lifestyle.

Operation: Military Kids (OMK)
Website: *www.operationmilitarykids.org*

OMK offers services to children facing the challenges of parental deployment, including participation in recreational and social activities with other children impacted by deployment.

Education and Employment

Employer Support of the Guard and Reserve (ESGR)
Website: *www.esgr.org/site*

ESGR aims to promote employer support and advocacy for service members, by making employers and employees aware of laws surrounding employment and rights of employees.

Vet Success
Website: *www.vetsuccess.gov*

This website provides tips and information to service members seeking employment. Information regarding how to build a resume and write a cover letter, as well as tips for interviews and completing job applications are offered.

Families and Couples

American Red Cross
Website: *www.redcross.org*

The American Red Cross website allows troops on active duty to communicate with their loved ones during crises, as well as provides military families with factual descriptions and verified information regarding these crises.

Families OverComing Under Stress (FOCUS)
Website: *www.focusproject.org*

FOCUS provides strategies to help military families understand and deal with the challenges of deployment and reintegration, communicate effectively, and create a family plan to help with future deployment. Online programs, as well as in-person trainings, are available.

Marine Corps Community Services (MCCS)
Website: *www.usmc-mccs.org/family*

MCCS provides a variety of services to help Marines and their families maintain strong relationships. Its programs target parent support; children, youth, and teens; and family readiness.

Military Spouse Magazine
Website: *www.milspousemag.com*

This magazine provides information and resources regarding difficulties associated with deployment, relationships, family, and finance to spouses of military personnel.

Strategic Outreach to Families of All Reservists (SOFAR)
Website: *www.sofarusa.org*

SOFAR provides free mental health services to assist families of Reserve and National Guard personnel to foster stabilization, prevent crises, and assist with reintegration after deployment.

Veterans and Families Foundation
Website: *www.veteransandfamilies.org/home.html*

This nonprofit organization was developed to strengthen the homecoming safety net for veterans. It aims to provide information for families to facilitate the prevention and early intervention of difficulties related to reintegration.

Well Spouse Association
Website: *www.wellspouse.org*

This website provides emotional support for partners of chronically ill or disabled individuals. This association brings individuals facing similar circumstances together and offers services such as support groups, newsletters, online chat forums, and respite weekends.

Grief and Loss

Children's Grief Education Association (CGEA)
Website: *www.childgrief.org*

CGEA is dedicated to supporting and educating children and families who have lost a loved one. Sections of the website are dedicated to grieving military families.

GriefNet.org
Website (adults): *www.griefnet.org*
Website (children): *www.kidsaid.com*

This website hosts an Internet support group for grieving adults and children dealing with the loss of a loved one.

MilitaryConnection.com: Grief and Resources
Website: *www.militaryconnection.com/military-spouses/grief-and-resources.asp*

This website provides online grief resources for spouses and children of fallen service members.

Tragedy Assistance Program for Survivors (TAPS)
Website: *www.taps.org*

TAPS provides support for individuals dealing with the loss of a military loved one. Programs include peer-based support, casework assistance, and crisis intervention.

Posttraumatic Stress Disorder

Women's Trauma Recovery Program (WTRP)
Website: *www.womenvetsptsd.va.gov*

This intensive program is designed to treat women in the military who have experienced traumatic events, including military sexual trauma and combat-related trauma.

Transitioning to and from Deployment

National Guard Bureau Joint Services Support
Website: *www.jointservicessupport.org*

This website offers a variety of support programs and resources to assist military personnel and their families with the challenges of reintegration, financial strain, mental health issues, and transitioning to and from deployment.

Survivingdeployment.com
Website: *www.survivingdeployment.com*

This website provides families of deployed military personnel resources to help them understand and overcome family challenges that arise due to deployment.

Transition Assistance Program (TAP)
Website: *www.turbotap.org*

TAP offers transition resources for military personnel regarding reintegration after deployment.

Veterans Resource Central
Website: *www.veteransresourcecentral.org*

This website offers career path guidance for military personnel and their families by providing resources to help with career transitions.

Yellow Ribbon Program
Website: *www.yellowribbon.mil*

The Yellow Ribbon Program provides National Guard and service members, as well as their families, information and resources to assist with their deployment-related needs.

Traumatic Brain Injury and Other Physical Injury

Defense and Veterans Brain Injury Center (DVBIC)
Website: *www.dvbic.org*

This center provides services to military personnel dealing with TBI and their families. It provides TBI assessments and treatments, and provides educational materials about TBI.

SELF-HELP AND INFORMATIONAL BOOKS

Alcohol and Substance Abuse

Carr, A. (2005). *The easy way to stop drinking.* New York: Sterling.
Fletcher, A. M. (2001). *Sober for good: New solutions for drinking problems: Advice from those who have succeeded.* Chicago: Houghton Mifflin/Harcourt.
Tate, P. T. (1996). *Alcohol: How to give it up and be glad you did* (2nd ed.). Tucson, AZ: See Sharp Press.

Children and Adolescents

Andrews, B. (2007). *I miss you!: A military kid's book about deployment.* Amherst, NY: Prometheus Books.
Ehrmantraut, B. (2005). *Night catch.* Aberdeen, SD: Bubble Gum Press.
Fritz, S., Johnson, P., & Zitzow, T. (2009). *You and your military hero: Building positive thinking skills during your hero's deployment.* Edina, MN: Beaver's Pond Press.
Graham, M. J. E. (2009). *While you were away: Absence journal for teens.* Ottawa, ON: Egerton Graham Consulting.
Hoyt, C. R. (2005). *Daddy's in Iraq, but I want him back.* Bloomington, IN: Trafford.

Kilgore, M. (2010). *Where is my mommy?: A book about children's fears.* Seattle: Parenting Press.

LaBelle, J. (2009). *My dad's deployment: A deployment and reunion activity book for young children.* St. Paul, MN: Elva Resa.

LaBelle, J. (2009). *My mom's deployment: A deployment and reunion activity book for young children.* St. Paul, MN: Elva Resa.

McElroy, L. T. (2005). *Love, Lizzie: Letters to a military mom.* Park Ridge, IL: Albert Whitman.

Pelton, M. (2004). *When dad's at sea.* Park Ridge, IL: Albert Whitman.

Penn, A. (2006). *The kissing hand.* Terre Haute, IN: Tanglewood Press.

Redman, M. (2008). *The wishing tree.* St. Paul, MN: Elva Resa.

Robertson, R. (2005). *Deployment journal for kids.* Saint Paul, MN: Elva Resa.

Sederman, M. (2002). *Magic box: When parents can't be there to tuck you in.* Washington, CA: Magination Press.

Sherman, M. D. (2006). *I'm not alone: A teen's guide to living with a parent who has a mental illness.* Edina, MN: Beaver Pond.

Sherman, M. D., & Sherman D. M. (2009). *My story: Blogs by four military teens.* Edina, MN: Beaver Pond.

Thomas, J. (2010). *What will I play while you are away?* Charleston, SC: CreateSpace.

Tomp, S. (2005). *Red, white, and blue goodbye.* London: Bloomsbury.

Couples and Families Facing Deployment

Armstrong, K., Best, S., & Domenici, P. (2006). *Courage after fire: Coping strategies for returning soldiers and their families.* Berkeley, CA: Ulysses Press.

Friedman, M. J., & Slone, L. B. (2008). *After the war zone: A practical guide for returning troops and their families.* Cambridge, MA: Da Capo Press.

Hightower, K., & Scherer, H. (2007). *Help! I'm a military spouse—I get a life too! How to craft a life for you as you move with the military* (2nd ed.). Dulles, VA: Potomac Books.

Kay, E. (2002). *Heroes at home: Help and hope for America's military families.* Ada, MI: Bethany House.

Matsakis, A. (2007). *Back from the front: Combat trauma, love, and the family.* Brooklandville, MD: Sidran Press.

Depression

Burns, D. (1989). *The feeling good handbook.* New York: Penguin Books.

Copeland, M. E., & McKay, M. (2002). *The depression workbook: A guide for living with depression and manic depression* (2nd ed.). Oakland, CA: New Harbinger.

Greenberger, D., & Padesky, C. (1995). *Mind over mood: Change how you feel by changing the way you think.* New York: Guilford Press.

Orloff, J. (2010). *Emotional freedom: Liberate yourself from negative emotions and transform your life.* New York: Three Rivers Press.

Domestic Violence

Kubany, E. S., McCaig, M. A., & Laconsay, J. R. (2004). *Healing the trauma of domestic violence: A workbook for women*. Oakland, CA: New Harbinger.

Grief and Loss

Huntley, T. (1991). *Helping children grieve when someone they love dies*. Minneapolis, MN: Augsberg Fortress.
Noel, B., & Blair, P. D. (2008). *I wasn't ready to say goodbye: Surviving, coping and healing after the sudden death of a loved one*. Naperville, IL: Sourcebooks Incorporated.

Posttraumatic Stress Disorder

Allen, J. (2004). *Coping with trauma: Hope through understanding*. Washington, DC: American Psychiatric Association.
Mason, P. (2002*). Recovering from the war: A guide for all veterans, family members, friends and therapists*. High Springs, FL: Patience Press.
Matsakis, A. (1996). *I can't get over it: A handbook for trauma survivors* (2nd ed.). Oakland, CA: New Harbinger.
Rothbaum, B. O., & Foa, E. B. (2004). *Reclaiming your life after rape: A cognitive behavioral therapy for PTSD workbook*. New York: Oxford University Press.
Schiraldi, G. (2009). *The posttraumatic stress disorder sourcebook: A guide to healing, recovery, and growth* (2nd ed.). New York: McGraw-Hill.
Williams, M. B., & Poijula, S. (2002). *The PTSD workbook: Simple effective techniques for overcoming traumatic stress symptoms*. Oakland, CA: New Harbinger.

Transitioning to and from Deployment

Dumler, E. G. (2006). *I'm already home . . . again*. Euless, TX: Frankly Speaking.
Graham, M. J. E. (2009). *While you were away: 101 tips for families experiencing absence or deployment*. Ottawa, ON: Egerton Graham Consulting.
Moore, B. A., & Kennedy, C. H. (2010). *Wheels down: Adjusting to life after deployment*. Washington, DC: American Psychological Association.
Pavlicin, K. M. (2003). *Surviving deployment: A guide for military families*. St. Paul, MN: Elva Resa.
Petty, K. (2009). *Deployment: Strategies for working with kids in military families*. St. Paul, MN: Redleaf Press.

UNITED STATES MILITARY BRANCHES

Air Force
Website: *www.af.mil*

Air Force Reserve Command
Website: *www.afrc.af.mil*

Air National Guard
Website: *www.ang.af.mil*

Army
Website: *www.army.mil*

Army National Guard
Website: *www.arng.army.mil*

Coast Guard
Website: *www.uscg.mil*

Coast Guard Reserve
Website: *www.uscg.mil/reserve/*

Marines
Website: *www.usmc.mil*

Marines Reserve
Website: *www.usmc.mil/unit/marforres*

Navy
Website: *www.navy.mil*

Navy Reserve
Website: *www.navyreserve.com*

RESOURCES FOR OTHER COUNTRIES

Canada

National Defence and the Canadian Forces
Website: *www.forces.gc.ca/site/index.asp*
Website: *www.forces.gc.ca/site/fam/index-eng.asp*

Navy
Website: *www.navy.forces.gc.ca*

Army
Website: *www.army.forces.gc.ca*

Air Force
Website: *www.airforce.forces.gc.ca*

Veterans Affairs Canada
Website: *www.veterans.gc.ca*

Military Family Resource Centre of the National Capital Region
Website: *www.familyforce.ca/sites/NCR/EN*
Provides information and support for Canadian Forces families.

United Kingdom

Ministry of Defence
Website: *www.mod.uk*

Army
Website: *www.army.mod.uk*

Navy
Website: *www.royal-navy.mod.uk*

Air Force
Website: *www.raf.mod.uk*

Australia

Department of Defence
Website: *www.defence.gov.au*

Navy
Website: *www.navy.gov.au*

Army
Website: *www.army.gov.au*

Air Force
Website: *www.airforce.gov.au*

APPENDIX B

United States Military Ranks

Enlisted

Grade	Army	Marine Corps	Air Force	Navy
E-1	Private	Private	Airman Basic	Seaman Recruit
E-2	Private 2	Private First Class	Airman	Seaman Apprentice
E-3	Private First Class	Lance Corporal	Airman First Class	Seaman
E-4	Corporal/Specialist	Corporal	Senior Airman	Petty Officer Second Class
E-5	Sergeant	Sergeant	Staff Sergeant	Petty Officer Second Class
E-6	Staff Sergeant	Staff Sergeant	Technical Sergeant	Petty Officer First Class
E-7	Sergeant First Class	Gunnery Sergeant	Master Sergeant	Chief Petty Officer
E-8	First/Master Sergeant	First/Master Sergeant	Senior Master Sergeant	Senior Chief Petty Officer
E-9	Sergeant Major	Master Gunnery Sergeant/Sergeant Major	Chief Master Sergeant	Master Chief Petty Officer

Officers

Grade	Army	Marine Corps	Air Force	Navy
O-1	Second Lieutenant	Second Lieutenant	Second Lieutenant	Ensign
O-2	First Lieutenant	First Lieutenant	First Lieutenant	Lieutenant Junior Grade
O-3	Captain	Captain	Captain	Lieutenant
O-4	Major	Major	Major	Lieutenant Commander
O-5	Lieutenant Colonel	Lieutenant Colonel	Lieutenant Colonel	Commander
O-6	Colonel	Colonel	Colonel	Captain
O-7	Brigadier General	Brigadier General	Brigadier General	Rear Admiral (lower half)
O-8	Major General	Major General	Major General	Rear Admiral (upper half)
O-9	Lieutenant General	Lieutenant General	Lieutenant General	Vice Admiral
O-10	General	General	General	Admiral
O-11	General of the Army		General of the Air Force	Fleet Admiral

APPENDIX C

Military Structure and Unit Sizes

The unit sizes presented below are approximations. Military unit sizes are constantly adapting and changing. Thus, the information presented below is only a guideline to military structure.

U.S. Army

Unit	Approximate personnel	Composition
Army	100,000+	2-5 Corps
Corps	20,000–40,000	2–5 Divisions
Division	10,000–18,000	3 Brigades
Brigade	3,000–5,000	3+ Battalions
Battalion	500–600	3–5 Companies
Company	100–200	3–5 Platoons
Platoon	16–40	3–4 Squads
Squad	4–10	—

U.S. Marine Corps

Unit	Approximate personnel	Composition
Regiment	6,000	5 Battalions
Battalion	1,200	5 Companies
Company	240	4 Platoons
Platoon	60	4 Squads
Squad	15	3 Fire Teams

U.S. Air Force

Unit	Composition
Major Command	A major command (MAJCOM) is a major subdivision of the Air Force. It consists of two basic types: operational and support.
Numbered Air Force	Two or more wings are usually grouped with auxiliary units to form a Numbered Air Force (NAF).
Wing	The basic unit for generating and employing combat capability. There are three basic types of wings: operational, air base, and specialized mission.
Group	Usually consists of two to four squadrons and a group headquarters.
Squadron	The basic fighting unit of the U.S. Air Force. A squadron usually consists of two or more flights.
Flight	Two or more airplanes form a flight.
Party	Usually a two-airman team.

U.S. Navy

The structure of the United States Navy is complex, comprising fleets made up of different ship arrangements. Due to this complexity, the presentation of its structure has been omitted.

APPENDIX D

U.S. Department of Veterans Affairs Organizational Structure

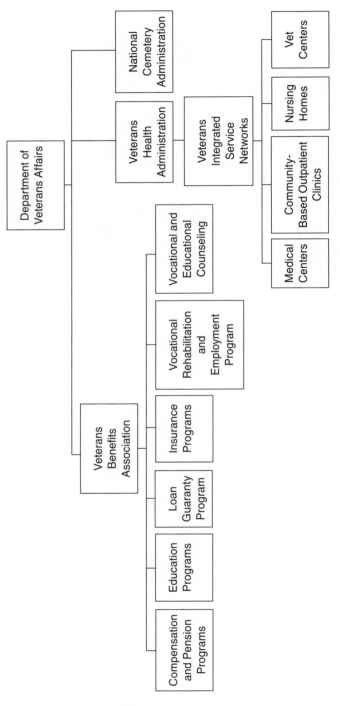

APPENDIX E

Common Terms and Abbreviations

ABM—antiballistic missile
ACC—Air Combat Command (USAF)
AEW—airborne early warning
AFB—Air Force base (US)
APC—armored personnel carrier
ARMY—U.S. Army
AWACS—Airborne Warning and
    Control System (Boeing E-3 Sentry)
AWOL—absent without leave
BOLO—be on the lookout
CAT—crisis action team
CO—commanding officer
DMZ—demilitarized zone
DO—Director of Operations
DoD—U.S. Department of Defense
EOD—explosive ordinance disposal
ETS—expiration of term of service
FOB—forward operating base
FUBAR—"fouled" up beyond all
    recognition/repair
GPMG—general purpose machine gun
HEAP—high explosive antipersonnel
HQ—headquarter(s)
IED—improvised explosive device
IFF—identification, friend or foe
KIA—killed in action
LAV—light armored vehicle
LZ—landing zone
MG—machine gun
MIA—missing in action

MOS—military occupational specialty
MP—military police
MRAV—multirole armored vehicle
NAS—naval air station
NATO—North Atlantic Treaty
    Organization
NCO—noncommissioned officer
PCS—permanent change of station
QRF—quick response force
RECON—reconnaissance
ROE—rules of engagement
RP—rocket propelled
RPG—pocket propelled grenade
SAM—surface-to-air missile
SEALs—SEa, Air and Land (USN)
    teams
SNAFU—situation normal, all
    "fouled" up
TDY—temporary duty
UAV—unmanned aerial vehicle
UN—United Nations
USAF—U.S. Air Force
USAFE—U.S. Air Force in Europe
USMC—U.S. Marine Corps
USN—U.S. Navy
VA—U.S. Department of Veterans
    Affairs
VTOL—vertical takeoff and landing
WIA—wounded in action
XO—executive officer

Index

Note. "f" indicates a figure; "t" indicates a table.